D0218541

Task Analysis

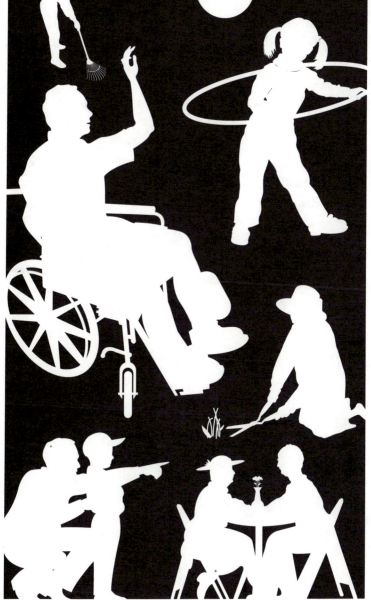

An Occupational Performance Approach

Diane E. Watson,
MBA, OTR/L, BCP
University of Scranton

Foreword by:
Lela A. Llorens,
PhD, OTR, FAOTA

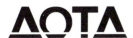 The American
Occupational Therapy
Association, Inc.

For information address: The American Occupational Therapy Association, Inc., 4720 Montgomery Lane, PO Box 31220, Bethesda, MD 20854-1220.

Disclaimers
"This publication is designed to provide accurate and authoritative information in regard to the subject matter covered. It is sold or distributed with the understanding that the publisher is not engaged in rendering legal, accounting, or other professional service. If legal advice or other expert assistance is required, the services of a competent professional person should be sought."
—From the Declaration of Principles jointly adopted by the American Bar Association and a Committee of Publishers and Associations.

It is the objective of the American Occupational Therapy Association to be a forum for free expression and interchange of ideas. The opinions expressed by the contributors to this work are their own and not necessarily those of either the editors or the American Occupational Therapy Association.

Director of Nonperiodical Publications: Frances E. McCarrey
Managing Editor of Nonperiodical Publications: Mary C. Fisk
Designer: Editech Services, Inc.

Printed in the United States of America

ISBN: 1-56900-065-4

TABLE OF CONTENTS

TABLE OF CONTENTS

DEDICATION

To my grandparents and in loving memory of
Gladys Mary and Evelyn Louisa.

FOREWORD

Occupational therapy as a health profession embraces the use of activities and tasks as significant in achieving therapeutic goals in the treatment and rehabilitation of persons with occupational dysfunction resulting from disease or disability. Activities and tasks are used in therapy to facilitate communication; develop relationships; increase self-esteem through successful participation; and assess and develop specific sensory, motor, psychological, social, and cognitive skills for learning, organizing work, and solving problems. The activities and tasks used in therapy may include painting, quilt making, spinning a top, playing games, house cleaning, grocery shopping, driving, accessing a computer, and other daily life occupations. Functional adaptation to resolve or compensate for deficit, dysfunction, or disability is the expected outcome of therapy.

Many schemata have been proposed for analysis of tasks and activities; however, to date there is no definitive agreement on any one model. The focus on task analysis guided by a theoretical frame of reference as represented in this volume is most timely and will make it possible for students, educators, and clinical practitioners to view and prescribe or implement the use of activities and tasks more systematically. Furthermore, it has the potential to provide data for research, which will enhance the body of knowledge in the profession.

A theoretical model that encompasses the sensory, motor, psychosocial, and cognitive functions provides a comprehensive framework from which to view activities and tasks and a place from which to begin to prescribe therapy. Occupational performance refers to "the accomplishment of tasks related to self-care/self-maintenance, work/education, play/leisure, and rest/relaxation" (Llorens, 1991, p. 46) that is critical to such functional roles as worker, parent, mate, peer, student, and family

member. Role performance is predicted on the development and/or redevelopment of skills needed for successful functioning following serious illness or as a result of disability or deficit.

Christiansen (Christiansen & Baum, 1991) differentiated between **activities** and **tasks** by defining a **task** "as a set of activities sharing some purpose recognized by the task performer" (p. 29). Tasks have "dimensions related to their complexity, their degree of structure... and their purposes...and whether they entail cooperation or competition and whether...[they are] public or private" (p. 29) as having a vital influence on performance. **Activity**, on the other hand, is viewed as a more general term that "refer[s] to all purposeful behaviors" (p. 28). Diane Watson has defined **task analysis** within this text as "the process of analyzing the dynamic relationship between people and their [everyday] occupations and environments." The complexity to which Christiansen refers is depicted in the Occupational Performance Analysis Form and the various teaching exercises that have been designed to assist the student to learn to analyze tasks and activities in the context of role performance within physical, social, and cultural environments. Watson accurately recognizes that the Occupational Performance Analysis Form cannot fully "capture the interactive and transactional relationship between people and their tasks and environments." Similarly, the analysis of definitive tasks cannot fully capture the role performance of the individual within her or his environment. However, it is necessary to know as much as possible about the many tasks and activities in which clients/patients engage. Activity and task analysis make it possible for the therapist to acquire this knowledge. The application of knowledge acquired through activity and task analysis must be tempered by individual communication with patient/client so that therapy is individualized and appropriate activities and tasks are prescribed. Information provided by the client/patient together with what is known about specific tasks and activities can result in an appropriate match between the patient's/client's role performance needs and selected therapy activities and tasks to produce an outcome that will enhance the patient's/client's quality of life.

This textbook emphasizes the need for "doing" in becoming an occupational therapist (Fidler & Fidler, 1978). The doing focus is valuable for learning the skill of task analysis. It is incumbent upon those who use this book, however, to ensure that the knowledge and skills learned in this process are not only *applied* in the practice of occupational therapy but that they are also clearly articulated *verbally*. Ability to verbally articulate the connection between **task and activity analysis** and **task and activity use** in occupational therapy will empower students in their communication with patients, colleagues, and the public regarding the therapeutic usefulness of activities and tasks.

Successful practice of occupational therapy is dependent upon the skill with which the therapist can use the information gained in the analysis and synthesis of knowledge of human behavior and activities and relationships for application within a theoretical framework. The inclusion of role performance in the theoretical framework for therapy will assist patients/clients to solve problems of dysfunction, deficit, and/or disability for functional adaptation in their daily life tasks and activities.

Lela A. Llorens, PhD, OTR, FAOTA
Professor Emerita, San Jose State University
Consultant in Occupational Therapy and
Gerontology

References

Christiansen C., & Baum, C. (Eds.). (1991). *Occupational therapy: Overcoming human performance deficits.* Thorofare, NJ: Slack.

Fidler, G. S., & Fidler, J. W. (1978). Doing and becoming: Purposeful action and self-actualization. *The American Journal of Occupational Therapy, 32:* 305–310

Llorens, L. A. (1991). Performance tasks and roles throughout the life span. In C. Christiansen & C. Baum (Eds.). *Occupational therapy: Overcoming human performance deficits.* Thorofare, NJ: Slack.

PREFACE

As clinical practitioners we seek to use meaningful and purposeful activities to create rehabilitation experiences that are valued by clients. In parallel with this tradition, *Task Analysis: An Occupational Performance Approach* attempts to create a meaningful and purposeful context for teaching task and activity analysis to create a learning experience that is valued by students.

Task analysis, within this text, refers to the dynamic and interdependent relationships between people and their chosen occupations and performance contexts. Task analysis is presented here as a process of inquiry, analysis, and reasoning. Occupational therapy practitioners use task analysis to develop and justify evaluation and intervention strategies in all areas of practice. In keeping with Llorens (1993) and others (Cynkin, 1979; Trombly, 1995), this text uses the term **activity analysis** to refer to the process of analyzing an activity to determine whether its inherent properties elicit motivation and fulfill a client's needs in occupational performance and performance components. The readings and assignments in this text have been designed to actively engage students in pursuing the knowledge and skills to be proficient in both types of analysis.

"Generic activity analysis frameworks" address the domains of concern to occupational therapy, but such frameworks can become exercises with "no discernible purpose" when they do not assist in the process of designing activities for evaluation and intervention (Mosey, 1981, p. 115). To avoid this educational tragedy, this text incorporates the occupational performance approach and the case method. The occupational performance approach provides a framework for students to structure the task analysis process and learn the domains of concern to the occupational therapy practitioner. The case method creates a meaningful and purposeful context for designing activities for evaluation and intervention.

The hypothetical clients portrayed in this text range in age from 4 to 89 years and their occupational performance issues challenge students to analyze:

1. Activities of daily living such as bathing (Dawn case), eating (Rhonda case), dressing (Rena case), driving (Jeff case), functional mobility (Wayne and Minnie case), socialization (Ali, Barb, Carl, and Dana case), toilet hygiene (Dawn case), and sexual expression (Gladys case).
2. Work and productive activities such as home management (Nelson case), care of others (Rena case), educational activities (Sidney case), job site analysis (Daniel case), and functional capacity evaluation (Rick case).
3. Play or leisure pursuits including playground activities (Bob case) and sports (Jeff case).

Cases span clinical contexts that include children's day-care centers (Bob case), schools (Sidney case), transition services (Daniel case), home health (Gladys case), outpatient physical rehabilitation (Rick case), outpatient behavioral health (Ali, Barb, Carl, and Dana case), inpatient physical rehabilitation services (Nelson case), inpatient behavioral health (Laurie case), and skilled nursing facilities (Bert and Maureen case). The cases provide a meaningful context for students to learn the use of assistive technology devices (Sidney case), crafts (Bert and Maureen case), computers (Greg case), and narratives (Laurie case). Students will be exposed to new activities, crafts, and games, and will research the range of purposeful activities used in contemporary practice. Assignments offer a meaningful context for students to learn to cook (Sylvie and Laureal case), sew (Rick case), and design and build adapted equipment (Rick case). A proposed course module (Appendix N), section overviews, and supplemental learning resources are provided to assist instructors and students in planning their learning experience.

Although the clinical cases presented in this text are hypothetical, the issues are representational. The realism of the cases used provides a context for occupational therapy students to practice the cognitive steps and professional behaviors required of clinical practitioners. The learning experiences are developmental, collaborative, and integrative, and assignments provide ample opportunity for students and educators to determine the focus and intensity of instruction. The case method approach parallels occupational therapy's traditional use of purposeful activity to promote clients' learning, insight, skills, and independent performance, as well as the belief that meaningful engagement sanctions diversity and flexibility in learning and adaptation (Watson, 1996). Exposing students to client case scenarios, and providing them with opportunities to practice resolving clinical issues, should develop their narrative, interactive, procedural, and conditional clinical reasoning (Van Leit, 1995).

References

Cynkin, S. (1979). *Occupational therapy: Toward health through activities.* Boston: Little, Brown.

Llorens, L. A. (1993). Activity analysis: Agreement between participants and observers on perceived factors in occupation components. *American Journal of Occupational Therapy, 13,* 198–211.

Mosey, A. C. (1981). *Occupational therapy: Configuration of a profession.* New York: Raven Press.

Trombly, C. A. (1995). Purposeful activity. In C. A. Trombly (Ed.), *Occupational therapy for physical dysfunction* (pp. 237–253). Baltimore: Williams & Wilkins.

Van Leit, B. (1995). Using the case method to develop clinical reasoning skills in problem-based learning. *American Journal of Occupational Therapy, 49,* 349–353.

Watson, D. E. (1996). *Clinical cases for learning pediatric occupational therapy: A problem-based approach.* San Antonio, TX: Therapy Skill Builders.

ACKNOWLEDGMENTS

The conceptual origins of this project must be credited to the faculty of the Department of Occupational Therapy at the University of Alberta who, over 10 years ago, taught me about client-centered practice and the dynamic relationships between people and their activities and environments. Sharon Brintnell, MSc, BOT, OT(C); Sylvia Wilson, MSc, OT(C); and their Occupational Performance Analysis Unit still influence my thoughts and touch my life today. Many other therapists and scholars have influenced the conceptual foundation of this text and their work is summarized in the introductory chapters. Also, the educators at the Western Business School at the University of Western Ontario must be acknowledged for introducing me to the potential of problem-based learning by role-modeling their version of the case method.

The University of Scranton, Dr. Jack Kasar, OTR/L, and the occupational therapy class of 1998 are acknowledged for their contributions to the development and implementation of a task analysis course. This text contains submissions from occupational therapy students: Rachel Budney, Alison Devers, Megan Early, Susan Finora, Erin Panciera, Karin Sandstrom, and Carolyn Silva. Acknowledgments are extended to my course advisers: Michael Goodling, OTR/L; Amy Frantz, MS, OTR/L; Lila Nappi, OTR/L; Neil Penny, MS, OTR/L; Dr. Paul Petersen, OTR/L; Rhonda Waskiewicz, OTR/L; and Karl Young, OTR/L. The adolescent case "Barb" is Neil Penny's creation. Acknowledgments are extended to our youngest contributors Rachel and Hanna.

Versions of this manuscript have been reviewed by many experts in their area of specialty. They have also considered the applicability of the readings and assignments to educational programs for certified occupational therapy assistants, registered occupational therapists, and Canadian certified occupational therapists. Acknowledgments to Jennifer Angelo, PhD, FAOTA, ATP; Linda F. Fazio, PhD, OTR, FAOTA; Joy Hammel, PhD, OTR/L, FAOTA; Leslie L. Jackson, MEd, OTR; Anne Morris, EdD, OTR; Neil Penny, MS, OTR/L; Sherry Pfister, AAS, COTA/L; Rhonda Waskiewicz, OTR/L; Shirley A. Wells, MPH, OTR; and Rhona Reiss Zukas, MOT, OTR, FAOTA. I am particularly grateful to Lela A. Llorens, PhD, OTR, FAOTA, for formative feedback during the development of this manuscript and for her contribution to the foreword. Anonymous reviewers from the Canadian Occupational Therapy Foundation are acknowledged for their comments regarding an initial draft of this manuscript. Finally, I am particularly grateful to my husband Gregg Landry, BS, OT(C), for editorial assistance and continuous, daily support of "my projects."

The ideas, inspirations, and recommendations of Maureen Muncaster, MA, Acquisitions Editor at the American Occupational Therapy Association (AOTA), contributed to the quality and timely completion of this project. Mary Fisk, MA, at AOTA and Kathy Kelly at Publications Professionals contributed their literary talents, and Hank Isaac provided the graphic design for the cover and pages.

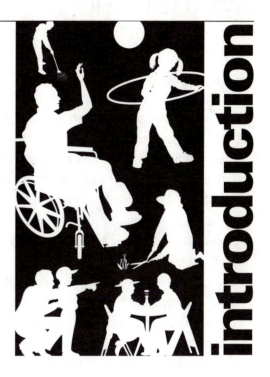

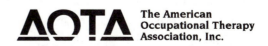

The American
Occupational Therapy
Association, Inc.

INTRODUCTION

Occupational therapy practitioners[1] provide services directed at improving the health, performance, and quality of life of individuals and communities. This vision is accomplished in practice through the use of **task analysis** and **activity analysis,** both of which are key process skills (Mosey, 1981; Trombly, 1995). Practitioners use task analysis to analyze the dynamic relationships between individuals and their occupations, including roles, tasks, and activities, and their performance contexts. Analysis of individuals involves consideration of their past experiences, interests, goals, and values, as well as their sensorimotor, cognitive, psychosocial, and psychological skills and abilities. Analysis of performance contexts is concerned with temporal variables and individuals' cultural, physical, and social environments. Activity analysis, as distinguished from task analysis, is used to assess activities, crafts, or games to determine whether they motivate and fulfill clients' occupational performance needs and enhance their performance components (Llorens, 1993). Both task analysis and activity analysis are integral to screening, evaluation, program planning, intervention, and reevaluation process.

Task Analysis: An Occupational Performance Approach will provide student therapists with the opportunity to (a) learn the historical and contemporary use of purposeful activities with people to promote health and well-being; (b) develop the knowledge and skills required to perform task and activity analyses and participate in the occupational therapy evaluation and intervention; (c) analyze activities of daily living, work and productive activities, and play and leisure pursuits of clients of all age groups; and (d) create a resource guide for use when entering clinical practice. This text presents an occupational performance approach to analysis and uses the *Uniform Terminology* of the American

Occupational Therapy Association (1994). The historical use of occupation, task and activity analysis, and the development of the occupational performance approach are reviewed in the introductory chapter titled "Historical and Contemporary Perspectives." Application of an occupational performance approach to task analysis is illustrated in the chapter titled "The Contribution of Occupational Therapy to Health." Section One contains a number of chapters that provide information and assignments to enable occupational therapy students to develop their knowledge and skills in task analysis using an occupational performance approach.

Sections Two, Three, Four, and Five provide opportunities to practice applying task analysis within the evaluation and intervention process using the specific cases of children, adolescents, adults, and seniors. Each chapter contains learning assignments and resources to aid students and instructors in structuring the depth and breadth of the learning experience. Section Six includes a number of examples of completed Occupational Performance Analysis—Short Forms. The Appendices include a number of documents relevant to task analysis from the American Occupational Therapy Association.

An individual's occupational performance profile is a product of the dynamic relationship between the individual and his or her occupations and environments. Discrepancies between past and present occupational performance profiles help establish the need for therapeutic intervention, and understanding a client's profile is essential to initiating and managing the therapy process. Although the clients, families, and therapists described in this text are hypothetical, the situations portrayed are realistic and representative. Using task analysis for these clinical cases reinforces the utility of newly

---

[1]Occupational therapy practitioner refers to both registered occupational therapists and certified occupational therapy assistants.

acquired information and the role of clinical practitioners in promoting health. Understanding task analysis can also strengthen one's ambition to practice occupational therapy: the satisfaction derived from rehearsing the cognitive steps and professional behaviors of clinical practitioners should not be underestimated.

Occupational therapy practitioners engage their clients in purposeful and therapeutic activities that translate theories and principles into concrete activities that promote function and adaptation (Trombly, 1995). Occupational therapy students will use activity analysis to design intrinsically rewarding, meaningful, and purposeful activities. The three chapters titled "Children's Cultural Crafts and Games"; "Adolescent Activities, Crafts, and Games"; and "Adult Activities, Crafts, and Games" introduce a number of therapeutic activity ideas. Students may choose to use these activities when designing intervention for client cases.

Task analysis is one of the essential skills used by all occupational therapy practitioners. After learning how to conduct a task analysis by completing the readings and assignments in Section One, students can refine this skill by applying it to client clinical scenarios. The case method approach used in *Task Analysis: An Occupational Performance Approach* parallels occupational therapy's traditional use of purposeful activities to promote learning, insight, skills, and independent performance and the belief that meaningful engagement sanctions diversity and flexibility in learning and adaptation (Watson, 1996).

Upon completion of the readings and assignments in this text, the occupational therapy student will

1. Describe the historical relevance of occupation to the occupational therapy profession.

2. Illustrate and explain an occupational performance theoretical model.

3. Identify, describe, and apply some of the theories underlying the use of purposeful activity.

4. Define and compare the constructs of (a) impairments, disabilities, and handicaps; (b) roles, tasks, and activities; (c) occupation, occupational performance, and function; (d) meaningful and purposeful activity; and (e) independence.

5. Identify and define the domains of concern to the occupational therapy practitioner as defined in *Uniform Terminology for Occupational Therapy*.

6. Explain the concept of person-activity-environment (PAE) fit, identify the variables that affect PAE fit, and describe the relevance of PAE fit to the process of occupational therapy evaluation and intervention.

7. Explain the term **task analysis** and describe its use during client screening, evaluation, program planning, intervention, and reevaluation.

8. Explain and give examples of how task analysis is used to contribute to the health and wellness of individuals and communities.

9. Analyze the activities of daily living, productive work, play, and leisure pursuits of pediatric, adolescent, and adult client cases to understand their previous or current occupational performance profiles and begin to predict potential future profiles.

10. Develop clinical observation and task analysis skills by applying logical thinking, critical analysis, creativity, and problem solving; evaluate client cases; and select and design purposeful, therapeutic activities to address intervention goals and priorities.

11. Describe the relevance of habituation, lifestyle, and a balance of occupations to health and wellness.

12. Develop and apply skills in teaching and working with others through small group tasks, collaborative team projects, group discussions, and oral presentations.

13. Conclude that an individual's roles, tasks, and developmental issues change across the life span; and that participation in selected tasks and meaningful activities can restore, reinforce, and enhance role functioning, adaptation, health, and wellness.

References

American Occupational Therapy Association. (1994). *Uniform terminology for occupational therapy* (3rd ed.). Bethesda, MD: Author.

Llorens, L. A. (1993). Activity analysis: Agreement between participants and observers on perceived factors in occupation components. *Occupational Therapy Journal of Research, 13,* 198–211.

Mosey, A. C. (1981). *Occupational therapy: Configuration of a profession.* New York: Raven Press.

Trombly, C. A. (1995). Purposeful activity. In C. A. Trombly (Ed.), *Occupational therapy for physical dysfunction* (4th ed., pp. 237–253). Baltimore: Williams & Wilkins.

Watson, D. E. (1996). *Clinical cases for learning pediatric occupational therapy; A problem-based approach.* San Antonio, TX: Therapy Skill Builders.

TASK ANALYSIS: HISTORICAL AND CONTEMPORARY PERSPECTIVES

"Man, through the use of his hands, as they are energized by mind and will, can influence the state of his own health" (Reilly, 1962, p. 3).[1]

Chapter Objectives

1. Describe the historical relevance of occupation to the occupational therapy profession.
2. Recite the characteristics of a purposeful activity.
3. Define and compare the terms **impairment**, **disability**, and **handicap**.
4. Illustrate and explain one occupational performance model.
5. Recite the occupational performance areas, performance component domains, and environmental contexts of performance.
6. Illustrate and explain the concept of person-activity-environment fit.
7. Define and compare the difference between **task analysis** and **activity analysis**.

Occupation: Our Heritage

The belief that activity engagement has healing power has its roots in the arts and crafts movement of the late 19th century and in the philosophies of the profession's founders. Early occupational therapy theorists acknowledged the unity between mind and body and the link between engagement, self-fulfillment, and health (Atwood, 1907; Meyer, 1922; Moher, 1907). Goal-directed activities were used for their diversional, therapeutic, vocational, and motivational qualities to instill craftsmanship and industry, and encourage adjustment to disability. Consider the following proposed definition of occupational therapy from 1921: "Occupational therapy is defined as any activity, mental or physical, definitely prescribed and guided for the distinct purpose of contributing to and hastening recovery from disease or injury" (Hall, 1922, p. 61).

Throughout the 20th century occupational therapists have been developing their skills in activity analysis to select and design goal-directed, therapeutic activities. In the early 1910s, Gilbreth (1911) introduced the concept of job analysis through motion studies. Characteristics of the worker, the worker's surroundings, and motion requirements of the job were considered and adaptations were made to improve efficiency. Friedman (1916) recommended that health professionals who seek to match patients with a vocation consider the physical, mental, and psychological requirements of the particular occupation.

Occupational therapists and educators incorporated activity analysis into practice and educational programs during World War I (Creighton, 1992). Joint position, action, and muscle strength were of primary interest. By the 1920s, Haas (1922) had suggested a system of activity analysis and rating. Classification according to therapeutic benefit of activity occurred between 1920 and the 1940s, and through the 1960s analyses included physical requirements and emotional and social properties (Creighton, 1992). Then, during the 1970s and 1980s a number of frames of reference influenced methods of analysis, requiring therapists to recognize sensorimotor, cognitive, biomechanical, volitional, and habituation parameters (Creighton, 1992). Activities were used to assess, diagnose, and treat clients to develop or restore their independence in self-care, work, and leisure.

By analyzing the features, characteristics, and qualities of activities, therapists now realize that they can grade and adapt tasks according to the

---

[1]From "Occupational Therapy Can Be One of the Great Ideas of the 20th Century Medicine," by M. Reilly, 1962, *American Journal of Occupational Therapy, 16*, p. 3. Copyright 1962 by the American Occupational Therapy Association. Reprinted with permission.

client's residual capabilities or prescribe activities as therapeutic modalities (Hinojosa, Sabari, Rosenfeld, 1983; Kidner, 1930). **Purposeful activities** are therapeutic when they (a) are relevant, meaningful, and goal-directed; (b) elicit coordination among sensorimotor, cognitive, psychological, and psychosocial systems; and (c) promote mastery and feelings of competence (American Occupational Therapy Association [AOTA], 1993; Fidler & Fidler, 1978; Trombly, 1995a). Therapeutic activities were used to provide feedback to clients and therapists about performance and promoted development and feelings of competence and mastery (Breines, 1984; Fidler, 1981).

Contemporary definitions of the profession continue to echo the value placed on engagement in occupations, performance of tasks and roles, and promotion of mastery:

> Occupational therapy is the art and science of directing an individual's participation in selected tasks to restore, reinforce, and enhance performance; facilitate learning of those skills and functions essential for adaptation and productivity; diminish or correct pathology; and promote and maintain health. Reference to occupation in the title is in the context of individuals' goal-directed use of time, energy, interest, and attention. Its fundamental concern is the development and maintenance of the capacity throughout the life span to perform with satisfaction to self and others those tasks and roles essential to productive living and to the mastery of self and the environment (AOTA, 1995a, p. 89; AOTA, 1995b, p. 105).

> Occupational therapy is the art and science which utilizes the analysis and application of activities specifically related to occupational performance in the areas of self care, productivity and leisure.

> Through assessment, interpretation, and intervention, occupational therapists address problems impeding functional or adaptive behaviour in persons whose occupational performance is impaired by illness or injury, emotional disorder, developmental disorder, social disadvantage or the aging process. The purpose is to prevent disability and to promote, maintain or restore occupational performance, health, and spiritual well-being. Furthermore, occupational therapy services can be directed through health, educational and social service systems (Canadian Association Occupational Therapist [CAOT], 1991, p. 140).[2]

An Occupational Performance Approach to Theory and Practice

"The focus of practice will shift from reducing impairment through purposeful activity to preventing handicap through occupational engagement" (Polatajko, 1994, p. 591).[3]

Occupational engagement is increasingly being used to treat impairments, reduce disabilities, and prevent handicaps (Polatajko, 1994). An **impairment** is a loss, abnormality, or disturbance of an anatomical, physiological, mental, or emotional structure or function that may be temporary or permanent (Nagi, 1991; World Health Organization [WHO], 1980). Functional limitations manifest at the level of the person (e.g., seeing, walking); **disability** refers to "any restriction or lack (resulting from an impairment) of ability to perform an activity in the manner or within the range considered normal" (Nagi, 1991; WHO, 1980, p. 143). Disabilities may be temporary or permanent, reversible or irreversible, progressive or regressive and are

[2]From *Guidelines for the Client-Centerd Practice of Occupational Therapy,* Health Canada, 1983. Reproduced with permission of the Minister of Public Works and Government Services Canada, 1996.
[3]From "Dreams, Dilemmas, and Decisions for Occupational Therapy Practice in the New Millennium: A Canadian Perspective," by H. J. Polatajko, 1994, *American Journal of Occupational Therapy, 48,* p. 591. Copyright 1994 by the American Occupational Therapy Association. Reprinted with permission.

"characterized by excesses or deficiencies of customarily expected activity performance and behavior" (WHO, 1980, p. 143). **Handicap** represents a disadvantage experienced by an individual as a result of an impairment and disability "that limit or prevent fulfillment of a role that is normal (depending on age, sex, and social and cultural factors) for that individual" (WHO, 1980, p. 183).[4] Handicaps are characterized by discord between an individual's performance and the expectations of self or others.

Occupational therapy practitioners' contribution to health, therefore, includes treatment of impairments and intervention directed at people and/or environments to minimize disability and prevent handicap. The **occupational performance approach** provides one model for practice that enables therapists to accomplish this vision. The **occupational performance** approach focuses on the interactive and transactional relationship between people and their occupations and environments because health is shaped by the continuous and simultaneous interaction between these factors (AOTA, 1994; CAOT, 1993; Law et al., 1996).

Occupational Performance Analysis in Theory

In the early 1970s the American Occupational Therapy Association proposed that the role, function, and domain of concern of occupational therapy personnel was occupational performance, which includes performance areas and performance components (AOTA, 1973; AOTA, 1974). Occupational performance models have been proposed by Mosey (1981), Reed and Sanderson (1980), AOTA (1994), the Canadian Association of Occupational Therapists (1991), Christiansen and Baum (1991), Law et al. (1996), and Pedretti (1995).

Uniform Terminology for Occupational Therapy provides occupational therapy practitioners with a generic outline of the scope of practice. It also suggests that the tool that determines successful performance is **person-activity-environment fit** (AOTA, 1994). Occupational therapy services create a fit, or match, between the person, the activity, and the environment by aligning "the skills and abilities of the individual; the demands of activity; and the characteristics of the physical, social, and cultural environments" (AOTA, 1994, p. 277) (see Figure 1). The domains of concern in designing the fit include performance areas, performance components, and performance contexts. **Performance areas** are the broad categories of tasks that are part of a typical day, including activities of daily living, work and productive activities, and play or leisure activities. **Performance components** are the human abilities required for successful engagement in performance areas, including sensorimotor, cognitive, psychological, and psychosocial systems. **Performance contexts** are the situations or factors that influence desired and successful engagement, including temporal (chronological age, developmental age, place in the life cycle, and health status) and environmental (physical, social, and cultural) aspects.

Figure 1. Person-Activity-Environment Fit.

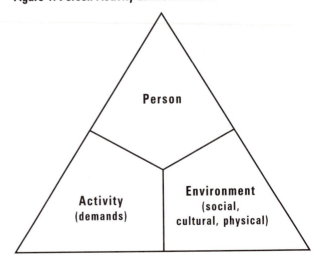

[4]From "International classification of impairments, disabilities, and handicaps" by the World Health Organization, 1980, *Task Analysis, An Occupational Performance Approach*, p. 143, 183. Reprinted with permission. 1996.

The Model of Occupational Performance (Figure 2) purports that health, well-being, and occupational performance in the areas of self-care, productivity, and leisure are predicated on a balanced integration of spiritual, physical, mental, and sociocultural components of individuals within the social, cultural, and social environmental context (CAOT, 1990). The model provides a guide to assist occupational therapists in restoring, maintaining, and developing function and to prevent dysfunction in individuals (CAOT, 1991).

Figure 2. Interacting Elements of the Individual in a Model of Occupational Performance (*original depiction*).

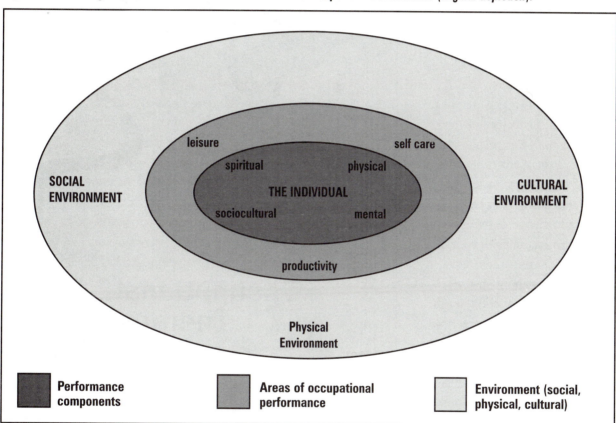

From *Occupational Therapy Guidelines for Client-Centred Mental Health Practice* by Canadian Association of Occupational Therapists, 1993. Reproduced with permission of the Minister of Public Works and Government Services Canada, 1996.

The 1993 proposal for revision of the Model of Occupational Performance (Figure 3) rearranges the concentric circles to conceptualize the multidimensional, simultaneous, and dynamic interaction between the environmental elements that influence an individual's occupational performance (CAOT, 1993). The revised model proposes that occupational performance is affected in an "ever-changing way" by an individual's performance components and context. The contexts of concern to therapists and clients include the political, economic, legal, physical, cultural, and social environments. The principles of this model include an acknowledgment of (a) the tendency of individuals to reflect on the nature and meaning of their life, (b) the need for the occupational therapist to elicit and sustain volition as a basis for action, (c) the value of the therapeutic partnership between a client and therapist, (d) the importance of the teaching-learning process, and (e) the ethical framework that guides the occupational therapist's sense of responsibility and morality.

Figure 3. Interacting Elements of the Individual in a Model of Occupational Performance: Revised.

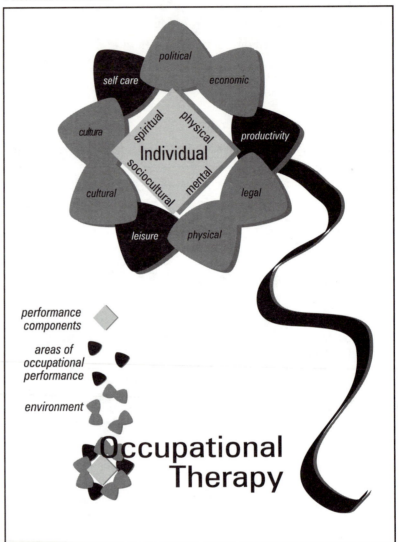

From *Occupational Therapy Guidelines for Client-Centred Mental Health Practice* by Health Canada, 1993. Reproduced with permission of the Minister of Public Works and Government Services Canada, 1996.

Figure 4. An Overview of the Person-Environment-Performance Framework.

ENVIRONMENT
   PHYSICAL, SOCIAL, AND CULTURAL FACTORS
      (Examples: People, objects, architecture, organizations, traditions, and public policy)

   PERFORMANCE
   ACTIVITIES, TASKS, AND ROLES OF OCCUPATIONS
      (Including requirements of work, play/leisure, and self-maintenance)

      PERSON
         Personality
         Motivations and Goals
         Experiences
         Beliefs about Self and Environment

         Abilities and Skills
         Intrinsic Performance Enablers
            • Cognitive
            • Psychological
            • Sensory
            • Neuromotor
            • Physiological
            • Pharmacologic

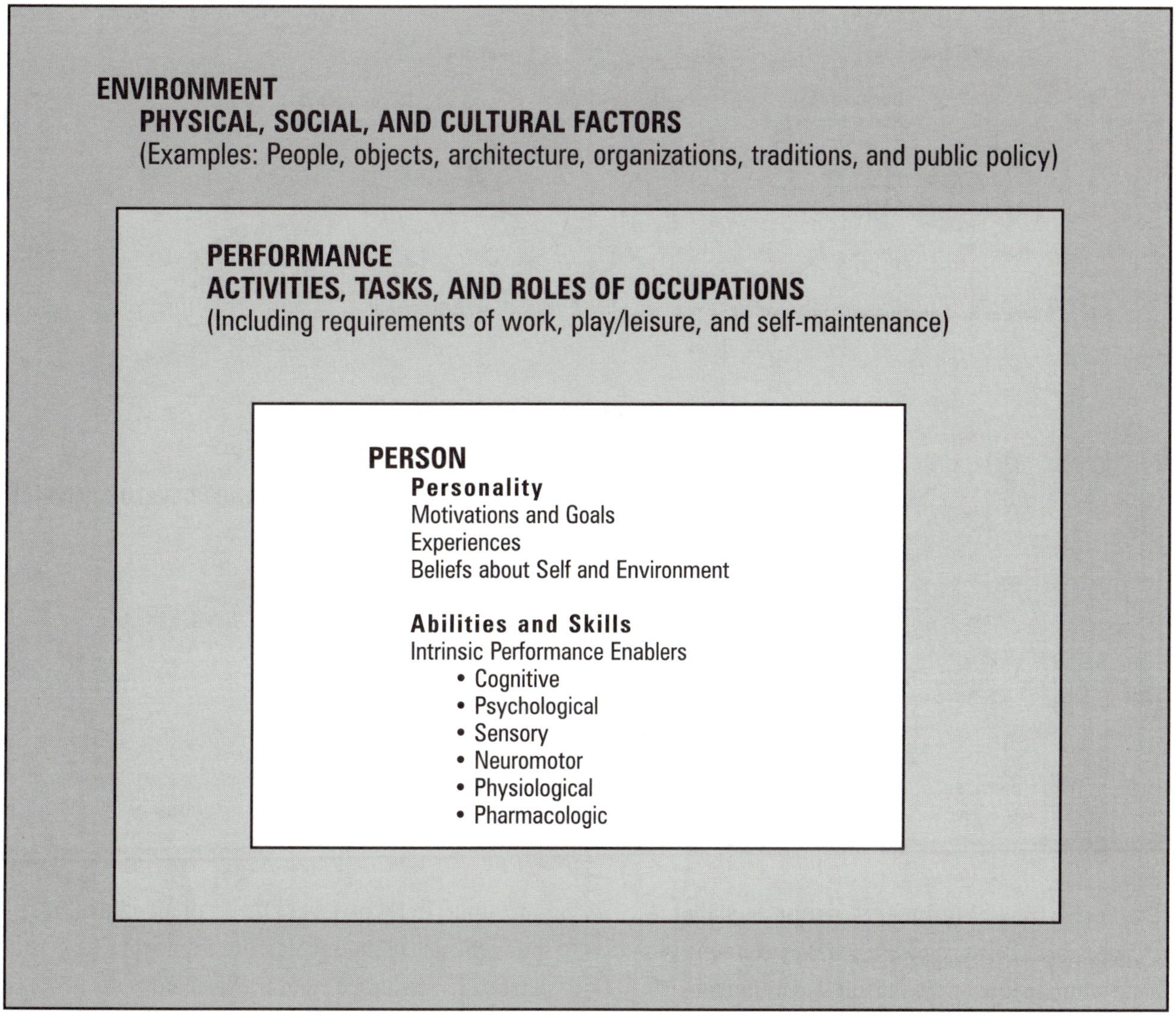

From *Occupational Therapy: Overcoming Human Performance Deficits,* by C. Christiansen and C. Baum, 1991, Thorofare, NJ: Slack. Reproduced with permission.

The Person-Environment-Performance Framework (Figure 4) also addresses this relationship between people, environments, and performance (Christiansen & Baum, 1991). Personality characteristics (motivations, goals, experiences, and beliefs about self and environment) and intrinsic enablers (psychological, cognitive, neuromotor, sensory, and physiological) are the human subsystems of interest to occupational therapy practitioners. Performance is understood in terms of the activities, tasks, and roles of occupation, as influenced by physical, social, and cultural environmental factors.

Figure 5. Depiction of the Person-Environment-Occupation Model of Occupational Performance Across the Life Span.

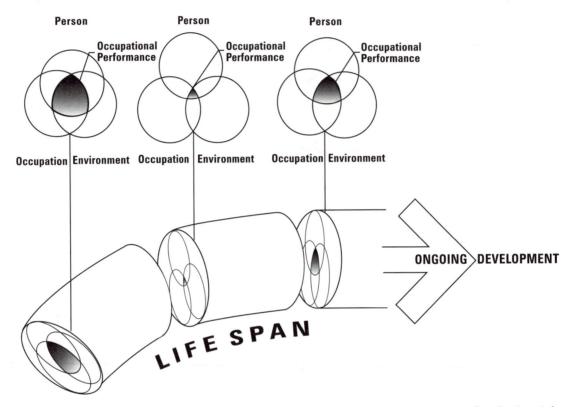

From "The Person-Environment-Occupation Model: A Transactive Approach to Occupational Performance," by M. Law et al., 1996, *Canadian Journal of Occupational Therapy, 63,* pp. 9-23. Copyright 1996 by the Canadian Association of Occupational Therapists (CAOT). Reproduced with permission of CAOT Publications.

The Person-Environment-Occupation Model of Occupational Performance (Figure 5) contains the same components as the Person-Environment-Performance Framework for defining health and the role and function of occupational therapists (Law et al., 1996). The person, environment, and occupation are represented by separate but interconnected spheres. Overlap among the spheres represents occupational performance. The closer the overlap between people and their environments and occupations, the more harmonious or compatible the interaction and the more optimized the occupational performance. The relationships of the components vary across time and can be described by the changing patterns and routines of individuals. Law et al. (1996) suggest that occupational therapists

must understand people in terms of attributes (performance components), life experiences, personality styles, cultural background, self-concepts, and personal competencies. The model recognizes the importance of the cultural, socioeconomic, institutional, physical, and social components of the environment.

Occupational Performance Analysis in Practice

The occupational performance approach has been recommended as a model for all clinical practice areas because it represents the domains of concern to occupational therapy (AOTA, 1994; CAOT, 1991). Recent publications have applied the approach to clinical practice in mental health

(CAOT, 1993); pediatrics (Case-Smith, Allen, & Pratt, 1996); and physical disabilities (Pedretti, 1996). This text draws on these conceptual foundations and proposes that therapists who seek to understand occupational performance must analyze three variables: (a) the occupation, (b) the person, and (c) the performance context. Using this type of holistic analysis in clinical practice increases the scope of assessment options and intervention strategies available to therapists beyond the use of activities to treat impairments (Dunn, Brown, & McGuigan, 1994; Law et al., 1996; Letts et al., 1994).

Task analysis, within this text, refers to the process of analyzing the dynamic relationship between individuals and their occupations and environments. Occupational therapy practitioners use task analysis as a tool in the evaluation *and* intervention processes. Analysis of individuals requires consideration of their past experiences, volition, and habits, as well as of their sensorimotor, cognitive, psychosocial, and psychological performance components. Analysis of occupations encompasses roles, tasks, and activities. Analysis of contexts encompasses temporal variables and cultural, physical, and social environments.

Activity analysis is the process of determining if an activity, craft, or game motivates and fulfills a client's occupational performance needs and enhances performance components (Llorens, 1993). Analysis is used to (a) determine whether an activity has therapeutic potential or value, and (b) select and design an activity to treat an impairment or functional limitation (Trombly, 1995b). Despite examples in the literature regarding different approaches to activity analysis, research suggests that there may not be consensus among therapists (Tsai, 1994; Neistadt McAuley, Zecha, & Shannon, 1993) and students (Llorens, 1993) in identification of components.

Although an occupational performance model of task analysis predominates, other frames of reference may be used to enhance understanding of specific performance components and contexts. Concepts from the Model of Human Occupation will aid in analysis of occupational therapy clients' volition and habituation. Sensorimotor theories and the Cognitive Disabilities Model will be used to enhance understanding of sensory, motor, and cognitive performance components. The biomechanical approach will aid in analysis of neuromusculoskeletal and physical environmental demands of the work place.

Assignment

1. Define these terms:
   Activity analysis
   Impairments
   Disabilities
   Handicaps
   Occupation
   Occupational performance analysis
   Person-activity-environment fit
   Performance areas
   Performance components
   Performance contexts
   Purposeful activity
   Task analysis

2. Read the introduction and person-activity-environment fit section of *Uniform Terminology for Occupational Therapy* (AOTA, 1994). Also read the article by Law et al., (1996). *The Person-Environment-Occupation Model: A Transactive Approach to Occupational Performance.*

3. Research one of the models described in this chapter or one of the articles compiled by Fleming Cottrell (1996) to prepare a 15-minute class presentation on the use of purposeful activity to enhance occupational performance.

The information that follows will (a) provide students and instructors with resources to enhance the learning experience and (b) assist the student in completing the assignment.

Learning Resources

Fleming Cottrell, R. P. (Ed.). (1996). *Perspectives on purposeful activity: Foundation and future of occupational therapy.* Bethesda, MD: American Occupational Therapy Association.

Law, M., Cooper, B., Strong, S., Stewart, D., Rigby, P., & Letts, L. (1996). The Person-Environment-Occupation Model: A transactive approach to occupational performance. *Canadian Journal of Occupational Therapy, 63,* 9–23.

Study Questions

1. Describe the use of task and activity analysis in occupational therapy in the 1910s; 1920s to 1940s; 1970s to 1980s.
2. Define **activity analysis.** Define **task analysis.** How do task analysis and activity analysis differ? How are they similar or related?
3. List five characteristics or qualities of purposeful activities.
4. Draw and describe one of the following models: Model of Occupational Performance (CAOT, 1993), Person-Environment-Performance Framework (Christiansen & Baum, 1991), Person-Environment-Occupation Model of Occupational Performance (Law et al., 1996).
5. Describe what is meant by **person-activity-environment fit** (AOTA, 1994).
6. Bob's girlfriend chose not to go dancing with him because he could not stand up. Bob is a paraplegic and uses a wheelchair. Identify Bob's impairment, disability, and handicap.
7. What is meant by the term **performance component**? Compare the performance component categories between two occupational performance theoretical models.

References

American Occupational Therapy Association (AOTA). (1973). *The roles and functions of occupational therapy personnel.* Bethesda, MD: Author.

AOTA. (1974). *A curriculum guide for occupational therapy educators.* Bethesda, MD: Author.

AOTA. (1993). *Position paper: Purposeful activity.* Bethesda, MD: Author.

AOTA. (1994). *Uniform terminology for occupational therapy* (3rd ed.). Bethesda, MD: Author.

AOTA. (1995a). *Essentials and guidelines for an accredited educational program for the occupational therapist.* Bethesda, MD: Author.

AOTA. (1995b). *Essentials and guidelines for an accredited educational program for the occupational therapy assistant.* Bethesda, MD: Author.

Atwood, C. E. (1907). *The favourable influence of occupation in certain nervous disorders.* New York Medical Journal, *86,* 1101–1103.

Breines, E. (1984). An attempt to define purposeful activity. *American Journal of Occupational Therapy, 38,* 543–544.

Canadian Association of Occupational Therapists (CAOT). (1990). *Occupational therapy: Core identity.* Toronto, ON: Author.

CAOT. (1991). *Canadian occupational therapy guidelines for client-centred practice.* Toronto, ON: Author.

CAOT. (1993). *Occupational therapy guidelines for client-centred mental health practice.* Toronto, ON: Author.

Case-Smith, J., Allen, A. S., & Pratt, P. N. (1996). *Occupational therapy for children* (3rd ed.). Baltimore: Mosby.

Christiansen, C., & Baum, C. (Eds.). (1991). *Occupational therapy: Overcoming human performance deficits.* Thorofare, NJ: Slack.

Creighton, C. (1992). The origin and evolution of activity analysis. *American Journal of Occupational Therapy, 46,* 45–48.

Dunn, W., Brown, C., McGuigan, A. (1994). The ecology of human performance: A framework for considering the effect of context. *American Journal of Occupational Therapy, 48,* 595–607.

Fidler, G. S. (1981). From crafts to competence. *American Journal of Occupational Therapy, 35,* 567–573.

Fidler, G. S., & Fidler, J. (1978). Doing and becoming: Purposeful action and self-actualization. *American Journal of Occupational Therapy, 32,* 305–310.

Friedman, H. M. (1916, September 23). Occupational specialization in the defective. *New York Medical Journal,* 587–592.

Gilbreth, F. B. (1911). *Motion study.* New York: Nostrand.

Haas, L. J. (1922). Crafts adaptable to occupational need: Their relative importance. *Archives of Occupational Therapy, 1,* 443–445.

Hall, H. J. (1922). Occupational therapy in 1921. *The Modern Hospital, 18,* 61–63.

Hinojosa, J., Sabari, J., & Rosenfeld, M. S. (1983). Purposeful activities. *American Journal of Occupational Therapy, 37,* 805–806.

Kidner, T. B. (1930). *Occupational therapy: The science of prescribed work for invalids.* Stuttgart, Germany: W. Kohlhammer.

Law, M., Cooper, B., Strong, S., Stewart, D., Rigby, P., & Letts, L. (1996). The Person-Environment-Occupation Model: A transactive approach to occupational performance. *Canadian Journal of Occupational Therapy, 63,* 9–23.

Letts, L., Law, M., Rigby, P., Cooper, B., Stewart, D., & Strong, S. (1994). Person-environment assessments in occupational therapy. *American Journal of Occupational Therapy, 48,* 608–618.

Llorens, L. A. (1993). Activity analysis: Agreement between participants and observers on perceived factors in occupation components. *Occupational Therapy Journal of Research, 13,* 198–211.

Meyer, A. (1922). The philosophy of occupational therapy. *Archives of Occupational Therapy, 1,* 1–10.

Moher, T. J. (1907). Occupation in the treatment of the insane. *Journal of the American Medical Association, 158,* 1664–1666.

Mosey, A. C. (1981). *Occupational therapy: Configuration of a profession.* New York, NY: Raven Press.

Nagi, S. (1991). Disability concepts revisited: Implications for prevention. In A. M. Pope & A. R. Tarlov (Eds.), *Disability in America: Toward a national agenda for prevention.* Washington, DC: National Academy Press.

Neistadt, M. E., McAuley, D., Zecha, D., & Shannon, R. (1993). An analysis of a board game as a treatment activity. *American Journal of Occupational Therapy, 47,* 154–160.

Pedretti, L. (1996). *Occupational therapy: Practice skills for physical dysfunction.* St. Louis, MO: Mosby.

Polatajko, H. J. (1994). Dreams, dilemmas, and decisions for occupational therapy practice in the new millennium: A Canadian perspective. *American Journal of Occupational Therapy, 48,* 590–594.

Reed, K. L., & Sanderson, S. R. (1980). *Concepts of occupational therapy.* Baltimore: Williams & Wilkins.

Reilly, M. (1962). Occupational therapy can be one of the great ideas of the 20th century medicine. *American Journal of Occupational Therapy, 16,* 1–9.

Trombly, C. A. (1995). Occupation: Purposefulness and meaningfulness as therapeutic mechanisms. *American Journal of Occupational Therapy, 49,* 960–972.

Trombly, C. A. (1995b). Purposeful activity. In C. A. Trombly (Ed.), *Occupational therapy for physical dysfunction* (pp. 237–253). Baltimore: Williams & Wilkins.

Tsai, P. L. (1994). *Activity analysis and activity selection among occupational therapists: A survey.* Unpublished master's thesis, Boston University.

World Health Organization. (1980). *International classification of impairments, disabilities, and handicaps: A manual of classification relating to the consequences of disease.* Geneva: Author.

TASK ANALYSIS: THE CONTRIBUTION OF OCCUPATIONAL THERAPY TO HEALTH

Task analysis, using an occupational performance approach, is the process of analyzing the dynamic relationship between people and their occupations and environments.

Chapter Objectives

1. Define and describe the stages of the occupational therapy process from referral to discharge.
2. Explain how task analysis is used as an assessment and intervention tool to improve the health of individuals and communities.
3. Identify the domains of concern to occupational therapy practitioners.
4. Explain the concept **occupational performance profile**.

Contributing to the Health and Wellness of Individuals and Communities

Occupational therapy practitioners provide services directed at improving the health and quality of life of individuals and communities. Therapists contribute to the health of individuals by enabling, maintaining, or restoring occupational performance to enhance function, self-esteem, self-efficacy, and well-being (AOTA, 1994; CAOT, 1991; Trombly, 1995a). Occupational therapy practitioners contribute to the health and well-being of communities by promoting healthy lifestyles and enhancing performance, by enabling people to balance their patterns of occupation, and by creating environments that minimize disability and prevent handicap (CAOT, 1994; Polatajko, 1994). Practitioners accomplish this vision in practice through the use of task analysis for assessment and intervention (Mosey, 1981; Trombly, 1995b).

Service to Individuals

An occupational performance approach to task analysis is integral to the referral, screening, evaluation, program planning, intervention, reevaluation, and discharge processes. Figure 1 illustrates the Occupational Performance Practice Model for Service to Individuals. Upon receipt of a referral, registered occupational therapists initiate the screening process. Interviews or informal assessments may be conducted to determine a client's self-perceptions of current performance and areas of concern, satisfaction, and importance (Law et al., 1994). Therapists assist their clients in identifying discrepancies between past, present, and future role performances (Trombly, 1993). In some practice settings, registered occupational therapists work with parents, families, teachers, physicians, and caregivers to establish intervention goals and priorities on behalf of clients who are unable to advocate on their own behalf.

Figure 1. Occupational Performance Practice Model for Service to Individuals.

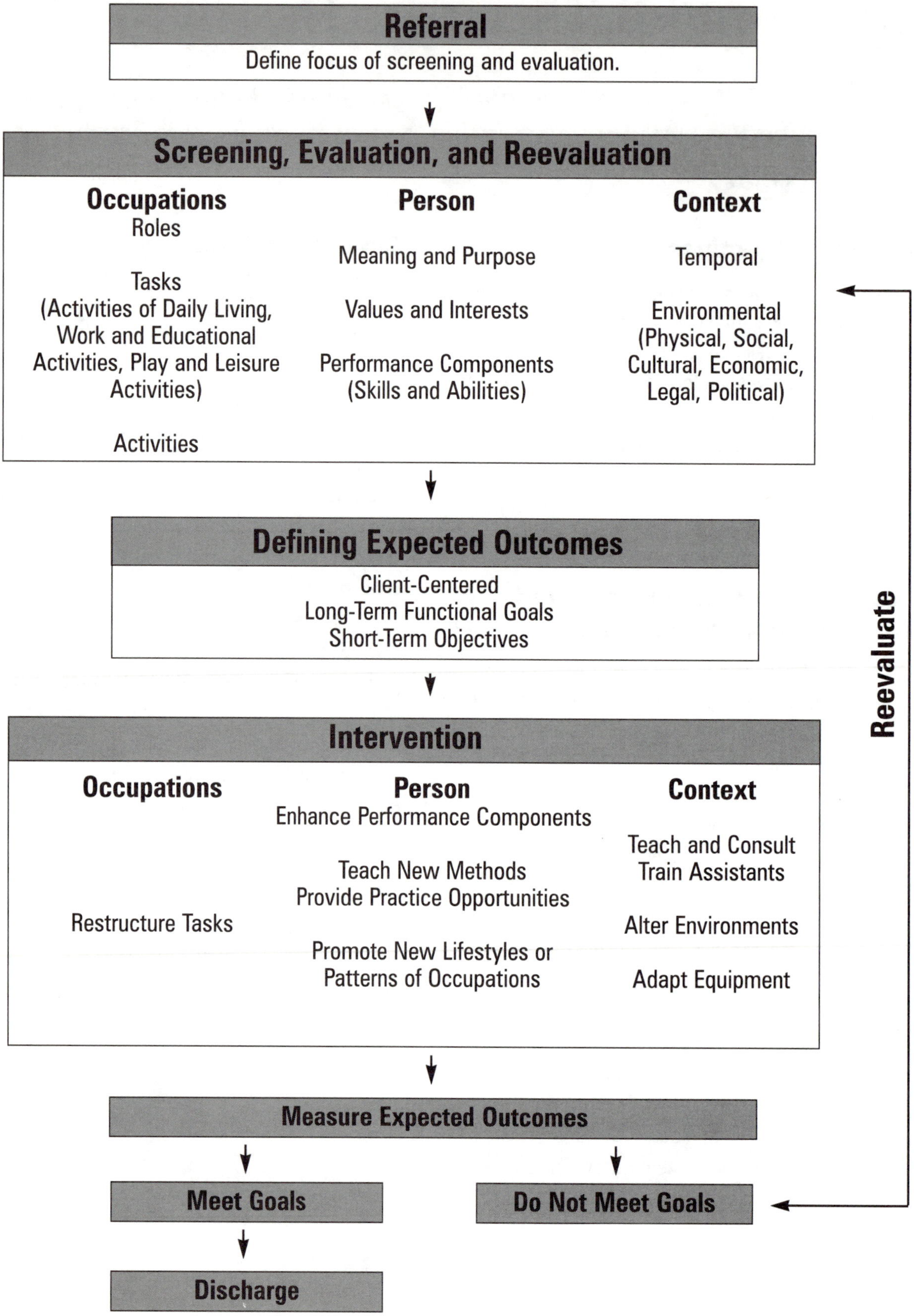

Referral

Define focus of screening and evaluation.

Screening, Evaluation, and Reevaluation

Occupations	Person	Context
Roles		
	Meaning and Purpose	Temporal
Tasks		
(Activities of Daily Living, Work and Educational Activities, Play and Leisure Activities)	Values and Interests	Environmental (Physical, Social, Cultural, Economic, Legal, Political)
	Performance Components (Skills and Abilities)	
Activities		

Defining Expected Outcomes

Client-Centered
Long-Term Functional Goals
Short-Term Objectives

Intervention

Occupations	Person	Context
	Enhance Performance Components	
		Teach and Consult Train Assistants
	Teach New Methods Provide Practice Opportunities	
Restructure Tasks		Alter Environments
	Promote New Lifestyles or Patterns of Occupations	Adapt Equipment

Measure Expected Outcomes

Meet Goals   **Do Not Meet Goals**

Discharge

Reevaluate

Task analysis is used during the screening process to determine which tasks a particular client must perform to assume a lifestyle that he or she values. Practitioners determine how an impairment or diagnosed condition influences present and future function and make predictions about potential gains in functional levels (Mattingly & Fleming, 1994). This determination (a) requires task analysis, (b) assists in structuring and streamlining the screening process, and (c) may help clients make informed decisions regarding the need for intervention.

> *After receiving a referral to see Ann,[1] a depressed single mother who recently had both arms amputated just below the elbow, the registered occupational therapist uses task analysis skills and experience to envision the types of functional tasks that might be difficult to perform with this particular impairment (e.g., buttoning a shirt) and what impact disability may have on psychosocial (i.e., role performance) and psychological (i.e., self-concept) well-being. This process streamlines the types of questions that occur during the screening process (e.g., "Are there tasks that you would do as a mother that you have difficulty performing? How has this change affected you?").*

Occupational therapy practitioners and clients collaborate during the evaluation process to determine the existence and level of disability in activities of daily living, work, and play or leisure and to identify intervention goals and priorities. Clients describe or demonstrate the meaningful tasks that they have difficulty doing but would like to perform. Practitioners use task analysis, clinical observations, and standardized assessments to evaluate client expectations, task performance, contextual parameters, and performance component capabilities to construct a client's occupational

performance profile. Conceptual frameworks and theoretical frames of reference give the analysis process direction and coherence (Mosey, 1981). Certified occupational therapy assistants contribute to the collection of assessment information under the supervision of a registered occupational therapist (AOTA, 1993).

> *Ann is discouraged with the amount of time and effort required for personal self-care and her lack of independence in this area. As a single mother of two very young boys, Ann does not want her children to assist her with personal care. The occupational therapy practitioner observes Ann dress and apply makeup and determines that she has not learned or developed proficiency with the prostheses. All of Ann's blouses have buttons, her cosmetic bag has a small zipper, and her makeup containers are very small and delicate, all requiring a higher level of dexterity and bilateral coordination than Ann currently has. Task analysis is used to determine the task parameters (i.e., small zippers and containers), contextual demands (i.e., recent injury, lack of spouse), and performance components (i.e., motor skill, interest in dressing independence) causing disability and frustration.*

Program planning occurs after the initial evaluation and requires the identification of a client's long-term goals and short-term objectives. Long-term goals relate to functional limitations in occupational performance areas that clients want addressed. Short-term objectives relate to the performance components or impairments that must be changed or the environmental parameters that must be altered in order to achieve the long-term goal (AOTA, 1994). Task analysis may be used to break down long-term goals into smaller, measurable units of activity. These goals direct intervention and

---

[1] The client cases within this text depict hypothetical events and are intended to serve as a basis for learning and/or group discussion. Any similarities to a real person or event are purely coincidental.

provide outcome measures to determine the effectiveness of the program plan.

Ann's current priorities relate to returning to her role as a mother, homemaker, and single parent. She also wonders about her ability to return to her job as a part-time receptionist. Ann and her therapist agree that improvements in current levels of independence in activities of daily living (dressing, personal hygiene, and socialization), productive activities (meal preparation, job performance), and leisure interests (playing with sons, baking, and sewing) are required to be successful in these roles. Her therapist uses task analysis to determine the areas of dressing that will be addressed first, to ensure that Ann attains success in progressively more difficult activities.

Occupational therapy practitioners provide intervention services directed at establishing a fit between occupational role and task parameters, client skills and abilities, and contextual demands (AOTA, 1994). Task analysis is used throughout the process to target intervention at occupations, people, and contexts. Figure 1 summarizes these intervention strategies and includes:

1. Intervention directed at occupation includes (a) designing and grading purposeful therapeutic activities to promote competency, mastery, and self-esteem; and (b) restructuring and adapting tasks.
2. Intervention directed at people includes (a) improving performance component skills and abilities; (b) teaching new methods or compensation strategies by providing practice opportunities; and (c) promoting new lifestyles, ways of living, or patterns of occupation.
3. Intervention directed at contexts includes (a) teaching or consulting, (b) training people to give assistance, (c) altering sociocultural and physical environments, and (d) adapting equipment.

Occupational therapy practitioners engage their clients in purposeful and therapeutic activities that translate theories and principles into concrete activities that promote function and adaptation (Trombly, 1995b). Activity analysis is used to design intrinsically rewarding, meaningful, and therapeutic activities that balance situational challenges with personal skills (Csikszentmihalyi, 1990). Purposeful activities are therapeutic when they (a) are relevant, meaningful, and goal-directed; (b) elicit coordination among sensorimotor, cognitive, psychological, and psychosocial systems; and (c) promote mastery and feelings of self-competence (AOTA, 1993; Fidler & Fidler, 1978; Trombly, 1995a).

During therapy sessions the occupational therapy practitioner offers a number of activity suggestions including baking, sewing, typing, or writing a letter. Ann decides to try baking cookies and sewing on the department's machine. During initial baking sessions, the therapist encourages Ann to practice manipulating all of the ingredients. As her fine motor dexterity improves, Ann progresses to practicing opening and closing containers. When Ann is still unable to open the package of chocolate chips, she is shown how to use adapted scissors.

After analyzing an activity for its potential to address client goals, the therapist may decide if adaptations are necessary to maximize therapeutic value (Trombly, 1995a). Therapists who are skilled at analysis are able to select the most appropriate activity from among those of interest to a particular client (Trombly, 1995b) or adapt an activity that a client has selected to optimize its therapeutic value. Although activity has been used as a treatment modality since the early years of occupational therapy practice, the use of therapeutic activity to improve performance components is "based on the assumption that the activity holds within itself a healing property that will change organic or behavioral impairments" (Trombly, 1995a, p. 964).

> *Ann relearns how to use the sewing machine with her prostheses by making a cosmetic bag with a drawstring and sewing Velcro® on the front of her shirts. Engagement in sewing improves her proficiency with the prostheses, and completion of these projects eliminates the need for Ann to master shirt button closures or a small cosmetic bag zipper. She gains independence with dressing, makeup management, and sewing; renews her confidence in independently engaging in self-care and leisure interests; and begins to envision her potential to return to her role as a mother and homemaker.*

Mattingly and Fleming (1994, p. 133) indicate that "therapists think about the whole condition; this includes the person, the illness, the meanings the illness has for the person, the family, and the social and physical contexts in which the person lives."[2] Occupational therapists use this process of conditional reasoning to envision a client's potential. Potential, however, is conditional on a client's participation in the construction of his or her vision for the future. Therapists enlist clients in this participatory process by providing meaningful choices during treatment and by structuring therapeutic activities to address multiple, simultaneous, and individualized goals. Activity and task analysis is used throughout the process to suggest appropriate treatment activities and to structure engagement to address multiple therapy goals. Clients are typically discharged when they achieve their goals or withdraw from services or when it is determined that they no longer benefit from intervention.

> *Through the therapy process Ann eventually gains greater independence in the occupational performance areas that give meaning to her life. She regains control over her patterns of occupations, returns to meaningful roles, and reestablishes a satisfying relationship with her children.*

Service to People in Communities

According to the United States Bureau of the Census, 19.4% of the population, or 48.9 million people, had disabilities in 1991 and 1992 (McNeil, 1993). This figure excludes those individuals who lived in nursing homes and other institutions (McNeil, 1993). Figure 2 portrays the percentage by age of people (population = 251.8 million) with a disability and with a severe disability in 1991 and 1992.

The incidence of people with significant and chronic disabilities is increasing (Public Health Service, 1992). Strauss and Corbin (1988) recommend that

Figure 2. Percentage of Population with a Disability and with a Severe Disability, by Age: 1991-1992.

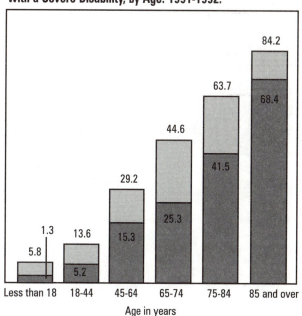

Percent with a disability
Percent with a severe disability

From "Americans With Disabilities: 1991-1992," by J. M. McNeil, 1993, *U.S. Bureau of the Census, Current Population Reports, P70-33.* Washington, DC: U.S. Government Printing Office.

---

[2]From Task Analysis: An Occupational Performance Approach. *"Therapists think about the whole condition,"* Mattingly & Fleming, 1994. Reprinted with permission.

health care professionals use a holistic, biopsychoso-cial view of the chronically sick person rather than focus on the disease process. They recommend promoting early detection and management, providing assistance to enable people to reorganize and manage their daily tasks, and helping individuals with chronic illness reconcile their psychosocial and personal identities. Health prevention and promotion efforts should focus on communities and individuals.

Service to Communities

The occupational performance approach to task analysis can be used to promote the health and well-being of communities. Registered occupational therapists and certified occupational therapy assistants at an advanced level of practice provide services to agencies, groups, and communities in areas of specific expertise (AOTA, 1993). Practitioners use task analysis to (a) identify discrepancies between desired and current levels of occupational performance in target populations; (b) determine the task parameters, contextual demands, and performance component impairments causing dysfunction or disability, if any; and (c) design intervention directed at promoting healthy lifestyles and educating communities to promote, establish, or develop programs that support these

goals. Figure 3 summarizes the Occupational Performance Practice Model for Service to People in Communities.

Occupational therapy practitioners consult with agencies such as day care services, employers, and nursing homes to design environments and structure tasks that enable children, adults, and seniors to engage in meaningful occupations in their communities. Therapists also collaborate with policy makers to ensure that the personal, sociocultural, and physical-environmental needs of individuals with disabilities are addressed in public policy.

Using Task Analysis to Guide Services to Individuals and Communities

The use of task analysis within an occupational performance approach is essential to the process of promoting the health and wellness of individuals and communities. Analysis skills allow occupational therapy practitioners to examine the roles, tasks, and activities of individuals and communities and to identify gaps between current and desired occupational performance and barriers to engagement. This examination and identification process ensures accurate analysis of need and effective selection of intervention strategies.

Figure 3. Occupational Performance Practice Model for Service to People in Communities.

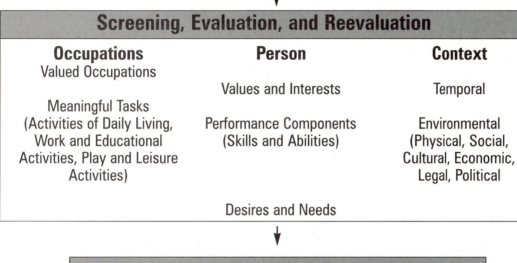

Referral

Define focus of screening and evaluation.

Screening, Evaluation, and Reevaluation

Occupations	**Person**	**Context**
Valued Occupations	Values and Interests	Temporal
Meaningful Tasks (Activities of Daily Living, Work and Educational Activities, Play and Leisure Activities)	Performance Components (Skills and Abilities)	Environmental (Physical, Social, Cultural, Economic, Legal, Political)

Desires and Needs

Defining Expected Outcomes

Vision
Values and Principles
Mission
Goals and Objectives

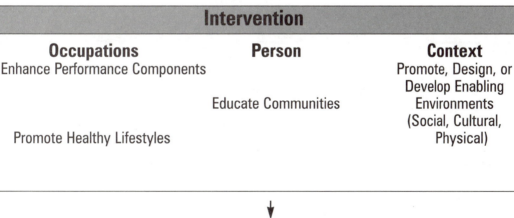

Intervention

Occupations	**Person**	**Context**
Enhance Performance Components		Promote, Design, or Develop Enabling Environments (Social, Cultural, Physical)
	Educate Communities	
Promote Healthy Lifestyles		

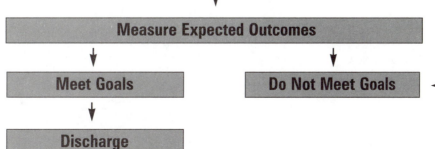

Measure Expected Outcomes

Meet Goals

Do Not Meet Goals

Discharge

Reevaluate

Study Questions

1. List the stages of the occupational therapy process in the correct chronological order beginning with referral.

2. Why do occupational therapy practitioners inquire into a client's past and present occupational performance profiles and participate in envisioning future profiles?

3. How do occupational therapy practitioners construct a particular client's occupational performance profile?

4. What services do occupational therapy practitioners offer individuals with (a) impairments, (b) disabilities, and (c) handicaps?

5. How is task analysis used to promote the health and wellness of communities?

References

American Occupational Therapy Association (AOTA). (1993). *Position paper: Purposeful activity.* Bethesda, MD: Author.

AOTA. (1993). Occupational therapy roles. *American Journal of Occupational Therapy, 47,* 1087–1099.

AOTA. (1994). *Uniform terminology for occupational therapy* (3rd ed.). Bethesda, MD: Author.

Canadian Association of Occupational Therapists (CAOT). (1990). *Position statement: Occupational therapy: Core identity.* Toronto, ON: Author.

CAOT. (1991). *Occupational therapy guidelines for client-centered practice.* Toronto, ON: Author.

CAOT. (1994). Position statement on everyday occupations and health. *Canadian Journal of Occupational Therapy, 61,* 294–295.

Csikszentmihalyi, M. (1990). *Flow: The psychology of optimal experience.* New York: Harper & Row.

Fidler, G., & Fidler, J. (1978). Doing and becoming: Purposeful action and self-actualization. *American Journal of Occupational Therapy, 32,* 305–310.

Law, M., Baptiste, S., Carswell, A., McColl, M. A., Polatajko, H., & Pollock, N. (1994). *Canadian Occupational Performance Measure* (2nd ed.). Toronto, ON: Canadian Association of Occupational Therapists.

Mattingly, C. & Fleming, M. (1994). *Clinical reasoning: Forms of inquiry in a therapeutic practice.* Philadelphia: F. A. Davis.

McNeil, J. M. (1993). Americans with Disabilities: 1991–1992 *U.S. Bureau of the Census. Current Population Reports, P70-33.* Washington, DC: U.S. Government Printing Office.

Mosey, A. C. (1981). *Occupational therapy: Configuration of a profession.* New York: Raven Press.

Polatajko, H. J. (1994). Dreams, dilemmas, and decisions for occupational therapy in the new millennium: A Canadian perspective. *American Journal of Occupational Therapy, 48,* 590–594.

Public Health Service. (1992). *Health people 2000: National health promotion and disease prevention objectives.* Boston: Jones and Bartlett.

Strauss, A. J., & Corbin, J. (1988). *Shaping a new health care system: The explosion of chronic illness as a catalyst for change.* San Francisco: Jossey-Bass.

Trombly, C. A. (1993). Anticipating the future: Assessment of occupational function. *American Journal of Occupational Therapy, 47,* 253–257.

Trombly, C. A. (1995a). Occupation: Purposefulness and meaningfulness as therapeutic mechanisms. *American Journal of Occupational Therapy, 49,* 960–972.

Trombly, C. A. (1995b). Purposeful activity. In C. A. Trombly (Ed.), *Occupational therapy for physical dysfunction* (4th ed., pp. 237–253). Baltimore: Williams & Wilkins.

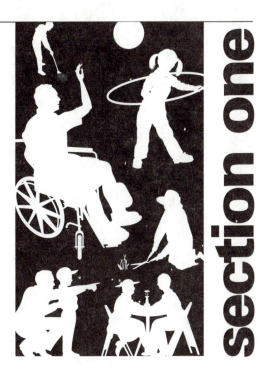

section one

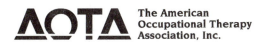

AOTA **The American**
Occupational Therapy
Association, Inc.

SECTION ONE: TASK ANALYSIS

"Generic activity analysis and synthesis is based on a conceptual framework drawn from the domain of concern of the profession. The full spectrum of all aspects of the domain of concern—performance components, age, occupational performance, environment—is taken into consideration" (Mosey, 1981, p. 115).[1]

Section One contains information and assignments to enable occupational therapy students to develop their knowledge and skills in task analysis using an occupational performance approach. Analysis of occupational performance focuses on the interactive and transactional relationship between people and their occupations and environments, because health is shaped by the continuous interaction between these factors (AOTA, 1989; Law et al., 1996). Analysis of the person considers past experiences, volition, and patterns of habituation, as well as sensorimotor, cognitive, psychosocial, and psychological performance components. Analysis of occupations involves delineating roles, tasks, and activities. Analysis of contexts encompasses temporal variables and cultural, physical, and social environments.

The chapter on "Occupational Performance Profiles" provides the opportunity for students to become familiar with domains of concern to occupational therapy practitioners. The terms **occupation, occupational performance,** and **function** are introduced and the hierarchy of roles, tasks, and activities is explained. Students will be introduced to the occupational performance assessments used by clinicians in practice. Completion of the required assignment will give students the opportunity to formulate an occupational performance profile and develop client interview skills. Students will recognize the diversity of occupational performance profiles and recognize that these profiles include occupations, people, and performance contexts. The Occupational Performance Profile Form is introduced in this chapter. This form will be used to understand client case profiles in subsequent chapters.

The "Occupational Performance Areas" chapter emphasizes the means by which occupational therapy practitioners facilitate clients' engagement in meaningful roles, tasks, and activities to enable clients to control and balance their patterns of occupation. Students will become familiar with the occupational performance areas of concern to practitioners by completing a weekly summary documenting their personal engagement in activities and tasks. These occupations are classified into the performance areas of activities of daily living, work and productive activities, and play or leisure pursuits. Being aware of the client's need to control and balance his or her pattern of occupation and the value of habits, routines, and lifestyle are emphasized. Students will learn to identify important and valued occupations and be aware of the diversity of profiles by assessing classmates.

Task analysis involves the assessment of clients' past experiences, volition, and patterns of habituation, as well as of performance components. Volition is the inner drive to explore, engage, and master, which is influenced by one's values and interests (Kielhofner, 1985). **Habituation** refers to our human tendency to construct and control patterns of occupations by establishing roles, habits, and routines (Kielhofner, 1985). The "Occupational Performance Profiles" chapter highlights the influences of past experience and volition. The concept of habituation is emphasized in the "Occupational Performance Areas" chapter.

---

[1]From *Occupational Therapy: Configuration of a Profession* (p. 115), by A. C. Mosey, 1994, New York: Raven Press. Copyright 1994 by Raven Press. Reprinted with permission.

Performance components are the varying abilities possessed by people that enable them to act and respond to the environment. The "Sensorimotor Performance Components" chapter delineates the sensory, perceptual, neuromusculoskeletal, and motor domains of concern to occupational therapy practitioners. The "Cognitive Performance Components" chapter delineates the cognitive domains of concern. The "Psychosocial Skills and Psychological Performance Components" chapter highlights the influence of these components on occupational performance. Completion of assignments within each chapter will require students to make judgments about the extent to which sensorimotor, cognitive, psychosocial, and psychological performance components are required to perform activities of interest to infants, children, and adults. Students will become familiar with the potential to use purposeful activities to assess and develop these performance component skills and abilities.

Occupational engagement occurs within a temporal and environmental performance context. The performance context includes the situations or factors that influence engagement in activities of daily living, work and productive activities, and play or leisure pursuits (AOTA, 1994). The "Temporal Aspects" chapter introduces the chronological, developmental, life cycle, and disability status variables that influence occupational performance. The "Physical Environment" chapter highlights the influence of the nonhuman environment on task engagement. Completion of an assignment will enable students to become familiar with the role of practitioners in adapting physical environments to develop skills and promote function. The "Social and Cultural Environment" chapter provides an assignment that will enable students to become aware of their sociocultural identity, potential personal bias, and the diversity of contexts within which people live. Being engaged in a group project

will demonstrate the potential use of activity groups in therapy. This chapter also introduces the role of occupational therapy intervention in the sociocultural and physical environmental domains to minimize disability and prevent handicaps.

The chapter on "Purposeful Modifications and Adaptations" emphasizes the role of occupational therapy practitioners in adapting activities and tasks to treat impairments, maximize independence, and promote role functioning. An assignment requires students to use the results of creative analysis to adapt task demands, environmental parameters, and a client's approach to alter the level of challenge in an activity.

Completion of the readings and assignments in Section One will prepare students to perform task analysis using an occupational performance approach. Two samples of thorough and complete task analyses is provided in the chapter titled "Occupational Performance Analysis Form." Sections Two, Three, Four, and Five will require students to apply task analysis to the evaluation and intervention process with children, adolescents, adults, and seniors. Section Six includes samples of the Occupational Performance Analysis - Short Form that have been completed by occupational therapy students.

References

American Occupational Therapy Association (AOTA). (1989). *Occupational therapy in the promotion of health and prevention of disease and disability.* Bethesda, MD: Author.

AOTA. (1994). *Uniform terminology for occupational therapy* (3rd ed.). Bethesda, MD: Author.

Kielhofner, G. (1985). *A Model of Human Occupation: Theory and application.* Baltimore: Williams & Wilkins.

Law, M., Cooper, B. A., Strong, S., Stewart, D., Rigby, P., & Letts, L. (1996). The Person-Environment-Occupation Model: A transactive approach to occupational performance. *Canadian Journal of Occupational Therapy, 63,* 9–23.

Mosey, A. C. (1981). *Occupational therapy: Configuration of a profession.* New York: Raven Press.

OCCUPATIONAL PERFORMANCE PROFILES

"We enable people to engage in those roles, tasks, and activities that have meaning to them on a day-to-day basis and that define their lives" (Trombly, 1993, p. 253). [1]

Chapter Objectives

1. Define the terms **occupation, occupational performance,** and **function.**
2. Rank behaviors into a hierarchy of roles, tasks, and activities.
3. Identify and list the domains of concern to the occupational therapy practitioner.
4. Conduct an interview to compose and write an occupational performance profile that contains information about the person and his or her occupations and environments.
5. Engage in a class discussion about the diversity of occupational performance profiles and the importance of a balance of the areas of occupation.
6. Identify some of the occupational performance interview assessments used by occupational therapy practitioners.

Understanding Clients' Occupational Performance Profiles

Occupational performance profiles are the product of the dynamic, interdependent, and transactional relationship between individuals, their occupations and roles, and the environments in which they live, work, and play (Law et al., 1996) (see Figure 1). Although initially separated in this textbook for learning purposes, these three variables are integrated when analyzing a client's past, present, and potential occupational performance profile.

Understanding clients' profiles, both past and present, is essential to initiating and managing the therapy process. Information on a client's occupational performance profile and his or her priorities and goals for intervention can be collected through

Figure 1. A Person-Environment-Occupation Model of Occupational Performance.

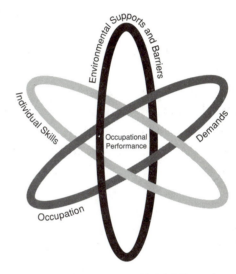

From "The Person-Environment-Occupation Model: A Transactive Approach to Occupational Performance," by M. Law, B. Cooper, S. Strong, D. Stewart, P. Rigby, & L. Letts, 1996. *Canadian Journal of Occupational Therapy, 63,* pp. 9-23. Copyright 1996 by the Canadian Association of Occupational Therapists (CAOT). Reproduced with permission of CAOT Publications.

the use of informal or standardized interviews, checklists, and schedules of activity patterns (Smith, 1993). Discrepancies between past and present occupational performance profiles establishes the need for intervention (Trombly, 1993). By envisioning and communicating a person's potential future functioning, therapists enlist clients' participation in the rehabilitation process (Fleming, 1994). Table 1 lists some of the assessments occupational therapy practitioners use to become familiar with a client's occupational performance profile.

By completing the assignments in this text students will develop skills in analyzing occupations, people, and contextual variables.

---

[1]From "Anticipating the Future: Assessment of Occupational Function," by C. A. Trombly, 1993, *American Journal of Occupational Therapy, 47,* p. 253. Copyright 1993 by the American Occupational Therapy Association. Reprinted with permission.

Table 1: Occupational Performance Interview Assessments

Occupational Performance Interview Assessments
Assessment of Occupational Functioning - Second Edition (Watts, Brollier, Bauer, & Schmidt, 1989)
Canadian Occupational Performance Measure (Law, Baptiste, Carswell, McColl, Opzoomer, Polatajko, & Pollock, 1994)
Goal Attainment Scaling (Ottenbacher & Cusick, 1990)
Occupational Case Analysis Interview and Rating Scale (Kaplan & Kielhofner, 1989)
Occupational Performance History Interview (Kielhofner, Henry, & Whalens, 1989)
Self-Assessment of Occupational Functioning and Children's Self-Assessment of Occupational Functioning (Baron & Curtin, 1990).

Analysis of Occupations

"**Occupations** are the ordinary and familiar things that people do every day" (AOTA, 1995a, p. 1015). Occupations have performance, contextual, and temporal dimensions and are multidimensional, multifaceted, and intrinsically necessary for health and well-being. Engagement is driven by the need for mastery, competency, self-identity, and group acceptance (AOTA, 1995a; Law et al., 1996; Polatajko, 1994). Occupational therapists contribute to their clients' health by enabling them to choose and engage in occupations that give their lives meaning and purpose (CAOT, 1993).

Function and **occupational performance** refer to "an individual's performance of activities, tasks, and roles during daily occupations" (AOTA, 1995b, p. 1016). Occupational performance can be classified as a hierarchy of roles, tasks, and activities (Christiansen & Baum, 1991). **Roles** occupy the highest level of the occupational performance hierarchy. They organize behavior, communicate expectations, and evolve across the life span (Christiansen & Baum). Roles add pleasure or enjoyment to life, contribute to achievement, and help maintain the self and family life (Trombly, 1995a). Life roles represent unique configurations of tasks, and some tasks fall into more than one role. **Tasks** contain an objective set of behaviors that are required to accomplish a goal (Dunn, Brown, & McGuigan, 1994). It is these tasks or **performance areas** that we classify into self-care/activities of daily living, work/productivity, and play/leisure. An individual's role and task configuration depends on individual skills, values, experiences, sociocultural mores and expectations, and contextual demands (Dunn et al., 1994; Trombly, 1995a). **Activities** are the basic units of occupational performance and consist of specific behaviors directed toward the completion of a task, whereas tasks are a set of activities that share some purpose.

Analysis of People

Analysis of people requires consideration of their past experiences, interests, values, goals, and routines, as well as of their sensorimotor, cognitive, psychological, and psychosocial performance components. The Model of Human Occupation (Kielhofner, 1985) provides a framework for understanding these factors. Behavior is seen as a product of the human system, the environment, and the task. Subsystems within individuals that influence their occupations include volition, habituation, and performance. These subsystems are arranged hierarchically such that higher subsystems govern lower ones and lower subsystems facilitate or constrain higher ones. **Volition** is the highest subsystem and is responsible for the inner drive to explore, engage, and master. It is influenced by personal causation, values, and interests, and is responsible for choosing to participate. **Personal causation** refers to the knowledge of one's own capacity for and perception of control over behavior and outcomes. **Habituation** is responsible for organizing behavior into roles, habits, and routines. The **performance** subsystem is responsible for producing action. Although Kielhofner (1985) includes perceptual-motor, process, and communication skills within the performance subsystem, the AOTA (1994) recommends that **performance components** include sensorimotor, cognitive, psychological, and psychosocial skills and abilities.

Analysis of Contexts

After identifying the occupations that clients wish or need to address, occupational therapy practitioners evaluate the features of performance context in which the tasks will be performed. Analysis of performance context should encompass temporal variables (chronological, developmental, life cycle, and disability status); and physical, social, and cultural environmental variables (AOTA, 1994). Although clients are interviewed and performance is observed during simulated tasks in clinical environments, independence in natural environments is difficult to predict (Brown, Moore, Hemman, & Yunek, 1996).

Individualizing Occupational Performance Profiles

The client-centered approach to assessment considers each person's unique occupational performance needs, abilities, and contexts (Pollock, 1993). Evaluation begins with an analysis of role competency and identification of clients' perceptions of needs, concerns, and priorities (Trombly, 1995b). In some practice settings, however, registered occupational therapists work with parents, families, teachers, physicians, and caregivers to establish intervention goals and priorities on behalf of clients who are unable to advocate on their own behalf. Occupational therapy practitioners prioritize goals by applying knowledge of which skills and abilities must precede the accomplishment of specific performance goals (Trombly, 1993).

Assignment

Materials

- Beads
- Canvas smock*
- Fabric paint
- Felt shapes
- Needle and thread
- Paper and pencil
- Sequins

*Canvas tote, waist apron, or cotton T-shirt can be used instead of smock.

1. Read the documents *Position paper: Occupation* (AOTA, 1995a) (Appendix I); *Occupational Performance: Occupational Therapy's Definition of Function* (AOTA, 1995b) (Appendix J) or the *Position Statement on Everyday Occupations and Health* (CAOT, 1993).
2. Divide into groups of two.

3. Define these terms:
   Occupations
   Occupational performance
   Function
   Roles
   Tasks
   Performance areas
   Activities
   Volition
   Habituation
   Performance components
   Performance context

4. Interview each other to determine your Occupational Performance Profiles. Your analysis will require that you ask about your partners' past experiences, volition, values, interests, roles, habituation, occupations, and performance contexts. Use the Occupational Performance Profile Form (Table 2) to document your interview results. A sample Occupational Performance Profile Form is provided for reference (Table 3). This form will be used to analyze and understand client case profiles in subsequent chapters. Additional copies of this form are available in Appendix G.

   Although clients often respond to informal interview questions regarding their roles and tasks with vague responses, identification of specific activities is required. For example, ask "What activities have been important to you in the past? What activities do you want to be able to perform in the future?" (Neistadt, 1996, p. 37).

Develop your own questions or use some of the questions within the *Assessment of Occupational Functioning* (Watts, Brollier, Bauer, & Schmidt, 1989), the *Occupational Performance History Interview* (Kielhofner, Henry & Whalens, 1989) or the *Occupational Case Analysis Interview and Rating Scale* (Kaplan & Kielhofner, 1989).

5. Reflect on your conversation with your partner and on the Occupational Performance Profile that you have completed to determine, prioritize, and visualize themes. It is these themes that you will be graphically reproducing on a canvas smock (see Figure 2).

Figure 2. Occupational Therapy Students with Canvas Smock Projects.

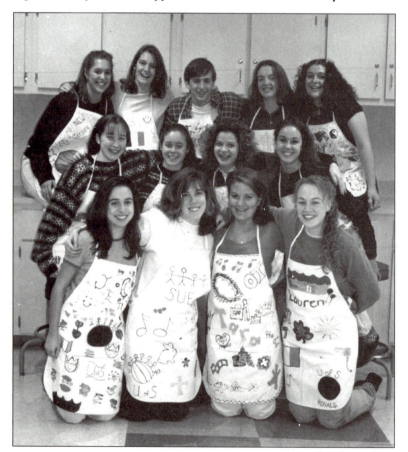

6. Plan your partner's smock design on paper before transferring your pattern and illustrations onto the canvas with pencil.

7. Sew on any beads, sequins, or appliques before using fabric paint.

8. Present the completed smock to your partner.

9. Reflect on your interview. What types of questions did you ask your partner? What questions did your partner ask you? Are these questions or answers important to the occupational therapy evaluation and intervention process?

10. Review the occupational performance profiles of other individuals. How similar or different are they from your own?

Table 2: Occupational Performance Profile Form

Occupations	Person	Context
<u>Roles</u>	<u>Values, Interests, and Goals</u>	<u>Temporal</u>
<u>Tasks and Performance</u>	<u>Performance Components</u>	<u>Social</u>
Activities of Daily Living	Sensorimotor Components	
Work and Productive Activities	Cognitive Integration and Cognitive Components	<u>Cultural</u>
Play or Leisure Activities	Psychosocial and Psychological Components	<u>Physical</u>

Table 3: Occupational Performance Profile Form—Example

Occupations	Person	Context
Roles *Daughter* *College student* *Sister* *Friend* *Roommate*	**Values, Interests, and Goals** *Become an occupational therapist.* *Practice therapy in my home community.* *Value honesty and close friendships.* *Value my independence.*	**Temporal** *20 years old*
Tasks and Performance **Activities of Daily Living** *Take care of own finances now.* *Drive home. Bike to class.* *Love to cook and bake.* *Clean apartment.*	**Performance Components** **Sensorimotor Components** *Not very coordinated anymore but enjoyed gymnastics when younger.* *Fast typist.* *Excellent visual memory.*	**Social** *Few local friends.* *Spend most of day with people in my major.* *See family once to twice per month. Large extended family.* *Two roommates—male and female.*
Work and Productive Activities *Spend most of the day in educational activities.* *Work part time on weekends at cafe.*	**Cognitive Integration and Cognitive Components** *Great long-term memory.* *Not a good problem solver.*	**Cultural** *Woman.* *Born and raised in northeastern USA. Hispanic heritage and some Hispanic family traditions. Catholic.*
Play or Leisure Activities *Play the flute.* *Go to movies on the weekend. Enjoy the theater.*	**Psychosocial and Psychological Components** *Pretty good self-concept and esteem, but stubborn.* *Optimistic.* *Goal-directed.* *Good listener.* *Assertive.* *Hate change.*	**Physical** *New apartment.* *Jesuit University.*

The information that follows will (a) provide students and instructors with resources to enhance the learning experience and (b) assist the student in completing the assignment.

Learning Resources

American Occupational Therapy Association (AOTA). (1995a). *Position paper: Occupation.* Bethesda, MD: Author.

AOTA (1995b). *Position paper: Occupational performance: Occupational therapy's definition of function.* Bethesda, MD: Author.

Canadian Association of Occupational Therapists. (1993). Position statement on everyday occupations and health. *Canadian Journal of Occupational Therapy, 61,* 294–295.

Kaplan, K. L., & Kielhofner, G. (1989). *Occupational Case Analysis Interview and Rating Scale.* Thorofare, NJ: Slack.

Kielhofner, G., Henry, A. D., & Whalens, D. (1989). *A user's guide to the Occupational Performance History Interview.* Bethesda, MD: American Occupational Therapy Association.

Watts, J. H., Brollier, C., Bauer, D. F., & Schmidt, W. (1989). The Assessment of Occupational Functioning: The second edition. In J. H. Watts & C. Brollier (Eds.), *Instrument development in occupational therapy* (pp. 61–88). New York: Haworth.

Study Questions

1. Define the term **occupation**. List five characteristics or qualities of occupations.
2. What is meant by the phrase **"patterns of occupation"**? Why is this concept important to the therapy process? How is this concept related to achieving balance in the areas of occupation?
3. Define **volition** and **habituation**. Why are these concepts important to the therapy process?
4. Draw a three-tiered hierarchy of **roles, tasks,** and **activities.** Define these terms.
5. Classify each of the following as a **role, task,** or **activity:**
   a. Wash dishes, home management, homemaker.
   b. Write papers, student, operate a computer.
   c. Friend, socialize, go to a movie.
6. Identify two occupational performance interview assessments.
7. When compiling a client's occupational performance profile, what domains are considered?

References

American Occupational Therapy Association (AOTA). (1994). *Uniform terminology for occupational therapy* (3rd ed.). Bethesda, MD: Author.

AOTA (1995a). *Position paper: Occupation.* Bethesda, MD: Author.

AOTA (1995b). *Position paper: Occupational performance: Occupational therapy's definition of function.* Bethesda, MD: Author.

Baron, K., & Curtin, C. (1990). *Self-Assessment of Occupational Functioning and Children's Self-Assessment of Occupational Functioning.* Chicago: University of Illinois.

Brown, C., Moore, W. P., Hemman, D., & Yunek, A. (1996). Influence of instrumental activities of daily living assessment method on judgements of independence. *American Journal of Occupational Therapy, 50,* 202–206.

Canadian Association of Occupational Therapists (CAOT). (1993). Position statement on everyday occupations and health. *Canadian Journal of Occupational Therapy, 61,* 294–295.

Christiansen, C., & Baum, C. (1991). *Occupational therapy: Overcoming human performance deficits.* Thorofare, NJ: Slack.

Dunn, W., Brown, C., & McGuigan, A. (1994). The ecology of human performance: A framework for considering the effect of context. *American Journal of Occupational Performance, 48,* 595–607.

Fleming, M. H. (1994). Conditional reasoning: Creating meaningful experiences. In C. Mattingly and M. H. Fleming (Eds.), *Clinical reasoning: Forms of inquiry in a therapeutic practice* (pp. 197–236). Philadelphia: F. A. Davis.

Kaplan, K. L., & Kielhofner, G. (1989). *Occupational Case Analysis Interview and Rating Scale.* Thorofare, NJ: Slack.

Kielhofner, G. (1985). *A Model of Human Occupation: Theory and application.* Baltimore: Williams & Wilkins.

Kielhofner, G., Henry, A. D., & Whalens, D. (1989). *A user's guide to the Occupational Performance History Interview.* Bethesda, MD: American Occupational Therapy Association.

Law, M., Carswell, A., McColl, M., Polatajko, H., & Pollock, N. (1994). *The Canadian Occupational Performance Measure.* Toronto, ON: CAOT.

Law, M., Cooper, B. A., Strong, S., Stewart, D., Rigby, P., & Letts, L. (1996). The Person-Environment-Occupation Model: A transactive approach to occupational performance. *Canadian Journal of Occupational Therapy, 63,* 9–23.

Neistadt, M. E. (1995, November). Assessing clients' priorities: Whose goals are they? *OT Practice,* 37–39.

Ottenbacher, K. J., & Cusick, A. (1990). Goal Attainment Scaling as a method of clinical service evaluation. *American Journal of Occupational Therapy, 44,* 519–526.

Polatajko, H. J. (1994). Dreams, dilemmas, and decisions for occupational therapy in a new millennium: A Canadian perspective. *American Journal of Occupational Therapy, 48,* 590–594.

Pollock, N. (1993). Client-centered assessment. *American Journal of Occupational Therapy, 47,* 298–301.

Smith, H. D. (1993). Assessment and evaluation: An overview. In H. L. Hopkins & H. D. Smith (Eds.), *Willard and Spackman's occupational therapy* (8th ed., pp. 169–191). Philadelphia: Lippincott.

Trombly, C. A. (1993). Anticipating the future: Assessment of occupational function. *American Journal of Occupational Therapy, 47,* 253–257.

Trombly, C. A. (1995a). Occupation: Purposefulness and meaningfulness as therapeutic mechanisms. *American Journal of Occupational Therapy, 49,* 960–972.

Trombly, C. A. (1995b). Planning, guiding, and documenting therapy. In C. A. Trombly (Ed.), *Occupational therapy for physical dysfunction* (pp. 29–40). Baltimore: Williams & Wilkins.

Watts, J. H., Brollier, C., Bauer, D. F., & Schmidt, W. (1989). The Assessment of Occupational Functioning: The second edition. In J. H. Watts & C. Brollier (Eds.), *Instrument development in occupational therapy* (pp. 61–88). New York: Haworth.

OCCUPATIONAL PERFORMANCE AREAS

"The Life Style Performance Model proposes that the outcome of occupational therapy intervention is to enable a way of living that allows persons to develop and bring into harmony a configuration of daily living activities that have personal, social, and cultural relevance for them and their significant others" (Fidler, 1996, p. 141).[1]

Chapter Objectives

1. Categorize daily life tasks and activities into three different occupational performance areas.
2. Define and describe the difference between **activities of daily living** and **instrumental activities of daily living.**
3. Describe the value of habituations and lifestyle and discuss their relevance to health.
4. Participate in a class discussion regarding patterns of occupation and the diversity of such patterns among people.
5. Define **health** and describe the value of a balance of occupations.
6. Explain the role of the occupational therapy practitioner in enabling clients to control and balance their patterns of occupation.

Enabling Clients to Control and Balance Their Patterns of Occupation

Throughout each day we engage in a number of routine tasks. People tend to construct patterns of occupation by establishing habits and routines. This tendency is called **habituation** (Kielhofner, 1985). These patterns, or habits, unfold with "remarkable regularity and without the necessity of deliberation" (Kielhofner, 1985, p. 30). They help us organize our time, produce patterns of efficient behavior, integrate society, and enable cultures to transmit and sustain customs (Kielhofner, 1985; Young, 1988). Individuals, through maturation and socialization, develop a configuration of activity patterns that characterize their lifestyle. This lifestyle, or way of

living, contributes to people's life satisfaction by enabling them to define and express their personal and social identity and develop self-regard (Fidler, 1996). Clients' values and interests influence the importance they attribute to participation or independence in these routine tasks.

Health and wellness are achieved through a balanced pattern of daily occupations (CAOT, 1994; Reed & Sanderson, 1983). Balance, however, does not imply an equal allocation of time to activities of daily living, work and productive activities, and play or leisure pursuits. For example, McKinnon (1992) suggests that self-perceptions of happiness and satisfaction have more to do with the quality of an individual's experiences than with his or her pattern of time use. Primeau (1996) proposes that a balance of affective experiences across one's occupations may be more important than a balance between work and play. Fidler (1996) asserts that individuals with healthy lifestyles achieve and maintain culturally relevant, age-specific harmony among activities that provide self-care and self-maintenance, intrinsic gratification, societal contribution, and interpersonal relatedness. The role of occupational therapy, therefore, is to enable people to balance their patterns of occupation by optimizing function in the occupational performance areas that give their lives meaning and purpose (AOTA, 1994; CAOT, 1994).

Uniform Terminology for Occupational Therapy (AOTA, 1994) provides a classification system for these routine tasks or occupational performance areas.

A. Activities of Daily Living
   1. Grooming
   2. Oral Hygiene
   3. Bathing/Showering
   4. Toilet Hygiene
   5. Personal Device Care
   6. Dressing
   7. Feeding and Eating
   8. Medication Routine
   9. Health Maintenance
   10. Socialization
   11. Functional Communication
   12. Functional Mobility
   13. Community Mobility
   14. Emergency Response
   15. Sexual Expression
B. Work and Productive Activities
   1. Home Management
      a. Clothing Care
      b. Cleaning
      c. Meal Preparation/Cleanup
      d. Shopping
      e. Money Management
      f. Household Maintenance
      g. Safety Procedures
   2. Care of Others
   3. Educational Activities
   4. Vocational Activities
      a. Vocational Exploration
      b. Job Acquisition
      c. Work or Job Performance
      d. Retirement Planning
      e. Volunteer Participation
C. Play or Leisure Activities
   1. Play or Leisure Exploration
   2. Play or Leisure Performance

Basic **activities of daily living** are self-care tasks, whereas **instrumental activities of daily living** are the more complex tasks that are necessary for maintaining independence in the home and community (Lawton & Brody, 1969). According to the United States Bureau of the Census, of people over the age of 15 in the United States during 1991 and 1992, 44 million had difficulty with or were unable to perform one or more functional activities, 19.5 million had a work disability, 11.7 million had some difficulty with one or more instrumental activities of daily living, and 7.9 million had difficulty with activities of daily living (McNeil, 1993). These figures exclude those individuals who lived in nursing homes and other institutions. Table 1 summarizes some of the findings of this national survey.

Table 1: Prevalence of Disability in Activities of Daily Living and Instrumental Activities of Daily Living in Persons 15 Years of Age or Older: 1991-1992*

	Percent of the Population	Number of People (millions)
Activities of Daily Living (ADL)		
Has difficulty with or needs personal assistance with one or more ADLs	4.1	7.919
Getting in or out of bed or a chair	2.7	5.280
Taking a bath or shower	2.3	4.501
Getting around inside the home	1.9	3.664
Dressing	1.7	3.234
Toileting	1.1	2.084
Eating	0.6	1.077
Instrumental Activities of Daily Living (IADL)		
Has difficulty with or needs personal assistance with one or more IADLs	6.0	11.694
Getting around outside the home	4.0	7.809
Doing light housework	3.2	6.313
Preparing meals	2.3	4.530
Keeping track of money and bills	2.0	3.901
Using the telephone	1.6	3.130

*Figures do not include those individuals who live in nursing homes and other institutions.

From "Americans With Disabilities: 1991-1992," by J. M. McNeil, 1993, U.S. Bureau of the Census, Current Population Reports, P70-33. Washington, DC: U.S. Government Printing Office.

Occupational therapy practitioners usually see clients during periods of crisis or major life changes, and helping clients to make these transitions is a crucial aspect of practice (Spencer, Davidson, & White, 1996). The relationship and interdependence between occupation and adaptation are fundamental principles in many occupational therapy theories. Occupation provides the means by which people adapt to their changing needs and conditions, while the desire to participate in occupation is the intrinsic force that leads to adaptation (Schkade & Schultz, 1992). According to Schkade and Schultz, occupations are characterized by active participation, provision of meaning to the person, and an output or product. **Adaptation** refers to the change in the functional state of the person as a result of the movement toward mastery over occupational challenges. **Occupational adaptation** is the outcome of the process by which people and their environments come together in occupation. Nelson (1988) proposes that adaptation occurs when occupation has any effect on an individual's developmental structure. This change occurs as a result of the dynamic relationship between external demands, perceived meaning and purpose, individual capacities, and engagement in occupation.

Assignment

1. Work individually to complete the Personal Patterns of Occupation form for documenting the tasks that make up your daily habit routine (Table 2).
   OR
   Complete the *Occupational Questionnaire* (Smith, Kielhofner, & Watts, 1986).
2. Use the occupational performance areas described in *Uniform Terminology for Occupational Therapy* (AOTA, 1994) to reference the list of routine tasks. For example, taking a shower is an Activities of Daily Living area *(A)* called Bathing/Showering *(3)*. This task is *A 3*.

Use a red pencil to circle those tasks that are important to you. Use a blue pencil to circle those tasks that you enjoy. Use a green pencil to circle the tasks and activities that enable you to perform your role as a student. What other roles do you assume? Use a different-colored pencil to highlight the tasks and activities that enable you to perform these roles.
OR
Use four different-colored pencils to highlight routine tasks. Use a red pencil to circle the tasks that are done for self-care and self-maintenance; a blue pencil to circle tasks done for intrinsic gratification; a green pencil to circle tasks done to contribute to society; and a yellow pencil to circle tasks that enhance interpersonal relatedness (Fidler, 1996).

The collage of colors on your Personal Patterns of Occupation form illustrates and documents your patterns of occupation.

Table 2: Personal Patterns of Occupation Form

MORNING	Monday	Tuesday	Wednesday	Thursday	Friday	Saturday	Sunday
7:00 - 8:00	Shower (A3) Eat (A7) Dress (A6)						
8:00 - 9:00							
9:00 - 10:00							
10:00 - 11:00							
11:00 - 12:00							

Table 2: Personal Patterns of Occupation Form

AFTERNOON	Monday	Tuesday	Wednesday	Thursday	Friday	Saturday	Sunday
12:00 - 1:00							
1:00 - 2:00							
2:00 - 3:00							
3:00 - 4:00							
4:00 - 5:00							
5:00 - 6:00							

Table 2: Personal Patterns of Occupation Form

EVENING	Monday	Tuesday	Wednesday	Thursday	Friday	Saturday	Sunday
6:00 - 7:00							
7:00 - 8:00							
8:00 - 9:00							
9:00 - 10:00							
Late Evening							

3. Share and compare your completed Personal Patterns of Occupation form with your class. How are students' profiles similar or different? Do different people classify the same task as self-care, work, or leisure? For example, is cooking a self-care, work, or leisure task? The reason that individuals may assign the same tasks to different occupational performance areas may have something to do with the meaning those tasks have for each person (Trombly, 1995).

4. How have your routine tasks and patterns of occupation evolved during the different phases and stages of your life?

5. How would this profile be different if you were (a) sick and required to spend the week in bed, (b) mentally or physically challenged, (c) permanently injured in an accident?

6. Assume that you have no control over permanent changes made to your patterns of occupation. Would this change affect your life satisfaction, personal and social identity, or health?

7. Assume that you are unhappy with the profile of your daily tasks and activities. Now assume that your occupational therapy practitioner indicated that you could once again take control over your patterns of occupations by choosing and engaging in activities that are meaningful to you. Would this affect your life satisfaction, personal and social identity, or health?

8. Are there things about this schedule that you would like to change to improve your current life satisfaction, personal and social identity, or health and well-being?

9. What is your definition of health? Does this definition include participation in a particular balance of occupations?

Optional:

10. Read and discuss the proposals and concepts put forth by Fidler (1996); Nelson (1996); Schkade and Schultz (1992); or Spencer, Davidson, and White (1996).

The information that follows will (a) provide students and instructors with resources to enhance the learning experience and (b) assist the student in completing the assignment.

Learning Resources

Fidler, G. (1996). Life style performance: From profile to conceptual model. *American Journal of Occupational Therapy, 50,* 139–147.

Nelson, D. (1996). Therapeutic occupation: A definition. *American Journal of Occupational Therapy, 50,* 775–782.

Schkade, J. K., & Schultz, S. (1992). Occupational adaptation: Toward a holistic approach for contemporary practice, Part 1. *American Journal of Occupational Therapy, 46,* 829–837.

Smith, N., Kielhofner, G., & Watts, J. (1986). The relationships between volition, activity pattern, and life satisfaction in the elderly. *American Journal of Occupational Therapy, 40,* 278–283.

Spencer, J., Davidson, H. A., & White, V. K. (1996). Continuity and change: Past experience as adaptive repertoire in occupational adaptation. *American Journal of Occupational Therapy, 50,* 526–534.

Study Questions

1. Categorize the following tasks as activities of daily living, instrumental activities of daily living, work and productive activities, or play or leisure pursuits.
   a. Shopping
   b. Bowling
   c. Making a sandwich
   d. Vacuuming
   e. Typing
   f. Dressing
   g. Banking
   h. Landscaping
2. What is meant by the terms **patterns of occupation, habituation,** and **lifestyle?** Are these concepts related to health and wellness? Why are these concepts important to the therapy process?
3. Describe your lifestyle and its effect on your daily life.

References

American Occupational Therapy Association. (1994). Uniform terminology for occupational therapy (3rd ed.). *American Journal of Occupational Therapy, 48,* 1047–1054.

Canadian Association of Occupational Therapists. (1994). Position statement on everyday occupations and health. *Canadian Journal of Occupational Therapy, 61,* 294–295.

Fidler, G. (1996). Life style performance: From profile to conceptual model. *American Journal of Occupational Therapy, 50,* 139–147.

Kielhofner, G. (1985). *A model of human occupation: Theory and application* (2nd ed.). Baltimore: Williams & Wilkins.

Lawton, M. P., & Brody, E. (1969). Assessment of older people: Self-maintaining and instrumental activities of daily living. *Gerontologist, 9,* 179–186.

McKinnon, A. (1992). Time use for self care, productivity, and leisure among elderly Canadians. *Canadian Journal of Occupational Therapy, 59,* 102–110.

McNeil, J. M. (1993). Americans with Disabilities: 1991–1992 *U.S. Bureau of the Census. Current Population Reports, P70-33.* Washington, DC: U.S. Government Printing Office.

Nelson, D. L. (1988). Occupation: Form and performance. *American Journal of Occupational Therapy, 42,* 633–641.

Primeau, L. A. (1996). Work and leisure: Transcending the dichotomy. *American Journal of Occupational Therapy, 50,* 569–577.

Reed, K., & Sanderson, S. (1983). *Concepts in occupational therapy* (2nd ed.). Baltimore: Williams & Wilkins.

Schkade, J. K., & Schultz, S. (1992). Occupational adaptation: Toward a holistic approach for contemporary practice, Part 1. *American Journal of Occupational Therapy, 46,* 829–837.

Smith, N., Kielhofner, G., & Watts, J. (1986). The relationships between volition, activity pattern, and life satisfaction in the elderly. *American Journal of Occupational Therapy, 40,* 278–283.

Spencer, J., Davidson, H. A., & White, V. K. (1996). Continuity and change: Past experience as adaptive repertoire in occupational adaptation. *American Journal of Occupational Therapy, 50,* 526–534.

Trombly, C. A. (1995). Occupation: Purposefulness and meaningfulness as therapeutic mechanisms. *American Journal of Occupational Therapy, 49,* 960–972.

Young, M. (1988). *The metronomic society: Natural rhythms and human timetables.* Cambridge, MA: Harvard University Press.

SENSORIMOTOR PERFORMANCE COMPONENTS

"The interaction of the sensory and motor systems through all their countless interconnections is what gives meaning to sensation and purposefulness to movement .... Without interaction with the physical environment, learning is very difficult" (Ayres, 1979, p. 46).[1]

Chapter Objectives

1. Identify and define the different sensory, perceptual, neuromuscular, and motor performance components and recognize their interdependence and contribution to occupational performance.
2. Analyze an activity and distinguish which sensory, perceptual, neuromuscular, and motor performance components are challenged during engagement.
3. Judge the extent to which different sensory, perceptual, neuromuscular, and motor skills and abilities are required to perform selected activities of interest to infants, children, and adults.
4. Evaluate the potential to use purposeful activities to develop skills, remediate impairments, and/or optimize performance.
5. Briefly describe the contribution of sensory integration and motor control theories to the task analysis process.

Purposeful Engagement to Assess and Treat Sensorimotor Performance Components

The **sensorimotor components** of occupational performance include all of the abilities and skills required to receive and process sensory information and to produce a desired response. When sensory, perceptual, and motor impairments cause or have the potential to cause disability, occupational therapy may be recommended. Task analysis is used during the evaluation and intervention process to determine the impact of impairments on occupational performance and to design therapeutic intervention aimed at minimizing the disabling effects of these impairments.

A number of methods are available to therapists for assessing the integrity of specific sensory, perceptual, and motor systems, but activity and task engagement are used to determine the impact of impairments on occupational performance. Sensory impairments affect the ability to receive, process, and integrate incoming information; perceptual impairments affect the ability to interpret this information; and motor impairments affect the production or expression of a desired response. When observing occupational performance, therapists must become skilled at determining whether dysfunction may be based on underlying sensory, perceptual, or motor impairments. Completion of standardized norm-referenced assessments may be appropriate.

Sensory, perceptual, and motor impairments that cause disability can be treated through the use of purposeful activities. Intervention is directed at treating impairments that are amenable to change and teaching compensation skills for more permanent impairments. Task and activity analysis is used during this intervention process for selecting and designing therapeutic activities to improve skills and abilities or for restructuring tasks and altering environments to promote independence and adaptation. Remedial approaches promote development or recovery of central nervous system impairments (Neistadt, 1990). For example, occupational therapists use the following activities for remedial purposes:

- Computer software programs are used with children and adults with learning disabilities or traumatic brain injuries to promote perceptual skill development and learning.

- Karate is used with children to improve strength, endurance, balance, coordination, problem solving, sequencing, self-esteem, social skills, and confidence (Harris, 1995; Hirsch Botzer, 1995).
- Horseback riding is used with children and adults with cerebral palsy to enhance physical and psychosocial functioning (Stancliff, 1996; Spink, 1993; MacKinnon, Noh, Laliberte, Lariviere, & Allan, 1995).
- T'ai chi is used to improve postural control in the well elderly (Tse & Bailey, 1992) and to maintain health in clients with rheumatoid arthritis (Kirsteins, Dietz, & Hwang, 1991).
- Therapeutic touch is used with many different clientele to promote psychological and psychosocial well-being (Sayre-Adams, 1995).

The functional or rehabilitative approaches seek to maximize independence (Neistadt, 1990). Therapeutic intervention focuses on providing clients with the opportunity to learn and practice new methods to compensate for their impairments. Intervention is directed toward restructuring tasks, altering environments, teaching others to provide assistance, or using adapted equipment to compensate for impairments in sensory, perceptual, and motor systems. Occupational therapy practitioners teach new methods and structure practice opportunities to ensure that clients incorporate these techniques into their lifestyle. For example, when a client is unable to judge a safe temperature for bath water because of a sensory impairment or unable to transfer into a bath tub because of a motor impairment, the occupational therapy practitioner may recommend the use of a thermometer or bath seat and may provide opportunities to transfer safely into a tub.

Sensory Awareness and Processing
Our senses provide a conduit through which we receive information about our environment and understand the inner workings of our bodies (Dunn, 1991). Once received, transmitted, integrated, and interpreted within the nervous system, sensory information is used for stimulus detection and to form accurate and reliable maps of ourselves and our environments (Ayres, 1979; Dunn, 1991). It is these maps that we use to remember how task performance occurred in the past and to adapt performance to current demands (Dunn, 1991). Sensory processing affects many areas of our lives, including social and emotional development, engagement in important occupations, and learning (Ayres, 1979).

Sensation is complex and multidimensional (Dunn, 1991). The tactile, proprioceptive, vestibular, visual, gustatory, and olfactory properties of activities can have calming, comforting, arousing, stimulating, or aversive effects on people (Haldy & Haack, 1995). The **tactile** system receives, transmits, and interprets somatosensory information from the skin including: light touch, pressure, temperature, pain, and vibration. The **proprioceptive** receptors in muscles, joints, and other internal tissues provide information about body position. The **vestibular** system receptors in the inner ear provide information regarding position and movement (linear and angular) of the head in space (AOTA, 1994). Together the proprioceptive and vestibular systems allow us to complete routine motor tasks without constant visual or auditory monitoring of performance (Haldy & Haack, 1995). The **visual** system provides acuity and awareness of color and pattern (AOTA, 1994) and is an important channel for learning. The **auditory** system interprets, discriminates, and localizes sound and is important to receptive language. The **gustatory** system provides taste information, and the **olfactory** system receives, transmits, and interprets odors (AOTA, 1994).

Impairments may occur at any point(s) in the process of sensory information reception, transmission, and interpretation. The remedial approach to intervention is directed at treating deficits that are amenable to change, while the adaptive approach to intervention aims at teaching compensation for impairments that are more permanent (Neistadt, 1990). For example, occupational therapists use purposeful activities, repetition, and practice to challenge clients' visual perceptual abilities and to develop skills because deficits in visual perception may be amenable to change because of neural plasticity. Intervention directed at developing skills through purposeful activity engagement is a domain of occupational therapy practice. Retinal detachment, however, is a permanent impairment that affects the eye's ability to receive visual information. When blindness causes disability, therapy is directed at teaching compensation.

Adjunctive modalities may be used by therapists to treat underlying sensorimotor impairments. Registered occupational therapists may design or recommend splints and use physical agent modalities as therapeutic agents to treat impairments that affect sensorimotor and occupational performance. For example, wrist splints may be used to reduce the effects of peripheral nerve entrapment in a client with carpal tunnel syndrome, whose weak hand muscles impair their independence in self-care and work tasks. While both purposeful activities and adjunctive modalities are intervention tools used to enhance occupational performance, the former will be the focus of this text.

The **sensory integration** frame of reference for intervention proposes that the process of sensory registration and integration for goal-directed action within the environment is essential for development, learning, and emotional well-being (Ayres, 1979). The typical child actively selects and organizes sensations to produce actions or adaptive responses to environmental demands. These adaptive

responses, in turn, assist in the organizational process so that future actions are more effective and efficient. In summary, sensory integration enables adaptive responses that promote the development of sensory integration (Parham & Mailloux, 1996). Integration of vestibular-proprioceptive-visual systems, for example, provides the foundation for the motor responses needed to ride a bicycle. Consider the following portrayal by A. J. Ayres (1979) and insert terms to identify these sensory systems. Two references have been provided in brackets:

Watch a child ride a bicycle and you will see how sensory stimulation leads to adaptive responses and adaptive responses lead to sensory integration. To balance himself and the bicycle, the child must sense the pull of gravity [vestibular] and the movements of his body [proprioception]. Whenever he moves off center and begins to fall, his brain integrates the sensations of falling and forms an adaptive response. In this case, the adaptive response involves shifting the weight of the body to keep it balanced over the bicycle. If this adaptive response is not made, or is made too slowly, the child falls off the bicycle. If he repeatedly cannot make the adaptive response because he does not get good, precise information from his body and gravity senses, he may avoid riding a bicycle.

Additional adaptive responses are needed to steer the bicycle so that it goes where the child wants it to go. To know where he and the bicycle are in relation to a tree, his brain must integrate visual sensations with body sensations and the pull of gravity. Then it must use those sensations to plan a path around the tree. The faster the bicycle goes, the greater the sensory stimulation and the more accurate the adaptive response must be. If the child rides into a tree, it means that his brain did not integrate the sensations, or it did not do so quickly enough. When a child gets off his bicycle after a successful ride, his brain knows more about gravity and the space around his body and how his body moves, and so riding a bicycle becomes easier each time. This is how sensory integration develops (Ayres, 1979, p. 14-15).[2]

Accurate analysis of the sensory, perceptual, and motor responses elicited through selected activities enables therapists to structure the environment to facilitate a child's sensory integration and the production of adaptive responses. This is one of the roles of therapists who use a sensory integrative frame of reference for intervention.

Assignment 1

1. Divide into groups of two.
2. Select and perform one infant, child, and adult activity from the suggestions listed below.

<u>Infants</u>: Play with a crib activity center or mobile. Finger feed banana pieces. Play with a textured, rubber toy that squeaks when squeezed. Crawl through a large barrel.

<u>Children</u>: Finger paint with paints, pudding, or a mixture of scented shaving foam and food coloring. Make a sponge art picture. Make a dough sculpture. Play with Sit and Spin® (Playskool) (see Figure 1). Play the Bunny Hop Game or the Mr. Thumbuddy Game (Miller, 1988). Jump on a trampoline. Play on a swing.

<u>Adults</u>: Design and use fabric paint to make a gift canvas smock. Type at a computer. Sculpt with clay media. Brush your teeth. Remove a jacket. Putt with a golf club. Throw balls into a basket.

Figure 1. Child on Sit and Spin.

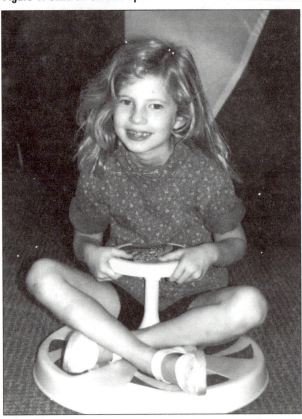

3. While engaging in the activity, determine which sensory systems are receiving, processing, and interpreting information for optimal performance. Document your observations in the Sensory Analysis Table (Table 1). Canadian students should use the table in Appendix D. Comments in the tactile area should include the type(s) of somatosensory stimulation: light touch, pressure, temperature, etc. Describe the body parts that require proprioceptive sense. Determine whether the vestibular stimulation is linear or angular. Use *Uniform Terminology for Occupational Therapy* (AOTA, 1994) to enhance your understanding of the definitions of these sensory processing performance components (Appendix E). Two examples have been completed for you.

4. Most tasks that we engage in during our daily lives challenge more than one sensory system. As a therapist it will be important to judge the degree of challenge. Develop your skills in this area by deciding "how much" each sensory system is challenged during engagement. Indicate your decision as follows:

N/A (Not Applicable): Sensory system performance component is not challenged.

Min (Minimal): Performance component is challenged or involved minimally.

Mod (Moderate): Performance component is challenged, but not to a great degree.

Max (Maximal): Performance component is challenged or involved to a great degree.

Support this decision with a brief statement.

5. Share your observations with your class.

Table 1: Sensory Analysis Table

	Infants	Children	Adults
	Rattle with mirror	Riding a tricycle	
Tactile	Min-Mod Texture of handle.	Min Texture of handles. Pressure from foot plates. Outside ambient temperature.	
Proprioceptive	Mod Force and velocity of arm movement.	Max Awareness of arm and leg Positions without looking.	
Vestibular	Min Head movement while sitting.	Max Linear movement of head through space, some angular if turn a corner.	
Visual	Mod-Max Bright, contrast colors. Picture of self reflected in the mirror.	Max Negotiate movement through cluttered environment.	

Table 1: Sensory Analysis Table

	Infants		Children		Adults
	Rattle with mirror		**Riding a tricycle**		
Auditory	Mod-Max Rattle movement causes noise.		Min If playing with friends.		
Gustatory	Min If placed in mouth.		N/A		
Olfactory	N/A		N/A Outdoor smells.		

Perceptual Processing

Perception is the process of organizing sensory impressions into meaningful information and patterns (AOTA, 1994; Quintana, 1995). Abreu and Toglia (1987) view perception as a dynamic process involving (a) sensory detection and registration; (b) analysis, interpretation, and organization of raw information; (c) comparison of stimuli with past experiences for hypothesis formation; and (d) a decision response.

Uniform Terminology for Occupational Therapy provides the following list and definitions of perceptual processing skills and abilities (AOTA, 1994) (Appendix E). **Stereognosis** is the process of identifying objects through the integration of proprioceptive, cognitive, and tactile information. **Kinesthesia** provides an awareness of weight, exertion, and direction of joint movement to enable us to make judgments about force and velocity. **Pain response** is the interpretation of noxious stimuli. **Body scheme** is the internal awareness of the body and the relationship of body parts to each other and to objects in the environment (AOTA, 1994; Quintana, 1995). **Right-left discrimination** is the differentiation of one side of the body from the other by understanding the concepts of right and left (AOTA, 1994; Quintana, 1995). **Form constancy** is the process of recognizing forms and objects as being the same in various environments, positions, and sizes (AOTA, 1994; Gardner, 1982). Form constancy helps us to develop stability and consistency in the visual world (Schneck, 1996). When picking out your clothes in the morning, for example, you will recognize a shirt whether it is hung in the closet or folded in a drawer. Form constancy enables you to recognize both visual images as shirts.

Position in space assists in the determination of spatial relationships of figures and objects to one's self and other forms and objects (AOTA, 1994). It enables us to make determinations of front, back, top, bottom, beside, behind, under, over, below, and so forth (Quintana, 1995). **Spatial relation**, however, determines the position of objects relative to each other (AOTA, 1994) and reflects the ability to determine the direction of forms (Gardner, 1982). For example, during daily activities spatial relations enable us to determine (a) the direction that the dial on the stove, washing machine, or water faucet is pointing; (b) the direction that the road or sidewalk in front of us is turning; or (c) the difference between the letters "b" and "d" or the numbers "6" and "9."

Visual-closure perception enables us to identify forms or objects from incomplete presentations (AOTA, 1994). Visual-closure allows us to make an assumption about what particular objects, shapes, or form are by matching current visual images with previously stored visual information (Schneck, 1996). During daily activities we use visual-closure perception to recognize objects that are partially covered by other objects, for example, recognizing a particular food product that is partially blocked by another item in the kitchen cupboard.

Figure-ground perception makes it possible to identify forms and objects by differentiating foreground from background. Finding a particular food product that is not obscured from view but is located in front of a cluttered background in the kitchen cupboard requires figure-ground. **Depth perception** enables us to determine relative distance of objects and sounds and is particularly important for accurate reach and for functional and community mobility. **Topographical orientation** is required to determine the location of objects and settings and the route to a destination (AOTA, 1994) and allows us to find our way around our homes and communities.

While some perceptual skills interpret information from a single sensory system, others occur in multiple sensory systems or require integration between systems.

Visual-closure perception is the interpretation of sensory information from which sense?

Kinesthesia requires extensive information from which sensory system?

Depth perception is the interpretation of sensory information from which system(s)?

Figure-ground perception is the interpretation of sensory information from which sensory system(s)?

Stereognosis requires the integration of cognitive information with which two sensory systems?

Assignment 2

1. Divide into groups of two. Review the passage on bicycle riding by A. J. Ayres (1979) and determine which perceptual skills are required to make adaptive responses.

2. Select and perform one infant, child, and adult activity from the suggestions listed below.

Infants: Play with a cribside activity center. Stack plastic rings on a dowel. Complete shape inset puzzles. Identify and label pictures in a storybook.

Children: Play hidden picture games. Play the Hide and Seek Game (Miller, 1988). Copy a sentence from a chalkboard. Draw a picture of yourself. Play hopscotch. Complete a six- to eight-piece puzzle.

Adults: Design and use fabric paint to make a gift canvas smock. Retrieve your jacket from a coat hanger. Find a pen and paper in a desk drawer and print your name. Make an origami figure. Lace a small leather project.

3. While engaging in the activity, determine which perceptual skills are required for optimal performance. Document your observations in the Perceptual Analysis Table (Table 2). Canadian students should use the table in Appendix D. Use *Uniform Terminology for Occupational Therapy* (AOTA, 1994) to enhance your understanding of the definitions of these perceptual performance components (Appendix E). While it may be difficult initially to differentiate various perceptual skills, with practice you will become very proficient at identifying these components. One example has been completed for you.

4. Most tasks in which we engage during our daily lives challenge more than one perceptual component. As a therapist it will be important to judge the degree of these combined challenges. Complete the Perceptual Analysis Table by deciding how much each perceptual component is challenged during engagement. Indicate your response as follows:

N/A (Not Applicable): Perceptual performance component is not challenged.

Min (Minimal): Performance component is challenged or involved minimally.

Mod (Moderate): Performance component is challenged, but not to a large degree.

Max (Maximal): Performance component is challenged or involved to a large degree.

Support this decision with a brief statement.

Table 2: Perceptual Analysis Table

	Infants	Children		Adults
		Riding a tricycle		
Stereognosis		*Min* *Recognize pedal with feet without looking.*		
Kinesthesia		*Max* *Force required in arms and legs to propel and turn tricycle and negotiate objects.*		
Pain Response		*Min* *For safety.*		
Body Scheme		*Mod-Max* *Awareness of arm, leg, and trunk position and movement at all times.*		

Table 2: Perceptual Analysis Table

	Infants	Children		Adults
		Riding a tricycle		
Right–Left Discrimination		*N/A* Requires directional sense, but not R/L discrimination.		
Form Constancy		*Mod* Identify objects despite their changing retinal image while moving on tricycle.		
Position in Space		*Max* Determine relative position of all objects in relation to one another and self as move tricycle between, behind, beside .		
Visual-Closure		*Min* Identify objects that are partially blocked from view.		

Table 2: Perceptual Analysis Table

	Infants	Children — Riding a tricycle	Adults
Figure-Ground		*Mod* — *Identify obstacles from a cluttered background to avoid them (e.g., see a crayon on a carpeted floor).*	
Depth Perception		*Max* — *Determine changing distances between self and objects to avoid collision.*	
Spatial Relations		*Mod* — *Determine the angle that an object is oriented or placed (e.g., angle of curb ahead or rotated position of a table).*	
Topographical Orientation		*Mod* — *Determine route to destination (e.g., home).*	

Neuromusculoskeletal and Motor Components

Uniform Terminology for Occupational Therapy lists the different neuromusculoskeletal and motor performance components that affect engagement in occupations (AOTA, 1994). Case-Smith (1996) suggests that (a) motor development and performance depends on the integrity of the neuromusculoskeletal components; (b) motor skills evolve in response to sensory input from the environment; and (c) motor skills and performance, in turn, influence cognitive and social development.

Neuromusculoskeletal Components

Reflexes are involuntary muscle responses that are elicited by sensory input. Activity and task engagement may elicit or inhibit reflexes. During initial analyses, therapists should indicate whether engagement elicits or inhibits primitive reflexes such as the grasp, positive supporting, and tonic labyrinthine reflexes. Although the neuromusculoskeletal system involves a number of reflexes, malfunctioning of these three primitive reflexes commonly influences the posture, movement, and performance of individuals served by occupational therapy practitioners. The grasp reflex causes flexion of the fingers when the palm of the hand is stimulated. The positive supporting reaction causes extension of the hip, knee, ankle, and foot when pressure is applied to the ball of the foot. The tonic labyrinthine reflex causes flexor tone to predominate when the body is pronated and extensor tone to predominate in supine. The postural reflexes will be analyzed under the performance component entitled postural control. As you become more familiar with primitive or postural reflexes, you will be able to incorporate them into your analyses.

Range of motion refers to movement of body parts through an arc. During engagement joints are maintained in a position or moved through a range of positions. Movement away from the anatomical

position in the sagittal plane is **flexion**, and movement in the sagittal plane to return to the anatomical position is **extension**. Movement away from the anatomical position in the frontal plane is **abduction**, and movement in the frontal plane to return to the anatomical position is **adduction**. During initial task analyses, document whether joints are positioned or move within the beginnings of ranges (initial degrees of flexion or abduction), in mid-range, or at end ranges. Completion of the optional Neuromusculoskeletal Analysis in the chapter titled "Worker Rehabilitation and the Biomechanical Approach" will require specification of exact joint positions and motions.

Muscle tone is the degree of tension or resistance in a muscle (AOTA, 1994). Muscle contractions can be classified as **isometric, isotonic, concentric,** or **eccentric.** Isometric contractions hold a joint position by maintaining tension throughout the muscle, while isotonic contractions shorten muscles and cause a change in joint position. Concentric contractions involve muscle tension and fiber shortening, while eccentric contractions involve muscle tension with fiber lengthening (Farber, 1991). Cocontraction refers to simultaneous contraction of antagonist musculature for the purposes of holding a joint or limb straight (Thomas, 1985). Analyses should specify the different types of contractions used in different joints during engagement.

Strength refers to the degree of muscle power. During engagement different amounts of muscle strength are used, depending on the influence of gravity or resistance of objects. Initial task analyses should document whether passive, active, active-assistive, or resistive muscle strength is required. Passive activities require minimal or no physical exertion. Active activities require muscle contraction or motion with no external assistance or resistance.

Active-assistive activities require muscle contraction and motion, but external assistance may be supplied. Resistive activities use gravity, weight, and tension to increase muscle strength (Levine & Bradley, 1991). Completion of the optional Neuromusculoskeletal Analysis in the chapter titled "Worker Rehabilitation and the Bio-mechanical Approach" will require specification of the exact amount of strength required in particular muscle groups.

Endurance requires sustained cardiac, pulmonary, and musculoskeletal exertion over time. Initial analyses should indicate the duration and amount of endurance required to complete the task. **Postural control** requires the use of righting, equilibrium, and protective reactions to maintain balance during functional movements. Righting reactions align segments of the body (i.e., head alignment with the body); equilibrium reactions return the body to a vertical position to correct for displacement; protective extension of the arm prevents the body from falling. **Postural alignment** refers to the biomechanical integrity or alignment among body parts. While postural alignment and control influence each other, the relationship is not always causal. In the prone lying position, for example, posture is aligned, but quite different amounts of postural control are required to lay on a bed in a bedroom or on a surfboard on the ocean. **Soft tissue integrity** refers to the anatomical and physiological condition of interstitial tissues and skin (AOTA, 1994).

Motor Components

Gross coordination is the controlled, goal-directed use of large muscle groups. **Crossing the midline** refers to movement of the limbs and eyes across the midsagittal plane of the body, such as reaching with trunk rotation. **Laterality** is the use of a preferred or dominant hand or foot for activities or tasks requiring a high level of skill. **Bilateral integration** requires coordination of both body sides. Laterality and bilateral integration can be used simultaneously or exclusively. For example, cutting a piece of paper requires simultaneous use of a dominant hand (i.e., laterality) to operate the scissors while both hands work together (i.e., bilateral integration) to manipulate and cut along a line on paper. Bilateral integration (exclusively) is required to push a lawn mower or grocery cart. Laterality (exclusively) is needed to pick up and eat a raisin.

Motor control refers to the use of functional and versatile movement patterns. Praxis refers to the ability and skill of planning movement. Ideation is the conceptual process of imagining purposeful movement; motor planning is an intermediary process between ideation and execution. Execution is a culmination of ideation and motor planning (Ayres, 1985; Walker, 1993). **Postural praxis** is the body's ability to assume novel positions. **Visual and constructional praxis** are required to copy novel designs with pencil on paper and to replicate a three-dimensional structure. Motor planning based on compliance with verbal instructions is **verbal praxis**, and processing the specific order of positions is **sequencing praxis.** Planning and executing oral motor movements is **oral praxis** (Ayres, 1989).

Fine coordination/dexterity requires the use of small muscle groups for controlled movements, particularly in object manipulation. During engagement different grasp patterns are used for different functions. Your task analysis should document these grasp patterns. Figure 2 illustrates seven different prehension and grasp patterns.

Visual-motor integration requires interaction of visual information with body movement during

Figure 2. Functional Grasp Patterns.

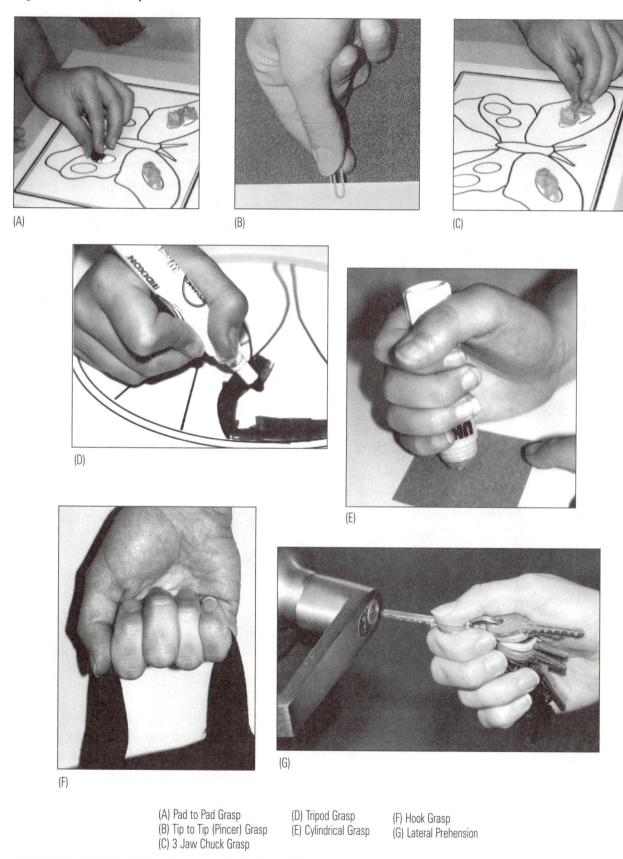

(A)

(B)

(C)

(D)

(E)

(F)

(G)

(A) Pad to Pad Grasp   (D) Tripod Grasp   (F) Hook Grasp
(B) Tip to Tip (Pincer) Grasp (E) Cylindrical Grasp   (G) Lateral Prehension
(C) 3 Jaw Chuck Grasp

performance. For example, tracing a line requires eye-hand coordination and walking along a balance beam requires eye-foot coordination. **Oral-motor control** is the coordination of oral and pharynacal musculature for controlled movements.

The hierarchical and neuromaturational theories of motor development (i.e., neurodevelopmental therapy) provide a framework for many of the assessment and treatment methods used by occupational and physical therapists. These theories assume that (a) aberrant muscle tone interferes with normal movement patterns, (b) movement progresses from primitive reflex pattern to voluntary, controlled movement, (c) movement control progresses in a cephalocaudal and proximodistal direction, and (d) the sequence of movement development is constant (Bobath, 1980; Piper and Darrah, 1994; Short-DeGraff, 1988). Assessment procedures and treatment activities, therefore, are selected and designed depending on their influence on reflexes, muscle tone, proximal postural control, and so forth.

The systems theory of motor development proposes that behavior is dependent on all factors that contribute to outcome (Piper and Darrah, 1994). These factors could include sensory, motor, and emotional inputs and the characteristics of the environment. Any change in these factors affects outcome. Assessment procedures, treatment activities, and intervention require analysis of the dynamic relationship between people, tasks, and environments.

Assignment 3

1. Divide into groups of two.
2. Review the passage on bicycle riding by A. J. Ayres (1979) and determine which neuromusculoskeletal and motor skills are required to make adaptive responses. In your estimation, which sensory system(s) enable the adaptive responses of postural control and visual motor integration?
3. Select and perform one infant, child, and adult activity from the suggestions listed below.

Infants: Crawl through a barrel. Walk up or down stairs. Eat a bowl of gelatin dessert or soup using a spoon. Finger feed banana pieces.

Children: String 1-inch beads. Cut out a circle. Write your name. Make a friendship bracelet. Walk across a balance beam. Play Twister® (Milton Bradley). Play the Simon Says Game (Miller, 1988). Perform the Tapping Feet Alternating While Making Circles with Fingers (Bruininks, 1978). Throw a ball at a target 5 feet away. Kick a ball at a target 5 feet away. Kick a rolling ball. Hit a baseball with a bat. Skip with a rope.

Adults: Design and use fabric paint to make a gift canvas smock. Type at a computer. Hammer a nail into wood. Make an origami figure. Remove a jacket. Brush your teeth. Iron a shirt. Lace a small leather project. Weave a small basket. Knit a small coaster. Roller blade. Putt with a golf club.

4. While engaging in the activity, determine the demands placed on the neuromuscular and motor systems for optimal performance. Document your observations on the Neuromusculoskeletal and Motor Analysis Table (Table 3). Use *Uniform Terminology for Occupational Therapy* (AOTA, 1994) to enhance your understanding of the definitions of these performance components (Appendix E). One example has been completed for you.
5. Complete the Neuromusculoskeletal and Motor Analysis Table by determining how much each component is challenged during engagement. Indicate as follows:

N/A (Not Applicable): Performance component is not challenged.

Min (Minimal): Performance component is challenged or involved minimally.

Mod (Moderate): Performance component is challenged, but not to a large degree.

Max (Maximal): Performance component is challenged or involved to a large degree.

Support this decision with a brief explanation.

6. Share your observations with your class.

7. Select one activity from this last exercise to engage your class in a discussion about the interactive relationship between sensation, perception, and motor systems.

Table 3: Neuromusculoskeletal and Motor Analysis Table

Neuromuscular	Infants	Riding a tricycle	Children	Adults
Reflex		Min-Mod Requires integration of the positive supporting reflex. Grasp reflex may be elicited and assist task during engagement.		
Range of Motion		Mod-Max End range of flexion in hands. Midrange flexion in shoulders, hips, and knees.		
Muscle Tone		Mod Isometric distal hand contractions, with isotonic elbow, shoulder, and knee contractions. Hip cocontraction to initiate propulsion.		
Strength		Mod Requires resistive strength in arms and legs.		

Table 3: Neuromusculoskeletal and Motor Analysis Table

	Infants	Children		Adults	
		Riding a tricycle			
Endurance		*Min-Mod* *Dependent on distance, weight of tricycle, and surface quality.*			
Postural Control		*Mod-Max* *Use head righting and equilibrium to maintain sit on tricycle seat.*			
Postural Alignment		*Mod* *Trunk in midline.*			
Soft Tissue Integrity		*N/A*			

Table 3: Neuromusculoskeletal and Motor Analysis Table

Motor	Infants	Children	Adults
		Riding a tricycle	
Gross Coordination		Mod Gross coordination of arms and legs to get on, off, and ride.	
Crossing the Midline		N/A Not required.	
Laterality		N/A Dominance not required.	
Bilateral Integration		Max Extensive information integration between arms to drive and legs to propel.	
Motor Control		Min-Mod Uses reciprocal leg movements similar to walking.	

Table 3: Neuromusculoskeletal and Motor Analysis Table

	Infants	Children		Adults	
		Riding a tricycle			
Praxis		*Mod-Max* *Postural praxis to get on and off for the first time and negotiate environment.*			
Fine Coordination/ Dexterity		*Min* *Cylindrical grasp.*			
Visual-Motor Integration		*Max* *Scan, track, and negotiate the environment during movement.*			
Oral-Motor Control		*N/A*			

The information that follows will (a) provide students and instructors with resources to enhance the learning experience and (b) assist the student in completing the assignment.

Learning Resources

Ayres, A. J. (1979). *Sensory integration and the child.* Los Angeles: Western Psychological Services.

Bruininks, R. H. (1978). *Bruininks-Oseretsky Test of Motor Proficiency: Manual.* Circle Pines, MN: American Guidance Services.

Miller, L. J. (1988). *Miller Assessment for Preschoolers: Manual.* San Antonio, TX: The Psychological Corporation.

Study Questions

1. Identify the seven sensory, 12 perceptual, eight neuromuscular, and nine motor performance components identified in *Uniform Terminology* (AOTA, 1994).

2. Identify and define five perceptual, neuromuscular, and motor performance components.

3. Using a hammer requires what type of finger muscular contractions? Elbow contractions?

4. Identifying the amount of force, exertion, and direction of joint motion needed to complete an activity requires which of the following performance components: proprioception, stereognosis, kinesthesia, or graphesthesia?

5. Riding in a car that is accelerating stimulates which sensory system?

6. Finding a dime in a deep pocket full of change requires which perceptual skill?

7. Which perceptual component is used to reach out and turn on a bedside table lamp at night?

8. Perception is the process of sensory transmission, interpretation, or awareness?

9. Walking forward on a balance beam requires which motor performance components?

10. What type of grasp pattern is required to open a locked door with a key?

11. Forming cookies with dough is an example of a passive, active-assistive, active, or resistive activity?

12. Crawling through a barrel requires hip flexion, extension, abduction, or adduction?

13. Which of the following activities would be most appropriate to develop postural control skills in an 8-year-old child: playing piano, playing hopscotch, or crawling through a maze?

14. Which of the following activities would be most appropriate to develop fine motor coordination in a 6-year-old child: playing piano, playing hopscotch, or crawling through a maze?

15. Write one paragraph describing the relationship between sensory integration and adaptive responses.

16. Write one paragraph describing the hierarchical approach to motor control.

References

American Occupational Therapy Association. (1994). *Uniform terminology for occupational therapy* (3rd ed.). Bethesda, MD: Author.

Abreu, B., & Toglia, J. (1987). Cognitive rehabilitation: A model for occupational therapy. *American Journal of Occupational Therapy, 41,* 439–448.

Ayres, A. J. (1979). *Sensory integration and the child.* Los Angeles: Western Psychological Services.

Ayres, A. J. (1985). *Developmental dyspraxia and adult onset dyspraxia.* Torrance, CA: Sensory Integration International.

Ayres, A. J. (1989). *Sensory integration and praxis tests.* Los Angeles: Western Psychological Services.

Bobath, K. (1980). *A neurophysiological basis for the treatment of cerebral palsy.* Philadelphia: Lippincott.

Bruininks, R. H. (1978). *Bruininks-Oseretsky Test of Motor Proficiency: Manual.* Circle Pines, MN: American Guidance Services.

Case-Smith, J. (1996). An overview of occupational therapy with children. In J. Case-Smith, A. Allen, & P. Pratt (Eds.), *Occupational therapy for children* (3rd ed., p. 17). St. Louis, MO: Mosby.

Dunn, W. (1991). Sensory dimensions of performance. In C. Christiansen & C. Baum (Eds.), *Occupational therapy: Overcoming human performance deficits* (pp. 231–258). Thorofare, NJ: Slack.

Farber, S. (1991). Neuromotor dimensions of performance. In C. Christiansen & C. Baum (Eds.), *Occupational therapy: Overcoming human performance deficits* (pp. 259–282). Thorofare, NJ: Slack.

Gardner, M. (1982). *Manual: Test of visual-perceptual skills (non-motor).* Burlingame, CA: Psychological and Educational Publications.

Haldy, M., & Haack, L. (1995). *Making it easy: Sensorimotor activities at home and school.* San Antonio, TX: Therapy Skill Builders.

Harris, G. (1995). The karate kids. *OT Week, 9*(45), 14–15.

Hirsch Botzer, M. (1995). Therapeutic karate with children aged 5-7. *World Federation of Occupational Therapy Bulletin, 32,* 20–23.

Kirsteins, A., Dietz, F., Hwang, S. (1991). Evaluating the safety and potential use of a weight-bearing exercise, T'ai Chi Chuan, for rheumatoid arthritis patients. *American Journal of Physical Medicine and Rehabilitation, 70*(3), 136–141.

Levine, R., & Bradley, C. (1991). Occupation as a therapeutic medium: A contextual approach to performance intervention. In C. Christiansen and C. Baum (Eds.), *Occupational therapy: Overcoming human performance deficits* (pp. 592–631). Thorofare, NJ: Slack.

MacKinnon, J., Noh, S., Laliberte, D., Lariviere, J., Allan, D. (1995). Therapeutic horseback riding: A review of the literature. *Physical and Occupational Therapy in Pediatrics, 15*(1), 1–15.

Miller, L. J. (1988). *Miller Assessment for Preschoolers: Manual.* San Antonio, TX: The Psychological Corporation.

Neistadt, M. E. (1990). A critical analysis of occupational therapy approaches for perceptual deficits in adults with brain injury. *American Journal of Occupational Therapy, 44*(4), 299–304.

Parham, L. D., & Mailloux, Z. (1996). Sensory integration. In J. Case-Smith, A. Allen, & P. Pratt (Eds.), *Occupational therapy for children* (3rd ed., pp. 307–356). St. Louis, MO: Mosby.

Piper, M. C., & Darrah, J. (1994). *Motor assessment of the developing infant.* Philadelphia: W. B. Saunders.

Quintana, L. (1995). Evaluation of perception and cognition. In C. A. Trombly (Ed.), *Occupational therapy for physical dysfunction* (pp. 201–224). Baltimore: Williams & Wilkins.

Sayre-Adams, J. (1995). *The theory and practice of therapeutic touch.* New York: Churchill Livingstone.

Schneck, C. (1996). Visual perception. In J. Case-Smith, A. Allen, & P. Pratt (Eds.), *Occupational therapy for children* (3rd ed, pp. 357–385). St. Louis, MO: Mosby.

Short-DeGraff, M. A. (1988). *Human development for occupational and physical therapists.* Baltimore: Williams & Wilkins.

Spink, J. (1993). *Developmental riding therapy: A team approach to assessment treatment.* Tucson, AZ: Therapy Skill Builders.

Stancliff, B. L. (1996). OTs recognize animals in therapy. *OT Practice, 2,* 12–13.

Thomas, C. (Ed.). (1985). *Taber's cyclopedic medical dictionary.* Philadelphia: F. A. Davis.

Tse, S., & Bailey, D. (1992). T'ai chi and postural control in the well elderly. *American Journal of Occupational Therapy, 46,* 295–300.

Walker, K. F. (1993). A. Jean Ayres. In R. J. Miller & K. F. Walker (Eds.), *Perspectives on theory for the practice of occupational therapy* (pp. 103–154). Gaithersburg, MD: Aspen.

COGNITIVE PERFORMANCE COMPONENTS

"Occupational therapy is a health profession that trains persons with cognitive, emotional, and physical limitations to be self-sufficient in the functional activities required for daily living as their capabilities allow" (AOTA, 1994, p. 1029).[1]

Chapter Objectives

1. Identify and define the different cognitive performance components.
2. Analyze an activity to distinguish which cognitive performance components are challenged during engagement.
3. Judge the extent to which different cognitive performance components are required to perform selected activities of interest to infants, children, and adults.
4. Evaluate the potential to use purposeful activities to develop cognitive skills and abilities.
5. Briefly describe how task analysis has been integrated into the Cognitive Disabilities Model.

Purposeful Engagement to Assess and Treat Cognitive Performance Components

Cognition refers to the acquisition and use of knowledge, the thinking process, the ability to use higher brain functions, and the ability to process, store, retrieve, and manipulate information (AOTA, 1994; Duchek, 1991; Quintana, 1995). When cognitive impairments cause or have the potential to cause disability, occupational therapy may be recommended.

Registered occupational therapists use standardized and informal testing to evaluate cognition, but activity and task engagement are used to determine the effect of impairments on occupational performance. When observing performance, occupational therapy practitioners use clinical observations and task analysis to validate the results of standardized assessment.

Occupational therapy intervention with individuals with cognitive disabilities is directed toward (a) developing or improving cognitive skills, or (b) adapting tasks and the performance context to compensate for impairments and match environmental demands with cognitive abilities. Remedial cognitive rehabilitation approaches to assessment and treatment are based on neuropsychology, informational processing, and learning theories. Task and activity analysis are used to select and adapt therapeutic activities to challenge a particular client's abilities and develop more advanced cognitive skills. Because the components of cognition are assumed to be hierarchically organized, treatment is directed at lower-order processes such as orientation and attention (Abreu & Toglia, 1987). The parameters, which may be graded to enhance the therapeutic value of a task to improve cognition, include environmental structure, task familiarity, directions for task completion, number of items, spatial arrangement of items, and response rate required (Wheatley, 1996).

Occupational therapy practitioners also offer services directed at enabling individuals to adjust to residual cognitive limitations that occur as a consequence of trauma, disorder, or disease. The Cognitive Disabilities Model is a frame of reference that uses task analysis to identify the performance patterns of individuals with different cognitive abilities (Allen & Allen, 1987). The model focuses on the management of permanent residual cognitive limitations and recommends that the role of the occupational therapy practitioner is to grade tasks and modify environments to compensate for impairments and optimize performance (Kielhofner, 1992). Task analysis is used within this frame of reference to determine the complexity of different tasks that are used for client assessment and management (Allen, Earhart, & Blue, 1992). The goal of analysis is to identify the steps that the client cannot perform and to adapt the process to enable clients to participate in the craft, activity, or task using residual capacities (Kielhofner, 1992). Therapists use crafts for their diversional qualities, to monitor the quality of task engagement, and to document changes in functional ability (Allen, Earhart, & Blue, 1992).

Uniform Terminology for Occupational Therapy lists the different cognitive performance components that effect engagement in occupations (AOTA, 1994). **Level of arousal** refers to the level of alertness and responsiveness to environmental stimuli. For example, different levels of arousal are required for watching television versus driving a motor vehicle. **Orientation** is the ability to identify person, place, time, and situation. Writing a check, for example, requires orientation to person, time, and situation. **Recognition** is the process of identifying familiar faces, objects, and materials.

Attention refers to our ability to focus mental effort, sustain this focus over time, and shift focus between simultaneous stimuli (Duchek, 1991). Focused attention enables us to respond to discrete auditory, visual, or tactile stimuli (Quintana, 1995). Sustained attention or **attention span** is required to focus on a task over time (AOTA, 1994; Quintana, 1995). Selective attention is the ability to focus on certain information to the exclusion of other information (Duchek, 1991). Alternating attention is the shifting of focus. Having divided attention enables us to respond simultaneously to multiple tasks (Quintana, 1995).

Initiation and termination of activity refers to the starting and stopping of a physical or mental activity at an appropriate time. Recalling information requires **memory**. Short-term memory retains information for temporary periods (30 seconds to 1 minute), and long-term memory involves intervals greater than a few minutes. Recent memory is required for recalling events that occurred within the last few hours to months, whereas remote memory is required for recalling past experiences like childhood (Duchek, 1991).

Sequencing enables us to place information, concepts, and actions in order and to determine "what comes next." **Categorization** is the identification of similarities and differences of information and is necessary to classify information or objects. Separating flatware into knives, forks, and spoons requires categorization. Organizing a variety of information to form thoughts and ideas is **concept formation.** Standing at the kitchen cupboards planning what to make for dinner requires concept formation. This conceptualization and planning involves organizing and integrating information such as time of day (breakfast, lunch, dinner), what types of food are usually served for this meal, which food items are available, the number of people eating, their food preferences, and so on.

Spatial operations involve the mental manipulation of objects. It is important to distinguish this skill from the perceptual performance components *position in space* and *spatial relations.* Position in space and spatial relations are perceptions and therefore are interpretations of visual information. Spatial operations are the cognitive manipulation of spatial information that first requires the individual to *determine* how to *manipulate the object.* The most important thing to remember is that the operations involve *manipulation of information.*

Problem solving refers to the process of (a) recognizing a problem, (b) defining the problem, (c) identifying possible solutions, (d) selecting a plan, (e) organizing steps in the plan, (f) implementing the plan, and (g) evaluating the outcome. **Learning** is the acquisition of new concepts and behaviors. **Generalization** is the application of previously learned concepts and behaviors to a variety of new situations (AOTA, 1994).

Deciding what to wear each day and getting dressed requires a number of cognitive components. The organization and synthesis of information about what appointments occur on any given day, what the weather is like, what articles of clothing are clean or dirty, and what "goes together" requires concept formation, orientation, and memory. Determining the order that garments are put on requires sequencing; determining how to manipulate a shirt or pants to put them on requires mental manipulation of objects, or spatial operations. If a button is missing on the shirt, problem solving will be required to (a) recognize and define the problem, (b) identify alternative solutions and select a plan, and (c) implement and evaluate a solution. Learning to sew on a button is one possible solution. Once learned, generalization of this new skill will enable a person to replace another missing button or do other sewing repairs.

Assignment

1. Divide into groups of two.
2. Select and perform one infant, child, and adult activity from the suggestions listed below.
   Infants: Play with nesting blocks. Place a circle, square, and triangle into a form board. Set up dishes and a doll for a pretend tea party.
   Children: Use a pattern to construct a three-dimensional object. Draw a clock that tells the current time. Build a fort. Print the letters of the alphabet. Tie shoelaces. Play a card game. Play a board game. Make a friendship bracelet.
   Adults: Write out a check to pay a utility bill. Write out a grocery list. Make a cup of coffee. Play a card game. Play a board game. Make an origami figure. Make a tile trivet. Weave a place mat or bookmark. Buy a soda from a machine.
3. While engaging in the activity, determine which cognitive components are required for optimal performance. Document your observations in the Cognitive Integration and Cognitive Components Analysis Table (Table 1). Canadian students should use the table in Appendix D. Use *Uniform Terminology for Occupational Therapy* (AOTA, 1994) to enhance your understanding of the definitions of these cognitive performance components (Appendix E). One example has been completed for you.
4. Most tasks in which we engage during our daily lives challenge more than one cognitive skill. As a therapist it will be important to judge the degree of challenge. Complete the Cognitive Integration and Cognitive Components Analyses Table by deciding how much each cognitive component is challenged during engagement. Indicate your response:

   N/A (Not Applicable): The cognitive performance component is not challenged.
   Min (Minimal): Performance component is challenged or involved minimally.
   Mod (Moderate): Performance component is challenged, but not to a large degree.
   Max (Maximal): Performance component is challenged or involved to a large degree.

   Support this decision with a brief explanation.
5. Share your observations with your class.

Table 1: Cognitive Integration and Cognitive Components Analysis Table

	Infants	Children	Adults
		Riding a tricycle	
Level of Arousal		*Max* *Required to respond to changing environmental obstacles.*	
Orientation		*Min* *Orientation of situation only.*	
Recognition		*Min-Mod* *Identify tricycle, objects, and obstacles.*	
Attention Span		*Mod* *Sustain attention for the ride. Divide attention between riding and environmental stimuli.*	
Initiation of Activity		*Min* *Initiate ride.*	

Table 1: Cognitive Integration and Cognitive Components Analysis Table

	Infants	Children Riding a tricycle	Adults
Termination of Activity		Min Terminate ride after appropriate amount of time.	
Memory		Mod Long-term recall how to get on and use, where to travel, and consequences of different routes (e.g., fall off curb)	
Sequencing		Min-Mod Get on and use. Plan route to specific destination.	
Categorization		N/A	
Concept Formation		N/A	

Table 1: Cognitive Integration and Cognitive Components Analysis Table

	Infants		Children	Riding a tricycle		Adults
Spatial Operations				*Max* *How to get on/off. How to maneuver tricycle around barriers, particularly moving obstacles.*		
Problem Solving				*Mod* *What course of action to take if stuck or cannot fit through a clearing.*		
Learning				*Min-Mod* *New learning will depend on previous experience on tricycle.*		
Generalization				*Mod* *Could generalize skill to riding a bicycle with or without training wheels.*		

Study Questions

1. List 10 of the 14 cognitive performance components.

2. Identify and define five cognitive performance components.

3. Which performance component refers to the cognitive process of forming and organizing information, thoughts, or ideas?

4. The ability to focus on certain information to the exclusion of other information is referred to as

   _____.

5. When paying a utility bill you must sign and date a check and write a return address on the envelope. Which cognitive performance component is challenged the most during engagement in this activity: attention, orientation, or initiation of activity?

6. Tying shoelaces challenges which of the following cognitive performance components: dexterity and praxis, sequencing and spatial operations, or orientation and categorization?

7. Which of the following activities could be used to enhance categorization and sequencing skills of a client who is attending a cognitive rehabilitation program: reading a novel, playing a card game of solitaire, or painting a picture?

8. Which frame of reference recommends that occupational therapy practitioners grade tasks and alter environments to compensate for client impairments and optimize performance?

References

Abreu, B. C., & Toglia, J. P. (1987). Cognitive rehabilitation: A model for occupational therapy. *American Journal of Occupational Therapy, 41,* 439–448.

Allen, C. K, & Allen, R. E. (1987). Cognitive disabilities: Measuring the social consequences of mental disorders. *Journal of Clinical Psychiatry, 48(5),* 185–190.

Allen, C. K., Earhart, C. A., & Blue, T. (1992). Occupational therapy treatment goals for the physically and cognitively disabled. Bethesda, MD: *American Occupational Therapy Association.*

American Occupational Therapy Association. (1994). *Uniform terminology for occupational therapy* (3rd ed.). Bethesda, MD: Author.

Duchek, J. (1991). Cognitive dimensions of performance. In C. Christiansen & C. Baum (Eds.), *Occupational therapy: Overcoming human performance deficits* (pp. 592–631). Thorofare, NJ: Slack.

Kielhofner, G. (1992). *Conceptual foundations of occupational therapy.* Philadelphia: F. A. Davis.

Quintana, L. (1995). Evaluation of perception and cognition. In C. A. Trombly (Ed.), *Occupational therapy for physical dysfunction* (pp. 201–224). Baltimore: Williams & Wilkins.

Wheatley, C. (1996). Evaluation and treatment of cognitive dysfunction. In L. W. Pedretti (Ed.), *Occupational therapy: Practice skills for physical dysfunction* (pp. 241–252). St. Louis, MO: Mosby.

PSYCHOSOCIAL AND PSYCHOLOGICAL PERFORMANCE COMPONENTS

"Tasks and activities as they are used in occupational therapy for patients with primary psychosocial problems are analyzed for those properties of the activity that fulfill specific psychosocial and psychodynamic needs"
(Llorens, 1973, p. 453).[1]

Chapter Objectives

1. Identify and define the different psychosocial and psychological performance components.
2. Analyze an activity to distinguish which psychosocial and psychological performance components are challenged during engagement.
3. Judge the extent to which different psychosocial and psychological performance components are required to perform selected activities of interest to infants, children, and adults.
4. Evaluate the potential to use purposeful activities to develop psychosocial and psychological performance components.
5. Become familiar with the potential to use social group activities as therapeutic agents to promote adaptation.
6. Define the terms **meaningful** and **purposeful** and explain their relevance to the therapy process.

Purposeful Engagement to Assess and Treat Psychosocial and Psychological Components

People possess attributes, skills, and abilities that make them unique as individuals and enable them to interact in society and to process emotions. These psychosocial and psychological components can be categorized in three domains: psychological, social, and self-management (AOTA, 1994).

Psychological

Psychological performance components include individual values, interests, and self-concept. **Values** are the ideas or beliefs that are important to self and others. **Interests** include the ability to identify the mental and physical activities that create pleasure and maintain attention. It is one's values, interests, and beliefs about personal causation that contribute to volition, according to the Model of Human Occupation. Volition is responsible for the inner drive to explore, engage, and master (Kielhofner, 1985). **Self-concept** refers to the value attributed to our physical, emotional, and sexual self (AOTA, 1994).

Occupational therapy practitioners assist clients in engaging in occupations that give meaning and purpose to their lives. An individual's values, interests, self-concept, experience, perceived needs, and sociocultural contexts shape the meaning and purpose he or she attributes to different tasks (Trombly, 1995; AOTA, 1993). The meaning of a task depends on personal interpretation of value or importance and can be described in terms of its presence or absence, degree, and type (Nelson, 1988; Trombly, 1995). **Purpose** refers to an individual's goals, such as to seek praise, satisfaction, money, or a particular effect on one's environment. Activities that have meaning and purpose to clients may enhance (a) motivation (Kircher, 1984; Hesse & Campion, 1983; Trombly, 1995); (b) personal satisfaction (Thibodeaux & Ludwig, 1988); (c) learning and adaptation (Yuen, 1988); and (d) motor skill development and performance (Hsieh, Nelson, Smith, & Peterson, 1996; Licht & Nelson, 1990; Yuen, 1988). To design effective and efficient evaluation and intervention, therapists must under-

---

[1]From "Activity Analysis for cognitive-perceptual-motor dysfunction by L. A. Llorens, 1973, *American Journal of Occupational Therapy, 27, p. 453.* Copyright 1973 by the American Occupational Therapy Association. Reprinted with permission.

stand the meaning and purpose that clients ascribe to different tasks.

Social

Psychosocial performance components enable people to interact with others, establish and maintain friendships and kinship bonds, cope with challenging situations, and manage their behavior (Case-Smith, 1996). The social performance components include role performance, social conduct, interpersonal skills, and self-expression (AOTA, 1994). **Role performance** involves identifying, maintaining, and balancing the functions one assumes or acquires in society. **Social conduct** refers to appropriate use of manners, personal space, eye contact, gestures, active listening, and self-expression. **Interpersonal skills** involve verbal and nonverbal communication to interact in a variety of settings. **Self-expression** refers to the use of a variety of styles and skills to express thoughts, feelings, and needs.

Self-Management

Self-management performance components include coping skills, time management, and self-control. **Coping skills** are required for identifying and managing stress and related factors. **Time management** refers to planning and participating in a healthy and satisfactory balance of self-care, work, leisure, and rest activities. Self-control is required to modify one's own behavior in response to environmental needs, demands, constraints, personal aspirations, and feedback from others.

Engaging Psychosocial and Psychological Components in Treatment

Participating in occupations in daily life contributes to the development and maintenance of psychosocial and psychological performance components. Occupational therapy practitioners use purposeful and meaningful activities to assess and treat psychosocial and psychological performance components. For example, aerobic exercise has been used with adolescents with depression and adults with chronic schizophrenia (Adams, 1995; Brollier, Hamrick, & Jacobson, 1994). A recreational kayaking program has been used with adults with traumatic brain injury to address self-concept, leisure satisfaction, and leisure attitude (Fines & Nichols, 1994). By engaging clients' minds, spirits, and bodies in tasks and occupations, therapists can optimize performance. This approach distinguishes occupational therapy from verbal therapies (CAOT, 1993).

The psychological components, including values, interests, and self-concept, of all occupational therapy clients must be considered when selecting and designing purposeful and meaningful therapeutic activities.

Assignment

1. Divide into teams of four to six persons.
2. Select and perform one child and one adult activity from the suggestions listed below.

Children: Have one group member teach your team how to play a musical instrument or work together to play a musical instrument for another team. Show your team how to play a game that you enjoyed in your childhood.

Adults: Participate in a solitary or team leisure game that is important to you. Design and host an aerobics class for other teams. Play a board game. Make cookies as a team. Host a talent or fashion show. Complete the Value Boxes exercise (Davis, 1994, p. 34), Values Priority exercise (Davis, 1994, p. 52), or the Environmental Crisis exercise (Davis, 1994, p. 55). Participate in one of the following

group activities: Earthquake Survival (Ballew &
Prokop, 1994), Lost at Sea (Pfeiffer & Company,
1989a), or Wilderness Survival (Pfeiffer &
Company, 1989b).

3. While engaging in the activity, determine the
demands placed on the psychosocial and psychological components for optimal performance.
Document your observations in the Psychosocial
and Psychological Analysis Table (Table 1).
Canadian students should use the table in
Appendix D. Use *Uniform Terminology for
Occupational Therapy* (AOTA, 1994) to enhance
your understanding of the definitions of these
performance components (Appendix E). One
example has been completed for you.

4. Most tasks that we engage in during daily life
challenge more than one psychosocial and
psychological component. As a therapist it will be
important to judge the overall degree of challenge.
Develop your skills in this area by deciding "how
much" each component is challenged during
engagement. Indicate as follows:

N/A (Not Applicable): The performance component
is not challenged.
Min (Minimal): Performance component is challenged or involved minimally.
Mod (Moderate): Performance component is challenged, but not to a large capacity.
Max (Maximal): Performance component is challenged or involved to a large capacity.

Support this decision with a brief statement.

5. Share your observations with your class.

Table 1: Psychosocial and Psychological Analysis

Psychological	Riding a tricycle			Children			Adults
Values	*Mod* *A child may value participation for personal gratification or social acceptance by peers.*						
Interests	*Min-Max* *A child's interest may be minimal to very important.*						
Self-Concept	*Mod-Max* *Accomplishment or participation influences self-concept if client is very interested or values riding a tricycle.*						

Table 1: Psychosocial and Psychological Analysis

Social	Children		Adults
	Riding a tricycle		
Role Performance	Mod One of the activities that children are expected to enjoy in our dominant culture.		
Social Conduct	Mod Dependent on social context. Need to respect others' space or tricycles.		
Interpersonal Skills	Min-Mod Dependent on social context.		
Self-Expression	Mod Riding provides the opportunity for creative expression and imaginative play.		

Table 1: Psychosocial and Psychological Analysis

Self-Management	Riding a tricycle	Children		Adults
Coping Skills	Mod-Max *Dependent on ability to ride, complexity of physical and social environmental demands where riding.*			
Time Management	N/A			
Self-Control	Mod *Dependent on complexity of physical and social environ-ment demands when riding.*			

The information that follows will (a) provide students and instructors with resources to enhance the learning experience and (b) assist the student in completing the assignment.

Learning Resources

Books and Periodicals

Davis, C. M. (1994). Values as determinants of behavior. In C. A. Davis (Ed.), *Patient practitioner interaction: An experiential manual for developing the art of health care* (2nd ed., pp. 37–60). Thorofare, NJ: Slack.

Activities

Ballew, A. C., & Prokop, M. K. (1944). *Earthquake survival: Leader's manual.* San Diego, CA: Pfeiffer & Company.

Pfeiffer & Company. (1989a). *Lost at sea: Simulation and leader's manual.* San Diego, CA: Author.

Pfeiffer & Company. (1989b). *Wilderness survival: Simulation and leader's manual.* San Diego, CA: Author.

Study Questions

1. List the three psychological, four social, and three self-management performance components.
2. Identify and define five of the psychosocial and psychological performance components.
3. What is the term that refers to one's ability to identify and manage stress?
4. What is the term that refers to the use of verbal and nonverbal communication to appropriately interact in a variety of social settings?
5. Therapists who facilitate group activities shape and role-model social conduct to develop what: clients' independence, self expression, or interpersonal skills?
6. Identify an activity that could be used with a student who is having difficulty with time management.
7. Explain why therapeutic activities should be meaningful and purposeful.

References

Adams, L. (1995). How exercise can help people with mental health problems. *Nursing Times, 91(36)*, 37–39.

American Occupational Therapy Association (AOTA). (1993). *Position paper: Purposeful activity.* Bethesda, MD: Author.

AOTA. (1994). *Uniform terminology for occupational therapy* (3rd ed.). Bethesda, MD: Author.

Brollier, C., Hamrick, N., & Jacobson, B. (1994). Aerobic exercise: A potential occupational therapy modality for adolescents with depression. *Occupational Therapy in Mental Health, 12(4)*, 19–29.

***Canadian Association* of Occupational Therapists. (1993).** *Occupational therapy guidelines for client-centred mental health practice.* Toronto, ON: Author.

Case-Smith, J. (1996). An overview of occupational therapy with children. In J. Case-Smith, A. Allen, & P. Pratt (Eds.), *Occupational therapy for children* (3rd ed.). St. Louis, MO: Mosby.

Fines, L., & Nichols, D. (1994). An evaluation of a twelve-week recreational kayak program: Effects on self-concept, leisure satisfaction and leisure attitudes of adults with traumatic brain injuries. *Journal of Cognitive Rehabilitation, 12(5)*, 10–15.

Hesse, K. A., & Campion, E. W. (1983). Motivating the geriatric patient for rehabilitation. *Journal of the American Geriatric Society, 31*, 586–589.

Hsieh, C., Nelson, D. L., Smith, D. A., & Peterson, C. Q. (1996). A comparison of performance in added-purpose occupations and rote exercise for dynamic standing balance in persons with hemiplegia. *American Journal of Occupational Therapy, 50*, 10–16.

Kielhofner, G. (1985). *A Model of Human Occupation: Theory and application.* Baltimore: Williams & Wilkins.

Kircher, M. A. (1984). Motivation as a factor of perceived exertion in purposeful versus nonpurposeful activity. *American Journal of Occupational Therapy, 38*, 165–170.

Licht, B. C., & Nelson, D. L. (1990). Adding meaning to a design copy task through representational stimuli. *American Journal of Occupational Therapy, 44*, 408–413.

Llorens, L. A. (1973). Activity analysis for cognitive-perceptual-motor dysfunction. *American Journal of Occupational Therapy, 27*, 453–456.

Nelson, D. L. (1988). Occupation: Form and performance. *American Journal of Occupational Therapy, 42*, 633–641.

Thibodeaux, C. S., & Ludwig, R. F. (1988). Intrinsic motivation in product-oriented and non-product-oriented activities. *American Journal of Occupational Therapy, 42*, 169–175.

Trombly, C. A. (1995). Occupation: Purposefulness and meaningfulness as therapeutic mechanisms. *American Journal of Occupational Therapy, 49*, 960–972.

Yuen, H. K. (1988). *The purposeful use of an object in the development of skill with a prosthesis.* Unpublished master's thesis, Western Michigan University, Kalamazoo, Michigan.

TEMPORAL ASPECTS

"The use of activities of interest to clients, and those which enhance their abilities to perform tasks appropriate to their health status and resources, form the core of occupational therapy's specialized subject matter"

(Canadian Association of Occupational Therapists [CAOT], 1991, p. 12).[1]

Chapter Objectives

1. Identify and define the different temporal performance contexts.
2. Analyze a client case scenario to identify the different temporal aspects of occupational performance.

Temporal Aspects of Occupational Performance Context

To evaluate clients and provide intervention services, occupational therapy practitioners must understand the reciprocal, interdependent, and transactional relationship between people and their environments. Therapists may "choose interventions based on an understanding of contexts, or may choose interventions directly aimed at altering the contexts to improve performance" (AOTA, 1994, p. 17). By creating a better match between individual skills and abilities and environmental demands, therapists facilitate client control and mastery over their occupations. (Law, 1991).

Therapists consider performance contexts during client evaluation when determining function and dysfunction relative to performance areas and performance components, and during intervention planning when determining the feasibility and appropriateness of treatment (AOTA, 1994).

Performance contexts include temporal aspects and the physical, social, and cultural environment (AOTA, 1994). The **temporal aspects** that influence performance include chronological, developmental, life cycle, and disability status. **Chronological** refers to an individual's age. When completing task

analyses, the therapist should refer to the age of the occupational therapy client and the age at which the task is typically performed. **Developmental** refers to the phase of maturation of the client or stage of maturation during which the task is typically performed.

Life cycle refers to important life phases, such as career or parenting cycles or the educational process (AOTA, 1994). When completing task analyses, therapists should document whether the task occurs in early childhood (birth to puberty), adolescence (puberty to 20 years of age), young adulthood (21-35 years of age), middle years (36-65), mature years (over 65), or across the life span (CAOT, 1991). Alternatively, the stage of life of the client should be considered according to developmental theorists such as Erik Erikson, Arnold Gesell, Robert Havighurst, Lawrence Kohlberg, or Jean Piaget.

Disability status is the "place in the continuum of disability, such as acuteness of injury, chronicity of disability, or terminal nature of illness" (AOTA, 1994, p. 285). When completing task analyses, the therapist should indicate the present location of the occupational therapy client on the continuum of disability and note whether the task is most appropriately performed during the acute, chronic, or terminal phase of illness.

Assignment

1. Read the client scenarios described in Table 1 and identify the temporal variables that influence occupational performance.

---

[1]From *Guidelines for the Client-Centred Practice of Occupational Therapy* (p. 12), by Health Canada, 1983, Toronto, ON: *Canadian Association of Occupational Therapists.* Reproduced with permission of the Minister of Public Works and Government Services Canada, 1996.

Table 1: Temporal Variables that Influence Occupational Performance

Client Scenario	
Albert is a 2-year-old boy who was diagnosed with spastic cerebral palsy at a young age. Although he is interested in all of the same toys and activities as his twin brother, his motor development and movement performance is not the same.	
Performance Context	
Temporal Aspects	Comments
1. Chronological	
2. Developmental	
3. Life Cycle	
4. Disability Status	

Client Scenario	
Mary is a 65-year-old woman who lives with her husband and is recently retired. Mary has arthritis and frequently complains of bilateral hip and knee pain. She broke her hip after slipping on ice while walking to her car and will be receiving inpatient rehabilitation services.	
Performance Context	
Temporal Aspects	Comments
1. Chronological	
2. Developmental	
3. Life Cycle	
4. Disability Status	

2. In preparation for the Physical and Sociocultural Environment chapters, read the article by Dunn, Brown, and McGuigan (1994), *The Ecology of Human Performance: A Framework for Considering the Effect of Context.*

The information that follows will (a) provide students and instructors with resources to enhance the learning experience and (b) assist the student in completing the assignment.

Learning Resources

Dunn, W., Brown, C., & McGuigan, A. (1994). The ecology of human performance: A framework for considering the effect of context. *American Journal of Occupational Therapy, 47,* 595–607.

Study Questions

1. List and define the four temporal variables of occupational performance context.
2. Rob is a 15-year-old boy who is mentally retarded. He attends high school and is learning how to write his full address and read small books. Identify the temporal variables that affect Rob's occupational performance.

References

American Association of Occupational Therapy. (1994). *Uniform terminology for occupational therapy* (3rd ed.). Bethesda, MD: Author.

Canadian Association of Occupational Therapists. (1991). *Occupational therapy guidelines for client-centred practice.* Toronto, ON: Author.

Law, M. (1991). 1991 Muriel Driver Lecture—The environment: A focus for occupational therapy. *Canadian Journal of Occupational Therapy, 58,* 171–179.

PHYSICAL ENVIRONMENT

"The purpose of practice is to alter the person's ability, the occupation, or the environment so that the person can achieve the necessary balance between ability and the environmental demands to enable occupational competence" (Polatajko, 1994, p. 592–593).[1]

Chapter Objectives

1. List the features of the physical or nonhuman environment that influence occupational performance.
2. Identify characteristics of the physical environment that may be altered to enable or enhance human performance of individuals with and without disabilities.
3. Analyze client case scenarios to identify the physical environmental variables that influence occupational performance.
4. Identify some of the physical barriers that limit functional and community mobility.
5. Use creative problem solving to resolve physical environmental access barriers for individuals with disabilities.

Physical Environmental Aspects of Occupational Performance Contex

Environmental variables of concern to occupational therapy practitioners include the physical, social, and cultural contexts. The **physical environment** includes the nonhuman aspects of performance contexts, including natural terrain, plants, animals, buildings, furniture, objects, tools, or devices (AOTA, 1994). The material objects within environments provoke curiosity, interest, motivation, and the desire to engage (Case-Smith, 1996). People have preferences for objects that hold personal meaning and tend to surround themselves with objects that reflect their patterns of occupation (Kielhofner, 1985). People value objects and possessions that enable them to express their values, interests, and feelings (Csikszentmihalyi & Rochberg- Halton, 1981). The stability and predictability of the nonhuman environment contribute to one's sense of security and self-understanding,

and interaction with this environment facilitates development and may be a source of pleasure, enjoyment, and relaxation (Mosey, 1981). Occupational therapy practitioners view the physical environment as an entity to be mastered and as a vehicle for promoting the development of sensorimotor, cognitive, psychosocial, and psychological performance components (Mosey).

Therapists who seek to understand and manage the physical-environmental features of occupational performance context use task analysis and clinical observations to determine if the nonhuman aspects of the environment enable or constrain performance. Criterion-referenced assessments may be administered. For example, a child with fine motor dexterity impairments may not be able to manipulate the same wind-up toy as his or her peers. A teenager who uses a wheelchair for community mobility may have difficulty entering a movie theater with stairs at the front entrance. A construction worker with a recent wrist injury may not have the strength required to use a manual screwdriver. A senior with limited near visual acuity may not be able to read the small print on a utility bill. The wind-up toy, movie theater entrance, manual screwdriver, and utility bill are all features of the physical or nonhuman environment that limit these individuals' ability to engage in meaningful and purposeful tasks.

When necessary, occupational therapy practitioners enable people to engage in meaningful roles, tasks, and activities by altering physical environments to compensate for impairments. Alterations in the physical environment may minimize disability for

---

individual clients or improve the occupational performance of communities. Recommending a string pull toy rather than a wind-up toy will enable a child with fine motor limitations to play, and consulting with large toy manufacturers about toy design will ensure that all children have access to play opportunities. Providing a ramp at one movie theater will enable people who use wheelchairs to gain access to the building. Suggesting the use of a power screwdriver will enable an injured worker to be more successful at work, and consulting with a large firm to help structure workplace environments that minimize employee injury promotes the health of an entire workforce. Providing a magnifying glass to a client with limited near visual acuity will enable him or her to read the utility bill, and advocating for companies to enlarge the print on their invoices will ensure that all individuals with limited near visual acuity can perform this same task independently.

Occupational therapy practitioners intentionally use the physical properties of objects, tools, or devices to remediate impairments, develop skills, or teach new methods. For example, a therapist who is providing treatment to a child with fine motor impairments may engage the child in play with toys that have particular physical characteristics. The child might (a) play with a toy that requires turning a large plastic dial, or (b) open large containers that have twist-off lids. After the child progresses to removing lids from small containers, this manipulative hand skill is generalized to wind-up toys. A therapist who is providing treatment to a worker with upper limb weakness resulting from a recent wrist injury may suggest that the client complete a leatherwork project using certain objects, tools, materials, and devices. Strength is improved by increasing the size and weight of the tools, the thickness of the leather used, the duration of time that the client participates in the activity, and so on. By analyzing and struc-

turing the physical environment of treatment, intervention is directed at remediating impairments, developing skills, or teaching new methods.

Assignment

1. Work individually or in small groups to complete Projects A and B. Project C is optional.

Project A

1. Complete Project A to learn about the architectural barriers in communities and the role of occupational therapy practitioners in modifying physical environments to compensate for impairments and enable independence.

2. Select a commercial or public building or home and recommend adaptations that will ensure that it is fully accessible to an individual who uses a wheelchair for functional and community mobility. Noll (1995) provides a guide that could be used to complete this project. Noll's guide recommends a three-step process: (a) identify meaningful tasks that must be performed in the home; (b) delineate the client's personal needs, preferences, and abilities; and (c) determine physical environmental supports and obstacles. This analysis process acknowledges the interactive relationship between people, tasks, and environments.

3. To identify physical environmental barriers, examine the approach to the house or building and maneuverability within various rooms. Ensuring accessibility to the house requires analysis of the driveway (e.g., location, slope, width); sidewalk (e.g., slope, surface quality, width); changes in elevation (e.g., height, distance); doorways (e.g., threshold type, width, door handle style, and weight); and safety features (e.g., lighting, locks). Use Table 1, ADA Accessibility Guidelines for Buildings and Facilities, to assist you with this process.

Table 1: ADA Accessibility Guidelines for Buildings and Facilities

Accessible Elements and Spaces	Inches	Millimeters
<u>Space Allowance and Reach Ranges</u>		
Wheelchair Pass Width—One Point	32	815
Wheelchair Pass Width—Continuous	36	915
Turning Space	60	1525
Maximum Forward Reach	48	1220
Maximum Side Reach	54	1370

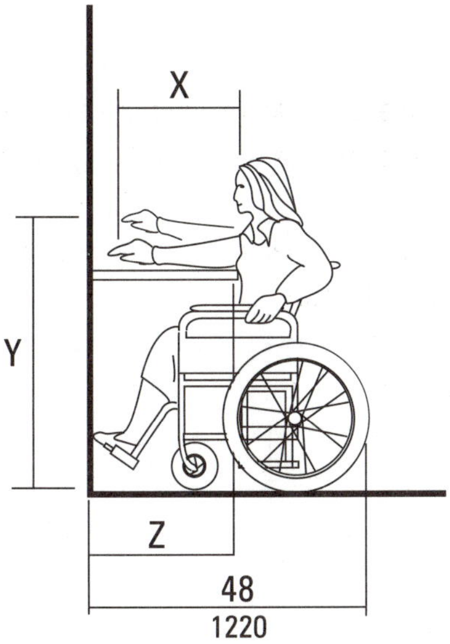

Figure 1. Maximum Forward Reach Over an Obstruction.

Note: x shall be $\leq$ 25 in. (635 mm); z shall be $\geq$ x. When x < 20 in. (510 mm), then y shall be 48 in. (1220 mm) maximum. When x is 20-25 in. (510-635), then y shall be 44 in. (1120 mm) maximum.

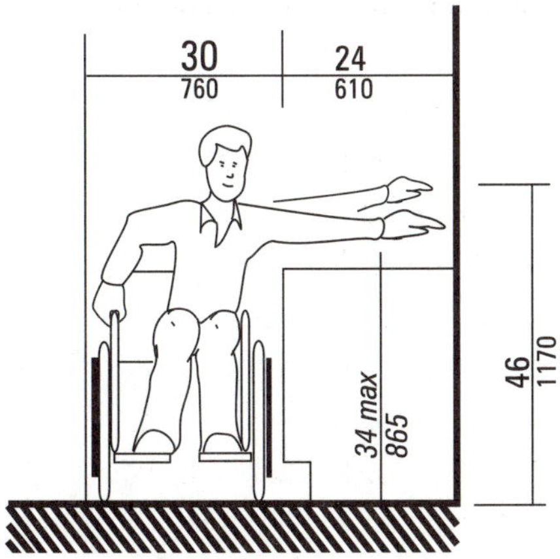

Figure 2. Maximum Side Reach Over Obstruction (inches and milimeters).

Table 1: ADA Accessibility Guidelines for Buildings and Facilities[1]

Accessible Elements and Spaces	Inches	Millimeters
<u>Changes in Level</u>		
Maximum ramp slope	1:12	1:305
Minimum ramp width	36	915
Maximum rise for any run	30	760
Minimum size of ramp landing	60	1525
Changes in level of 1/4 to 1/2 inches shall be beveled.		
Changes in level > 1/2 inch must be ramped.		
<u>Doorways</u>		
Minimum clear opening with door open 90°	32	815
Threshold heights—must be beveled if raised	3/4	13
Door handle shape shall be easy to grasp with one hand and not require tight grasp or pinch or twisting of the wrist. Floor or ground within required clearances shall be level and clear.		
<u>Toilet Stalls</u>		
Sink height above floor (minimum-maximum). Hot water and drain pipes under sinks shall be insulated to protect against contact. Lever-operated, push-type, and electronically controlled faucets are examples of accessible designs. Space size and arrangement and grab bar location should comply with Figure 3.	29–34	735–865

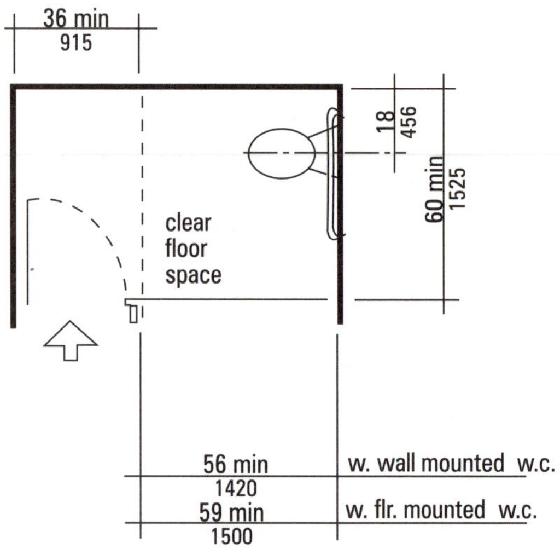

(a-1)
Standard Stall (end of row)

Figure 3. Standard toilet stall (inches and milimeters).

[1]Standards for Accessible Design, 56 Fed. Reg. 35605 (1991).

Project B

1. Complete Project B to identify the physical environmental variables that are used to remediate or compensate for impairments in occupational therapy clients.

2. Read the client scenarios described in Table 2 and identify the physical environmental variables that influence occupational performance.

Table 2: Physical Environmental Variables That Influence Occupational Performance

Client	Physical Environmental Variables
Albert is a 3-year-old boy who was diagnosed with spastic cerebral palsy and visual impairments. Although Albert is unable to sit on his own, he has a special chair with a lap tray that provides head and trunk support. Albert uses a strap across his pelvis and chest to keep him in this chair when he is upright. He is learning the concept of cause and effect. Albert uses a palmar grasp with objects and cannot isolate finger movements or use pincer prehension. During one treatment session with Albert you will give him a small, textured, high-contrast-color toy that squeaks when squeezed.	
Ben is a 25-year-old man who sustained a high-level, spinal cord injury. He uses a wheelchair for community mobility and has learned to drive his van with adapted hand controls. On a recent visit to the grocery store, Ben was unable to enter the building without assistance because the electric door opener was broken. Once in the store Ben could not reach items on the higher shelves and purchased only what he could carry in his lab or wheelchair tote bag.	
Mary is a 62-year-old woman with memory loss secondary to the early stages of Alzheimer's disease who enjoys cooking meals for her husband. She is unable to remember when the oven is on or how long food has been cooking on the stove. When Mary is shopping, she cannot remember what food items to purchase. Her husband suggested keeping a grocery list, but Mary creates and eventually misplaces multiple lists. You recommend using a kitchen timer, and appliances with automatic shut-off features (kettle, toaster, microwave). Mary now adds grocery items to a shopping list that is kept on an erasable bulletin board with an attached pen and is prominently mounted on the refrigerator.	

Project C

1. Project C is optional. Visit a local public service building such as a courthouse, grocery store, post office, shopping center, or library.
2. Identify physical environmental barriers or hazards to individuals with disabilities. Document and share your findings with others.
3. What role do occupational therapy practitioners have in minimizing or eliminating these barriers or hazards? What tasks and activities must be performed to accomplish this role?

The information that follows will (a) provide students and instructors with resources to enhance the learning experience and/or (b) assist the student in completing the assignment.

Learning Resources

Noll, T. (Ed.). (1995). *A consumer's guide to home adaptation.* Boston: Adaptive Environments Center. (Available from the American Occupational Therapy Association.)

Study Questions

1. List four features of the physical, nonhuman environmental context that influence human performance.
2. Identify three features of the physical environment that could affect the speed, efficiency, and accuracy of the task of typing on the computer.
3. Identify two ways that you could alter your environment to improve the effectiveness and efficiency of your study habits.
4. List some of the devices that occupational and physical therapists use to alter the environment and assist individuals with poor balance to walk or move about safely in the bathroom.

References

American Occupational Therapy Association. (1994). *Uniform terminology for occupational therapy* (3rd ed.). Bethesda, MD: Author.

Case-Smith, J. (1996). An overview of occupational therapy with children. In J. Case-Smith, A. S. Allen, & P. N. Pratt (Eds.), *Occupational therapy for children* (3rd ed.). St. Louis, MO: Mosby.

Csikszentmihalyi, M., & Rochberg-Halton, E. (1981). *The meaning of things.* Cambridge, MA: Cambridge University Press.

Kielhofner, G. (1985). *A Model of Human Occupation: Theory and application* (2nd ed.). Baltimore: Williams & Wilkins.

Mosey, A. C. (1981). *Occupational therapy: Configuration of a profession.* New York: Raven Press.

Polatajko, H. (1994). Dreams, dilemmas, and decisions for occupational therapy practice in the new millennium: A Canadian perspective. *American Journal of Occupational Therapy, 48,* 590–594.

SOCIAL AND CULTURAL ENVIRONMENTS

"Diversity is like a hand-stitched quilt pieced together with love, care, and understanding. The many colors, textures, shapes of the quilt form an image of artistic beauty and represent unity. Likewise, I believe, through diversity we can piece together college campuses, communities, and nations to create an atmosphere of understanding and respect for those who are different. Breaking down stereotypes and prejudices allows us to practice tolerance, which gives way to the healing of misunderstandings.... When taking the holistic approach, we as therapists must understand and respect each individual's culture, background, and beliefs in order to treat the patient as a 'whole person' with unique needs and concerns" (Barnes [as cited in Tessler, 1994]).[1]

Chapter Objectives

1. Identify and define the different environmental occupational performance contexts.
2. Analyze client case scenarios to identify the social and cultural performance contexts.
3. Complete a questionnaire and participate in a social group exercise to become aware of personal sociocultural identity and potential biases.
4. Participate in a class discussion about the diversity of social and cultural environments and the influence of sociocultural context on occupational performance.
5. Engage in a social activity to identify the characteristics of the group dynamic that influence the performance of group members.

The Social and Cultural Environmental Aspects of Occupational Performance Contexts

Occupation occurs within a performance context. Engagement in meaningful and purposeful tasks is bound not only by temporal variables (e.g., chronological and developmental age, life cycle, disability status) and by the physical environment but also by the social and cultural performance context. The **cultural environment** is the customs, beliefs, activity patterns, behavior standards, and expectations accepted by the society in which an individual is a member. This includes political aspects and opportunities for education, employment, and economic support (AOTA, 1994). Culture provides a framework that guides daily behavior and is an integral part of everyone's life (Krefting, 1991; Wells, 1994).

The **social environment** refers to the availability and expectations of significant others as well as the larger group influence on established norms, role expectations, and social routines. This human environment defines performance expectations, gives encouragement and support, and provides interaction opportunities (Case-Smith, 1996). People are social beings who establish and maintain kinship bonds, friendships, and relationships throughout local and regional communities. These familial relationships and social networks provide support, information, and emotional and material aid, and they shape identity (Davidson, 1991).

---

[1]From "Issues in Minority Affairs: OT Represented at Conference on Freedom," by E. Tessler, 1994, *OT Week 8*(49), pp. 8–9. Copyright 1994 by *OT Week*. Reprinted with permission.

Individuals are influenced by national, regional, community, and family cultural and social contexts (Krefting & Krefting, 1991). National and regional cultural influences include commonly held beliefs or activity patterns. The collective American cultural value of equal opportunity in education and employment, for example, is reflected in the proclamations of the Individuals with Disabilities Education Act (IDEA) (P. L. 101-476) and the Americans with Disabilities Act (ADA) (P. L. 101-366). An individual's leisure interests, for example, may be influenced by the region within which he or she lives. Swimming at the beach, mountain climbing, or hiking in the desert are examples of these regional influences. At the community level, distinctive commonalities may exist between people, including socioeconomic status, dialect, clothing, and so on. Community and individual demographic variables also affect the type and variety of health service options available to individuals, access to care, and utilization of health care services (Cheh & Phillips, 1993; Newbold, Eyles, & Birch, 1995; Saywell, Zollinger, Schafer, Schmit, & Ladd, 1993). The cultural influences of the family context are evident in ethnicity, family structure, delineation of power and responsibility, decision-making behaviors, style and frequency of worship, and others. Each person experiences a variety of cultural influences throughout their lives, creating differences at the individual level. Diversity is evident across all levels of cultural influence (Krefting, 1991; Krefting & Krefting, 1991).

The sociocultural environment (a) influences attitudes, customs, habits, and values; (b) determines beliefs about health, illness, and treatment; and (c) shapes the development of task and role performance (Davidson, 1991; Krefting, 1991). The sociocultural influences that guide client behaviors and decisions need to be identified and understood, as well as the cultural background of the therapists.

During the clinical interaction at least three cultures are involved: the culture of the provider, the culture of the client, and the culture of the health system (Wells, 1994). If the cultural differences between a therapist and client are not considered, both individuals may find that occupational therapy services are less satisfying (Wells).

Impairments and disabilities become handicaps when individuals are not able to meet the personal or social standards of role performance (World Health Organization, 1980). Therefore, it is important for therapists to help manage the expectation of others in the community (Christiansen, 1991). "We have as much responsibility to be agents of social change and institutional transformation as we have to help persons to change" (Kielhofner, 1993, p. 251).

Assignment

1. Divide into groups of four to eight people. Complete Project A to recognize the diversity of social and cultural environmental context and become aware of your personal sociocultural identity and its potential effect on the therapeutic relationship. Complete Project B to begin to identify the sociocultural environmental variables that influence occupational performance in clients.

Project A

1. Obtain large poster board, colored paper, scissors, pencils, markers or crayons, and glue. Each group member should select a piece of colored paper; then enlarge, trace, and cut the Sociocultural Identity Figure pattern (Figure 1).
2. Complete the Diversity Questionnaire (Figure 2).

Figure 1. Socio-Cultural Identity Figure.

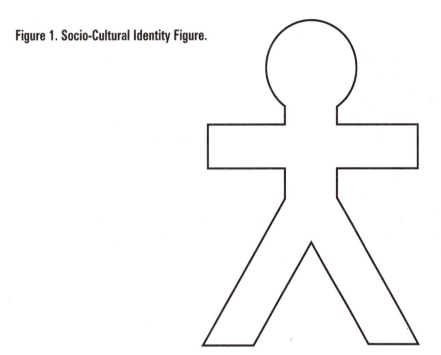

Figure 2. The Diversity Questionnaire.

Regional Influences

1. What values, interests, and beliefs do you share with people in your region of the world?

2. What behavior or lifestyle patterns do you share with people in your region that make you distinct from the global community (e.g., foods, gestures).

3. What values and attitudes do you share with other American occupational therapists? Review *Core Values and Attitudes of Occupational Therapy Practice* (AOTA, 1993).

Community Influences

4. In what community or neighborhood activities do you participate? Are you a silent member of a subculture?

5. In which organizations or social networks do you hold membership?

Family Influences

6. What values and beliefs do you hold in common with your family?

7. What family traditions do you value? Which of these traditions are unique?

8. What is your ethnic heritage? Do you have more than one heritage? How does this heritage influence your lifestyle, habits, values, and interests?

Individual Diversity

9. What roles, tasks, or activities do you value?

10. What personal experiences have influenced your life?

11. Who are the people that are important in your life?

12. Do you have individual values and beliefs that differ from those of your family or friends?

13. What type of lifestyle do you value?

14. Do you have a personal vision or life mission? What is it?

3. Use pencils, markers, and crayons to personalize your Sociocultural Identity Figure so that it represents your role in society and incorporates some of the themes or ideas generated from the Diversity Questionnaire. Include the regional, community, family, and individual cultural characteristics and the social relationships that influence your life and make you unique.

4. Group all of the figures together in a circle with their feet together and heads apart. Glue them onto the large poster board. You have created a community (Figure 3).

5. Discuss the symbols, illustrations, and themes portrayed on your figures with all of the community members (your classmates). Where two figures are holding hands, write down the similarities that only those two share. Within the circle created by the feet, write the cultural similarities shared by all group members. In the space above the heads of the figures describe the cultural differences that make each individual unique within the community.

6. After the poster is complete, reflect on this social group activity and discuss: How did you decide what to share with the group? Have you shared everything? If not, why? Are the things that you kept private more important to understanding you as an individual? Is this information relevant to establishing rapport and to understanding occupational therapy clients' needs and goals?

7. What characteristics do your community members have in common? What are the differences?

8. Is there more cohesiveness within the group after this experience than there was before? What is it about the social group process that changed the level of cohesiveness?

9. How can the knowledge you gained about the group process be used in a clinical context with clients or colleagues? What is the therapeutic value of this social group activity?

Project B

Read the occupational therapy client scenarios described in Table 1 and identify the sociocultural, political, economic, and institutional variables that influence their patterns of occupation.

Figure 3. Example of a Culturally Diverse Community.

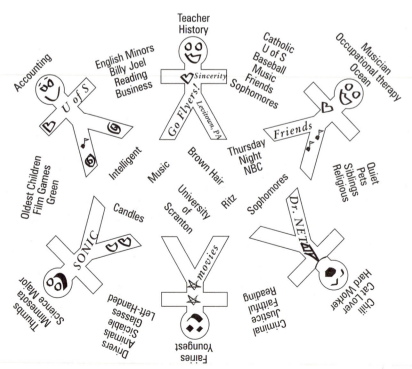

Table 1: Sociocultural Environmental Variables That Affect Occupational Performance

Client	Social Environment	Political Environment	Economic Environment	Institutional Environment
Albert is a 2-year-old boy who has been receiving early intervention services as mandated by the Individuals with Disabilities Education Act (IDEA). Occupational therapy services are currently provided in the home. Albert has a number of toys that his therapist uses during visits to teach his mother specific therapeutic activities and treatment principles. Albert's family lives in a rural area and has only one car. His father works in the city and frequently travels out of town. Funding for programs under IDEA is under debate in Congress and Albert's local community is reevaluating the cost-effectiveness of home-based treatment.				

Table 1: Sociocultural Environmental Variables That Affect Occupational Performance

Client	Social Environment	Political Environment	Economic Environment	Institutional Environment
Mary is a 72-year-old woman who has been living in a publically funded nursing home for 5 years. Mary would prefer to live with her husband of 52 years, but he is unable to manage her personal care needs. Mary has Alzheimer's disease and lives on a special unit with other individuals with dementias. Occupational therapy services are provided in group contexts.				

The information that follows will (a) provide students and instructors with resources to enhance the learning experience and (b) assist the student in completing the assignment.

Learning Resources

Books and Periodicals

Davis, C. M. (1994). Family history. In C. A. Davis (Ed.), *Patient practitioner interaction: An experiential manual for developing the art of health care* (2nd ed., pp. 17–36). Thorofare, NJ: Slack.

Krefting, L. (1991). The culture concept in the everyday practice of occupational and physical therapy. *Physical and Occupational Therapy in Pediatrics, 11,* 1–16.

Meier, K., & Stafford, J. (1995). *DiversiTRAIN: 25 diversity exercises to bridge cultural barriers.* Jacksonville Beach, FL: Talico.

Videos

Griggs Productions. *Valuing differences.* San Francisco: Author.

Wells, S. (1996). *Creating a multicultural approach and environment.* Bethesda, MD: American Occupational Therapy Association.

Study Questions

1. Identify and describe the three different environmental performance contexts.
2. Which environmental context considers the political, economic, and institutional climate of occupational performance and occupational therapy practice?
3. Identify the spheres of community influence on an individual's sociocultural identity.
4. Identify an activity that could be used in group therapy to familiarize members with the ethnic heritage of each individual.
5. Identify one ethnic heritage and identify the influence of the values and beliefs of this heritage on health, wellness, and independence.

References

American Occupational Therapy Association (AOTA). (1993). *Core values and attitudes of occupational therapy practice.* Bethesda, MD: Author.

AOTA. (1994). *Uniform terminology for occupational therapy* (3rd ed.). Bethesda, MD: Author.

Case-Smith, J. (1996). An overview of occupational therapy with children. In J. Case-Smith, A. S. Allen, & P. N. Pratt (Eds.), *Occupational therapy for children* (3rd ed.). St. Louis, MO: Mosby.

Cheh, V., & Phillips, B. (1993). Adequate access to posthospital home health services: Differences between urban and rural areas. *Journal of Rural Health, 9*(4), 262–269.

Davidson, H. (1991). Performance and the social environment. In C. Christiansen & C. Baum (Eds.), Occupational therapy: *Overcoming human performance deficits* (pp. 144–177). Thorofare, NJ: Slack.

Kielhofner, G. (1993). Functional assessment: Toward a dialectical view of person-environment relations. *American Journal of Occupational Therapy, 47,* 248–251.

Krefting, L. H. (1991). The culture concept in the everyday practice of occupational and physical therapy. *Physical and Occupational Therapy in Pediatrics, 11,* 1–16.

Krefting, L. H., & Krefting, D. V. (1991). Cultural influences on performance. In C. Christiansen & C. Baum (Eds.), *Occupational therapy: Overcoming human performance deficits* (pp. 102–140). Thorofare, NJ: Slack.

Newbold, K. B., Eyles, J., & Birch, S. (1995). Equity in health care: Methodological contributions to the analysis of hospital utilization in Canada. *Social Science and Medicine, 40(9),* 1181–1192.

Saywell, R. M., Zollinger, T. W., Schafer, M. E., Schmit, T. M., & Ladd, J. K. (1993). Children with special health care needs program: Urban/rural comparisons. *Journal of Rural Health, 9,* 314–325.

Tessler, E. (1994). Issues in minority affairs: OT represented at conference on freedom. *OT Week 8(49),* 8–9.

Wells, S. A. (1994). A multicultural education and resource guide for occupational therapy educators and practitioners. Bethesda, MD: *American Occupational Therapy Association.*

World Health Organization. (1994). *International classification of impairments, disabilities, and handicaps: A manual of classification relating to the consequences of disease.* Geneva: Author.

PURPOSEFUL MODIFICATIONS AND ADAPTATIONS

"An activity may be adapted by modifying or changing the equipment used, omitting or condensing steps in the sequence, altering the environment or altering the person's approach to the task" (Reed & Sanderson, 1980, p. 68).[1]

Chapter Objectives

1. Explain the reasons why occupational therapy practitioners modify and adapt activities.
2. Identify the variables that can be adapted to enable occupational performance.
3. Describe the roles of the therapist and client in therapeutic activity selection and design.
4. Grade and adapt a specific activity to increase or reduce the level of challenge to a specific performance component.

Purposeful Modifications and Adaptions

Occupational therapy practitioners use task analysis to (a) identify the variables within people, tasks, or environments that facilitate or hinder human performance and (b) determine strategies to recreate a match between people, occupations, and environments. "The purpose of practice is to alter the person's ability, the occupation, or the environment so that the person can achieve the necessary balance between ability and the environmental demands to enable occupational competence" (Polatajko, 1994, p. 592). Occupational therapists purposefully modify and adapt activities either to ensure independent performance or to develop or promote skill mastery.

Purposeful activities cannot be prescribed on the basis of analysis of their inherent characteristics alone; rather, by definition, prescription of purposeful activity is individual-specific. An occupational therapy practitioner grades or adapts a chosen activity for an individual to promote successful performance or elicit a particular response. Grading activities challenges the patient's

abilities by progressively changing the process, tools, materials, or environment of a given activity to gradually increase or decrease the performance demands. These incremental modifications are made in response to the individual's dynamic changes and provide opportunities for gradual development of skill and related therapeutic benefits. The grading of activities is accomplished by modifying the sequence, duration, or procedures of the task; the individual's position; the position of the tools and materials; the size, shape, weight, or texture of the materials; the nature and degree of interpersonal contact; the extent of physical handling by the occupational therapy practitioner during performance; or the environment in which the activity is attempted. Supportive or assistive devices or techniques may be used to enhance the effectiveness of an activity or to facilitate performance. Such techniques or devices are considered facilitative or preparatory to performance of purposeful activity and engagement in occupations (AOTA, 1993, p. 1081).

Tasks and activities are malleable and may be adapted by altering the task demands, environmental parameters, or the individual's approach or method. Modifying or adapting the equipment used and increasing, condensing, or omitting the steps in the sequence are strategies that alter task demands. Changing the physical and sociocultural context alters environmental demands, while teaching new methods alters the individual's approach to the task (Reed & Sanderson, 1980). Purposeful adaptations are performed either to reduce or increase the level of challenge or environmental demand to balance achievement with challenge, develop specific skills, or promote independence (see Table 1). "Therapists work with clients to structure activities so a balance between challenges and skills is achieved and activities progress in a spiraling fashion toward increased complexity" (Law, 1991, p. 175). The complex nature of occupational performance provides an infinite number of avenues for therapists to make purposeful adaptations to minimize disability by developing and remediating skills, or compensating for impairments.

For example, riding a tricycle can be modified or graded in the following ways:

1. **Adapting Task Demands:** The style of tricycle, height of seat, distance between the back tires, and the weight of the tricycle are features of the task equipment that influence the level of challenge to children who ride tricycles. If the level of challenge is too difficult for a weak child who would like to be independent in this task, an occupational therapy practitioner might recommend using a lightweight, plastic tricycle. If this same child is participating in treatment to enhance strength, the therapist might gradually increase the weight of the tricycle with beanbags to enhance strength while enabling independence in riding.

2. **Adapting Environmental Parameters:** The size and number of obstacles, terrain quality and slope, encouragement from parents, or competition with peers are physical and social environmental parameters that influence the level of challenge to individuals who ride tricycles. If the level of physical environmental challenge is too difficult for a child with visual and perceptual impairments, an occupational therapy practitioner might recommend that riding only be performed indoors on smooth, flat terrain with minimal obstacles. If this same individual is participating in treatment to enhance visual and perceptual skills, a therapist might design an obstacle course that gradually

increases in complexity and supervise or cue the child as he rides the tricycle around obstructions.

3. **Adapting Personal Approaches:** The method by which an individual mounts, rides, and dismounts a tricycle influences the level of challenge of riding a tricycle. If propelling a tricycle by the pedals is too difficult for the uncoordinated or apraxic child, an occupational therapy practitioner might recommend propulsion with the feet on the ground to promote independence. If this same individual is participating in treatment to enhance coordination and motor planning, the therapist may assist by placing the child's feet on the pedals and by giving a push start to add forward momentum. The therapist grades the amount of physical assistance provided as the child learns the new riding technique.

Occupational therapists structure activities to address or incorporate multiple, simultaneous, individualized goals and may use the same activity with different clients for very different reasons (Fleming, 1994). Therapists may also enlist a client's participation in the therapeutic process by providing meaningful activity choices during treatment. By inquiring into a client's prior interests and motivations, therapists identify and provide relevant and meaningful activity choices (Fleming). Ultimately, the client selects the therapeutic activity or occupation, and the therapist modifies or adapts the task or environment in ways that promote achievement of multiple, simultaneous, and individualized intervention goals. Engagement in activity is the means to achieving intervention goals. Task and activity analysis is used throughout the process to structure activities toward achievement of these individualized goals.

Assignment

1. Divide into groups of two.
2. Select and perform one child or adult activity from the suggestions listed below.
   Children: Walk across a balance beam. Paint a picture. Complete a paper craft project. Select and engage in a meaningful activity from your life.
   Adults: Design and use fabric paint to make a gift canvas smock. Make an origami figure. Cook a meal. Play basketball. Make a collage. Select and engage in an activity that has relevance and meaning in your own life.
3. Determine how the task, environment, or personal approach could be modified to alter the level of challenge to performance components. Document your ideas in Table 1.

Study Questions

1. What three variables can be changed to alter the level of challenge during engagement in an activity?
2. Why are occupational therapy practitioners skilled at purposeful adaptations and modifications?
3. Why was the word "purposeful" in this chapter title chosen to describe the task adaptations and modifications made by occupational therapy practitioners?
4. What role do clients play in the selection of therapeutic activities?
5. How could you modify or adapt a tricycle for a child with very poor postural control?

Table 1: Alterations to the Level of Challenge [1]

Sensory Awareness	Ride a Tricycle			
	Increase Challenge	Decrease Challenge	Increase Challenge	Decrease Challenge
Tactile	Ride barefoot. Texturize handles.	Ride with gloves, socks, and shoes on.		
Proprioceptive	↑ weight of tricycle with beanbags. Wear heavy clothes or weighted vest. Push someone else who is sitting on the tricycle. Ride up an incline.	↓ weight of tricycle.		
Vestibular	Ride down a ramp. Ride fast. Ride around a circular path.	Ride slowly.		
Visual	↑ # of obstacles. Low-contrast colors.	High-contrast colors. ↓ # of obstacles. Eliminate demonstration. Provide auditory cues for blind child to track.		

[1] If an adaptation dramatically changes the purpose of the task, indicate N/A: not applicable.

Key: ↑ = increase, ↓ = decrease, # = number

Table 1: Alterations to the Level of Challenge [1]

Ride a Tricycle

	Increase Challenge	Decrease Challenge	Increase Challenge	Decrease Challenge
Sensory Awareness				
Auditory	↑ amount of noise. Provide verbal instructions.	Quiet environment. Demonstrate task requirements.		
Gustatory	N/A	N/A		
Olfactory	N/A	N/A		
Sensory Processing				
Stereognosis	Do not watch feet while placing them on pedal.	Watch feet while placing them on pedal.		
Kinesthesia	Race another child. Ride up or down an incline.	Flat terrain. No obstacles.		
Pain Response	N/A	N/A		

[1]If an adaptation dramatically changes the purpose of the task, indicate N/A: not applicable.

Key: ↑ = increase, ↓ = decrease, # = number

Table 1: Alterations to the Level of Challenge [1]

	Ride a Tricycle			
	Increase Challenge	Decrease Challenge	Increase Challenge	Decrease Challenge
Body Scheme	↑ proprioceptive feedback as above.	↓ proprioceptive feedback as above.		
Right-Left Discrimination	Require child to turn right or left.	Uses signs with words right and left.		
Form Constancy	Vary types of obstacles.	Eliminate obstacles. Use same tricycle.		
Position in Space	↑ # and shapes of obstacles.	↓ # obstacles.		
Visual Closure	↑ # partially obscured from view.	↓ # obstacles.		
Figure-Ground	↑ # obstacles.	↓ # obstacles. Enhance color contrast between objects and the environment. Ensure that the seat and handlebars are a different color than the remainder of the tricycle.		

[1]If an adaptation dramatically changes the purpose of the task, indicate N/A: not applicable.

Key: ↑ = increase, ↓ = decrease, # = number

Table 1: Alterations to the Level of Challenge [1]

	Ride a Tricycle			
	Increase Challenge	Decrease Challenge	Increase Challenge	Decrease Challenge
Depth Perception	↑ #, size, and vary the distance between obstacles. Introduce moving obstacles (i.e., another child). Ride up or down an incline.	↓ # or eliminate obstacles.		
Spatial Relations	Change angle and rotation of obstacles.	Eliminate obstacles and changes in slope.		
Topographical Orientation	Ride to particular distant location.	Ride straight path and back.		
Neuromusculoskeletal				
Reflex	N/A	Difficult to eliminate.		
Range of Motion	Narrow handle bars. ↓ height of seat and distance to pedals.	Thick handle bars. ↑ height of seat and distance to pedals.		
Muscle Tone	↑ resistance to propulsion.	↓ resistance to propulsion.		

[1] If an adaptation dramatically changes the purpose of the task, indicate N/A: not applicable.

Key: ↑ = increase, ↓ = decrease, # = number

Table 1: Alterations to the Level of Challenge [1]

	Ride a Tricycle			
	Increase Challenge	Decrease Challenge	Increase Challenge	Decrease Challenge
Strength	*Ride up hill. Frequently stop and restart.*	*Ride down hill. Use standing position on pedals to initiate forward momentum. Therapist assists by pushing from behind.*		
Endurance	*↑ duration of ride. Maintain duration by increasing incline.*	*↓ duration of ride.*		
Postural Control	*Use tricycle with narrow wheel base. Get on with traditional one-leg method.*	*Provide postural support with seat back. Get on by squatting from the back of tricycle.*		
Postural Alignment	*N/A*	*N/A*		
Soft Tissue Integrity	*N/A*	*N/A*		

[1]If an adaptation dramatically changes the purpose of the task, indicate N/A: not applicable.

Key: ↑ = increase, ↓ = decrease, # = number

Table 1: Alterations to the Level of Challenge [1]

	Ride a Tricycle			
Motor	*Increase Challenge*	*Decrease Challenge*	*Increase Challenge*	*Decrease Challenge*
Gross Coordination	$\uparrow$ complexity of mount and dismount.	Use feet on the ground to propel.		
Crossing the Midline	N/A	N/A		
Laterality	Drive with one hand.	N/A		
Bilateral Integration	Frequent stop and restarts.	Use feet on the ground to propel. Drive with one hand. Give push start or use a pull string (i.e., tow) to assist momentum and demonstrate technique.		
Motor Control	Propel in reverse.	Give push start or use a pull string (i.e., tow) to assist momentum and demonstrate technique. Use foot straps to keep feet on pedals.		

[1] If an adaptation dramatically changes the purpose of the task, indicate N/A: not applicable.

Key: $\uparrow$ = increase, $\downarrow$ = decrease, # = number

119

Table 1: Alterations to the Level of Challenge [1]

Ride a Tricycle				
	Increase Challenge	**Decrease Challenge**	**Increase Challenge**	**Decrease Challenge**
Praxis	↑ # of obstacles. Auditory instructions or demonstration instructions only. Propel in reverse.	Combine auditory instructions and demonstration with physical guidance.		
Fine Coordination/ Dexterity	↑ size of handle bar.	↓ size of handle bar.		
Visual-Motor Integration	Ride tricycle along line path.	Ride in an open area without obstacles.		
Oral-Motor Control	N/A	N/A		
Cognitive Components				
Level of Arousal	↑ # of obstacles.	↓ # of obstacles.		
Orientation	Identify location and people.	N/A		
Recognition	Identify objects, people, and places.	N/A		

[1]If an adaptation dramatically changes the purpose of the task, indicate N/A: not applicable.

Key: ↑ = increase, ↓ = decrease, # = number

Table 1: Alterations to the Level of Challenge [1]

Ride a Tricycle

	Increase Challenge	Decrease Challenge	Increase Challenge	Decrease Challenge
Attention Span	↑ duration of ride. Vary presence, type, and frequency of distractions.	Minimize distractions.		
Initiation of Activity	Frequent stops and restarts.	Ride only.		
Termination of Activity	Frequent stops and restarts.	Ride only.		
Memory	"Ride around the room until you find the red beanbag and bring it back to me."	Ride only.		
Sequencing	"Ride around to find the red beanbag, bring it to me, and then find the blue beanbag and bring it to me."	Ride only.		
Categorization	"Ride around and collect all of the beanbags." "Now separate them into red and blue piles."	Ride only.		

[1] If an adaptation dramatically changes the purpose of the task, indicate N/A: not applicable.

Key: ↑ = increase, ↓ = decrease, # = number

Table 1: Alterations to the Level of Challenge [1]

Ride a Tricycle

	Increase Challenge	Decrease Challenge	Increase Challenge	Decrease Challenge
Concept Formation	Imaginative play. "Drive to the store to buy beanbags."	Ride only.		
Spatial Operations	$\uparrow$ #, type, and frequency of obstacles. Propel in reverse.	$\uparrow$ #, type, and frequency of obstacles. Ride straight line.		
Problem Solving	Create obstacle barriers. Introduce curbs.	Eliminate potential problems.		
Learning	Vary type of tricycles.	Preview or review new concepts.		
Generalization	Practice on different tricycles.	Use the same tricycle each trial.		
Psychosocial and Psychological				
Self-Concept	$\uparrow$ opportunity for success.	N/A		
Social Conduct	$\uparrow$ # of others. Perform with strangers. Cooperative or competitive game.	Perform alone. Parallel play.		

[1] If an adaptation dramatically changes the purpose of the task, indicate N/A: not applicable.

Key: $\uparrow$ = increase, $\downarrow$ = decrease, # = number

Table 1: Alterations to the Level of Challenge [1]

	Ride a Tricycle		Increase Challenge	Decrease Challenge
	Increase Challenge	Decrease Challenge		
Interpersonal skills	↑ requirements for conversations with others.	Perform alone.		
Self-Expression	Create imaginative game. Ride with costume.	Ride only.		
Coping Skills	Enhance challenge or reduce chance of success.	Reduce challenge and optimize opportunities for success.		
Time Management	Control time to destination.	N/A		
Self-Control	Create stressful situations.	Minimize stress and social interactions.		

[1] If an adaptation dramatically changes the purpose of the task, indicate N/A: not applicable.

Key: ↑ = increase, ↓ = decrease, # = number

References

American Occupational Therapy Association. (1993). Position Paper: Purposeful activity. *American Journal of Occupational Therapy, 47,* 1081–1082.

Fleming, M. H. (1994). Conditional reasoning. In C. Mattingly & M. H. Fleming (Eds.), *Clinical reasoning: Forms of inquiry in a therapeutic practice* (pp. 197–235). Philadelphia: F. A. Davis.

Law, M. (1991). 1991 Muriel Driver Lecture—The environment: A focus for occupational therapy. *Canadian Journal of Occupational Therapy, 58(4),* 171–179.

Polatajko, H. J. (1994). Dreams, dilemmas, and decisions for occupational therapy practice in a new millennium: A Canadian perspective. *American Journal of Occupational Therapy, 48,* 590–594.

Reed, K. L., & Sanderson, S. R. (1980). *Concepts of occupational therapy.* Baltimore: Williams & Wilkins.

USE OF THE OCCUPATIONAL PERFORMANCE ANALYSIS FORM

"Occupational therapy assessment involves examining performance areas, performance components, and performance contexts. Intervention may be directed toward elements of performance areas (e.g. dressing, vocational exploration), performance components (e.g. endurance, problem solving), or the environmental aspects of performance contexts" (American Occupational Therapy Association, 1994, p. 1047).[1]

Task analysis, within this text, refers to the process of analyzing the dynamic relationship between people and their occupations and environments. The **Occupational Performance Analysis Form** is a tool that will aid students' skill development in the task analysis process. This chapter provides two examples of completed forms. The first form has been completed for riding a tricycle, and the second form has been completed for morning personal care tasks. Blank copies of the form are available in Appendix A and C (American and Canadian versions). Notice that the form is divided into three parts titled occupation, person, and performance context. Part one, analysis of occupation, requires identifying and documenting the (a) applicable roles, occupational performance tasks, and specific activity; (b) steps required to perform; (c) materials, tools, and equipment; (d) safety precautions and contraindications; and (e) time required to complete. Part two, analysis of the specific client or any person engaging in the task or activity, requires identifying and documenting the (a) relevance and meaningfulness, (b) values and interests, and (c) performance components. Relevance, meaningfulness, values, and interests are separated from the psychological performance components and placed at the beginning of this section on the analysis form because they are significant in designing and using purposeful activity in therapy. Part three, analysis of performance context, requires information on temporal aspects and envi-

ronmental variables. The last page also provides the opportunity to identify and document (a) purposeful adaptations to the task, environment, or personal approach of a client; and (b) applicable assistive and adaptive equipment.

While the Occupational Performance Analysis Form provides a medium to structure task analysis, the dynamic nature of performance cannot be completely captured using this linear format. The interdependent relationship of performance components will become evident with experience using the form. For example, the relationship between sensation, perception, and motor performance is evident in both sample forms. Notice that riding a tricycle requires both visual motor integration and depth perception. These motor and perceptual skills, in turn, require vision. Documentation of a maximal level of challenge in visual motor integration and depth perception will necessitate a maximal level of challenge in vision. Notice that bathing and hygiene challenge body scheme and kinesthesia. These two perceptual skills, in turn, require proprioception.

The linear nature of the analysis form cannot completely capture the interactive and transactional relationships between people and their tasks and environments. This dynamic process will become particularly evident when applying the task analysis process to client case scenarios. Section One has provided information and learning exercises to

---

[1]From "Uniform Terminology for Occupational Therapy" (3rd ed.), by the American Occupational Therapy Association, 1994, *American Journal of Occupational Therapy, 48*, p. 1047. Copyright 1994 by the American Occupational Therapy Association. Reprinted with permission.

develop knowledge and skill in task analysis using the occupational performance approach. Section Two will provide an opportunity to apply task analysis to hypothetical pediatric occupational therapy clients. Sections Three, Four, and Five apply the process to adolescent and adult clientele.

Occupational Performance Analysis Form—Example

Occupation
Role: *Friend, Sister, Brother*
Task: *Leisure/play activities indoors/outdoors. Community and functional mobility around home, day care, and/or the community.*
Activity: *Ride a tricycle.* Steps Required to Perform: 1. *Get to the tricycle.* 2. *Get onto the tricycle.* 3. *Place feet onto pedals and propel.* 4. *Ride the tricycle and steer around various obstacles.* 5. *Get off the tricycle.*
Materials, tools, and Equipment (availability, cost, source . . .): *Tricycle ($20-$50). Can be purchased new or used.*
Safety Precautions and Contraindications: *The terrain may present hazardous conditions. Falling off a tricycle can be dangerous.*
Time to Complete: *A few minutes to 1 hour.*

The Person

Relevance and Meaningfulness: (historical or current personal and social relevance)

Children have likely used various toys throughout history to amuse themselves, learn, and develop. Tricycles can be purchased for children as gifts or given as "hand-me-downs" from siblings or friends. After riding tricycles children often graduate to bicycles with training wheels or two-wheeled bikes. On a personal level, riding a bicycle may hold meaning if this activity or its accomplishment is valued by oneself or others. The tricycle may hold significant meaning if it once belonged to a significant other (e.g., sibling), if it was a gift from a significant person (e.g., parent), or if it is a favorite color, model, etc.

Values and Interests:

Children may value or be interested in riding for personal gratification, imaginative play (e.g., pretend driving), social acceptance, or functional and community mobility purposes. Interest levels may vary between individuals.

For each performance component, determine the level of challenge required to perform. (Min = minimum, Mod = moderate, Max = maximum).	Level of Challenge			Comments (Indicate N/A if Not Applicable)
	Min	**Mod**	**Max**	
A. Sensorimotor Component 1. Sensory a. Sensory Awareness		X		*Requires awareness and integration of visual, vestibular, and proprioceptive information.*
b. Sensory Processing (1) Tactile	X			*Textured handles. Pressure from foot plates. Outdoor temperature.*
(2) Proprioceptive			X	*Awareness of arm and leg positions without looking.*
(3) Vestibular			X	*Linear movement of head through space, some angular if turn a corner.*
(4) Visual			X	*Negotiate movement through cluttered environment.*
(5) Auditory	X			*If playing with friends.*
(6) Gustatory				*N/A*
(7) Olfactory				*Outdoor smells?*

For each performance components, determine the level of challenge required to perform. (Min = minimum, Mod = moderate, Max = maximum).	Level of Challenge			Comments (Indicate N/A if Not Applicable)
	Min	Mod	Max	
c. Perceptual Skills (1) Stereognosis	X			Recognize pedal with feet without looking.
(2) Kinesthesia			X	Force required in arms and legs to propel and turn tricycle and negotiate objects.
(3) Pain Response	X			For safety.
(4) Body Scheme		X	X	Awareness of arm, leg, and trunk position and movement at all times.
(5) Right-Left Discrimination	X			Requires directional sense, but not right and left discrimination.
(6) Form Constancy		X		Identify objects despite their changing retinal image while moving on tricycle.
(7) Position in Space			X	Determine relative position of all objects in relation to one another and self as move between, behind, beside.
(8) Visual Closure	X			Identify objects that are partially blocked from view.
(9) Figure-Ground		X		Identify obstacles from a cluttered background to avoid them (e.g., see a crayon on a carpeted floor).
(10) Depth Perception			X	Determine changing distances between self and objects to avoid collision.
(11) Spatial Relations		X		Determine angle that an object is oriented or placed (e.g., angle of curb ahead or rotated position of a table.)
(12) Topographical Orientation		X		Determine route to destination (e.g., home).
2. Neuromuscular a. Reflex	X	X		Requires integration of positive supporting reflex. Grasp reflex may be elicited or assist engagement.

For each performance components, determine the level of challenge required to perform. (Min = minimum, Mod = moderate, Max = maximum).	Level of Challenge			Comments (Indicate N/A if Not Applicable)
	Min	Mod	Max	
b. Range of Motion		X	X	End range of flexion in hands. Midrange flexion in shoulders, hips, and knees.
c. Muscle Tone		X		Isometric distal hand contractions, with isotonic shoulder, elbow, and knee contractions. Hip cocontraction to propel.
d. Strength		X		Requires resistive strength in arms and legs. Legs greater than arms.
e. Endurance	X	X		Dependent on distance, weight of tricycle, and surface quality.
f. Postural Control		X		Postural stability to maintain sit on tricycle seat.
g. Postural Alignment	X			Trunk in midline.
h. Soft Tissue Integrity				N/A
3. Motor				
a. Gross Coordination		X		Gross coordination of arms and legs to get on, off, and ride.
b. Crossing the Midline				N/A Not required.
c. Laterality				N/A Dominance not required.
d. Bilateral Integration			X	Extensive information integration between arms to drive and legs to propel.
e. Motor control	X	X		Uses reciprocal leg movements similar to walking.
f. Praxis		X	X	Postural praxis to get on and off for the first time and negotiate environment.
g. Fine Coordination/Dexterity	X			Cylindrical grasp.
h. Visual-Motor Integration			X	Scan, track, and negotiate the environment during movement.
i. Oral-Motor Control				N/A

For each performance components, determine the level of challenge required to perform. (Min = minimum, Mod = moderate, Max = maximum).	Level of Challenge			Comments (Indicate N/A if Not Applicable)
	Min	**Mod**	**Max**	
B. Cognitive Integration and Cognitive Components				
1. Level of Arousal			X	*Required to respond to changing environmental obstacles.*
2. Orientation	X			*Orientation to situation only.*
3. Recognition	X	X		*Identify tricycle, objects, and obstacles.*
4. Attention Span		X		*Sustain for ride. Divided attention between ride and environmental stimuli.*
5. Initiation of Activity	X			*Initiate ride.*
6. Termination of Activity	X			*Terminate ride after appropriate time.*
7. Memory		X		*Long-term recall of how to get on and use, where to travel, and consequences of different routes (e.g., fall off curb).*
8. Sequencing	X	X		*Get on and use. Plan route to specific destination.*
9. Categorization				*N/A*
10. Concept Formation				*N/A*
11. Spatial Operations			X	*How to get on and off. How to maneuver tricycle around barriers, particularly moving obstacles.*
12. Problem Solving		X		*What course of action to take if get stuck or cannot fit through a clearing.*
13. Learning	X	X		*New learning dependent on previous experience on tricycle.*
14. Generalization		X		*Could generalize skill to riding bicycle with or without training wheels.*
C. Psychosocial Skills and Psychological Components				
1. Psychological a. Self-Concept		X	X	*Accomplishment or participation influences self-concept if client is very interested or values this activity.*

For each performance components, determine the level of challenge required to perform. (Min = minimum, Mod = moderate, Max = maximum).	Level of Challenge			Comments (Indicate N/A if Not Applicable)
	Min	Mod	Max	
2. Social				
a. Social Conduct		X	X	*Dependent on social context. Need to respect others' space or tricycle.*
b. Interpersonal Skills	X	X		*Dependent on social context.*
c. Self-Expression		X		*Riding provides the opportunity for creative expression and imaginative play (e.g., build obstacle course or pretend to drive).*
3. Self-Management				
a. Coping Skills		X	X	*Depending on ability to ride, complexity of physical and social environmental demands when riding.*
b. Time Management				*N/A*
c. Self-Control		X		*Depending on complexity of physical and social environmental demands when riding.*

Performance Context	
	Comments
A. Temporal Aspects	
1. Chronological	*Typically used between ages 2 1/2 and 5.*
2. Developmental	*Autonomy vs. shame and doubt (Erkson). Infancy and early childhood (Havighurst). Transition from sensorimotor to preoperational (Piaget).*
3. Life Cycle	*Play and early learning process.*
4. Disability Status	*N/A*
B. Environmental	
1. Physical	*Size, number, visibility, movement, and distance between obstacles. Competency with this activity increase mobility sphere.*
2. Social	*Number of friends/siblings around and what they are doing. Parallel play or competition.*
3. Cultural	*Popular activity in American and Canadian cultures. Tricycles are used by both sexes.*

Adaptations, Grading, and Structuring:

Activity or Task	Environment	Personal Approach
1. *Style of tricycle*	1. *Size and number of obstacles*	1. *Duration of the activity*
2. *Height of seat*	2. *Surface terrain*	2. *Method: mount/dismount*
3. *Distance between back tires*	3. *Surface slope*	3. *Propel via feet on ground*
4. *Size of tricycle*	4. *Friends or peers present*	4. *Distance expected*
5. *Weight of tricycle*	5. *Parent encouragement*	5. *Standing on back and propelling with one leg*

Assistive and Adaptive Equipment:

1. *Large/small, narrow/thick handlebars*

2. *Handlebar and/or foot pedal straps*

3. *Foot pedal blocks*

4. *Back and/or lateral support (with/without strap) on seat*

5. *Use of hand-propelled toddler vehicle instead*

Occupational Performance Analysis Form–Example
Rachel Budney, Occupational Therapy Student, Class of 1998

Occupation
Role: *Base requirement for all roles, i.e., family member, worker, friend.*
Task: *Activities of daily living, i.e., grooming, oral hygiene, bathing and showering, toilet hygiene, medication routine, and functional mobility.*

Activity: *Morning daily routine in bathroom, excluding dressing.*

Steps Required to Perform:

1. *Ambulate from the bathroom entrance, undress lower extremity garments, and transfer onto toilet.*

2. *Complete toilet hygiene activities and transfer off the toilet.*

3. *Remove clothes (robe) and transfer into tub for a bath.*

4. *Wash self and hair in the tub.*

5. *Transfer out of the tub, dry self, and put on robe.*

6. *Brush teeth.*

7. *Comb or brush hair.*

8. *Take medication, if applicable.*

Materials, tools, and Equipment (availability, cost, source . . .):

Clothes, toilet paper, shampoo soap, toothpaste, toothbrush, comb, towels, and medication. Most can be purchased at the nearest grocery store or drugstore. Medication will be obtained from a pharmacy.

Safety Precautions and Contraindications:

The temperature of the water must be recognized with regard to burns. Balance must be sufficient for bathing and completing toilet hygiene independently. Shampoo and soap can irritate eyes. The tub and floor may be slippery upon completion of bathing. The correct dosage of medication must be taken to avoid adverse reactions.

Time to Complete: *45 minutes to 1 hour.*

The Person

Relevance and Meaningfulness: (historical or current personal and social relevance)

Our society believes in independence in completing personal care activities and in attaining an acceptable physical presentation of the self. Upon successful completion of and satisfaction with appearance, one acquires a heightened self-esteem and pride. On a personal level this activity may hold significant meaning if it is conducted in one's own bathroom. A person may have personal preferences that he or she values about how a particular hygiene routine is conducted (e.g., hair style). The items used may also hold meaning if they are gifts from others (e.g., bath potions) or if they are preferred products (i.e., brand preferences).

Values and Interests:

People of all ages frequently value their outward physical presentation. One may value or be interested in bathing and grooming activities for personal gratification or for social acceptance among peers.

For each performance component, determine the level of challenge required to perform. (Min = minimum, Mod = moderate, Max = maximum).	Level of Challenge			Comments (Indicate N/A if Not Applicable)
	Min	**Mod**	**Max**	
A. Sensorimotor Component				
1. Sensory				
a. Sensory Awareness		X		*Requires awareness and integration of tactile, proprioceptive, and vestibular information.*
b. Sensory Processing				
(1) Tactile			X	*Cold, smooth, hard toilet seat. Texture of toilet paper. Temperature and texture of water. Texture of towel.*
(2) Proprioceptive			X	*Stepping into tub. Transferring from a sitting to standing position. Balancing and walking.*
(3) Vestibular		X		*Bending to remove clothes. Balancing in transferring from a sitting to standing position. Moving head while bathing and washing hair (linear and angular).*

For each performance components, determine the level of challenge required to perform. (Min = minimum, Mod = moderate, Max = maximum).	Level of Challenge			Comments (Indicate N/A if Not Applicable)
	Min	Mod	Max	
(4) Visual		X		Reading symbols and noticing colors on temperature controls in tub. Reaching for objects. Looking in mirror while brushing teeth and hair.
(5) Auditory	X			Toilet flushing. Tub filling with water. Running water in sink.
(6) Gustatory	X			Flavor of toothpaste.
(7) Olfactory	X			Scent of shampoo, soap, toothpaste.
c. Perceptual Skills				
(1) Stereognosis		X		Cleaning self after toileting. Rising shampoo from hair. Combing the back of hair.
(2) Kinesthesia			X	Pulling the proper amount of toilet paper. Turning the knobs at sink and in tub for water adjustment. Squeezing bottle of shampoo and tube of toothpaste.
(3) Pain Response	X			For safety with regard to water temperature and getting soap in eyes.
(4) Body Scheme			X	Stepping in and out of tub. Washing self in tub. Dressing without looking.
(5) Right-Left Discrimination	X			Dressing. May become confusing when looking in mirror.
(6) Form Constancy				Recognize hygiene and medicinal items in cupboard.
(7) Position in Space	X			Recognize location of different bottles and supplies in tub, on sink's counter, and in medicine cabinet.
(8) Visual Closure	X			Recognize medicine or shampoo from incomplete presentations.
(9) Figure-Ground	X			White soap in white soap dish. Determining the amount of water filling the tub.

For each performance components, determine the level of challenge required to perform. (Min = minimum, Mod = moderate, Max = maximum).	Level of Challenge			Comments (Indicate N/A if Not Applicable)
	Min	Mod	Max	
(10) Depth Perception		X		Height of step to get into tub. Amount of water filling the tub. Pouring water to use when taking medication. Spitting toothpaste into sink.
(11) Spatial Relations	X			Determine direction that the arrows on the water faucet are pointing.
(12) Topographical Orientation	X			Finding the way around the bathroom and locating proper items.
2. Neuromuscular				
a. Reflex			X	Integration of primitive reflexes is essential for balance and equilibrium reactions in this activity. Grasp reflex may help hold items.
b. Range of Motion			X	End range arms and hands. Midrange hips and knees.
c. Muscle Tone		X		Isometric and isotonic contractions vary around joints throughout this activity.
d. Strength			X	Flushing toilet. Turning on water in tub and at sink. Squeezing toothpaste tube and shampoo bottle. Opening medicine containers. Holding arms up while washing hair. Controlled ascent and descent at the toilet and tub.
e. Endurance		X		Sitting and balancing throughout bathing.
f. Postural Control			X	Balance while transferring from sitting to standing and while removing clothes. Control in ascents and descents. Drying self.
g. Postural Alignment			X	Trunk in midline for most of activity.
h. Soft Tissue Integrity	X			No open wounds–skin closure required.
3. Motor				
a. Gross Coordination		X		Ambulation and transfers. Adjustment of body position while dressing
b. Crossing the Midline		X		Brushing teeth. Drying self. Combing hair.

For each performance components, determine the level of challenge required to perform. (Min = minimum, Mod = moderate, Max = maximum).	Level of Challenge			Comments (Indicate N/A if Not Applicable)
	Min	**Mod**	**Max**	
c. Laterality			X	*Getting toilet paper. Flushing toilet. Cleaning self at toilet. Turning knobs in tub and at sink. Closing drain in tub. Brushing teeth. Combing hair.*
d. Bilateral Integration			X	*Undressing lower extremities. Washing body and hair. Drying self. Putting toothpaste on toothbrush. Opening medicine bottles.*
e. Motor Control		X		*Completing motions of entire activity with ease, especially transfers and applying toothpaste.*
f. Praxis		X		*Postural praxis to align body over the toilet and to enter or exit tub. Ideational praxis to recognize and determine purpose of everyday utensils.*
g. Fine Coordination/Dexterity			X	*Grasping and tearing toilet paper. Flushing toilet. Grasping medication tablets. Turning on water. Closing drain. Brushing teeth and combing hair.*
h. Visual-Motor Integration			X	*Aligning body with toilet. Putting toothpaste on toothbrush. Spitting into sink.*
i. Oral-Motor Control		X		*Brushing teeth and spitting into sink. Taking medication.*
B. Cognitive Integration and Cognitive Components				
1. Level of Arousal	X			*Required to respond to safety factors and to take medication competently.*
2. Orientation		X		*Time to take medication. Where things are located in the bathroom and the arrangement of the bathroom environment (orient to place).*
3. Recognition		X		*Distinguishing between hot and cold. Knowing when body is dry. Recognizing utensils, objects, and medication.*
4. Attention Span	X			*Sustain for bathing process.*
5. Initiation of Activity	X			*Sense the need to groom self or to use the toilet.*

For each performance components, determine the level of challenge required to perform. (Min = minimum, Mod = moderate, Max = maximum).	Level of Challenge			Comments (Indicate N/A if Not Applicable)
	Min	Mod	Max	
6. Termination of Activity	X			*Terminate toileting and bathing in appropriate amount of time.*
7. Memory			X	*Long-term recall of which way to turn the knobs on tub and sink. Taking medication. Short term of remembering to close the drain in tub to prevent leaking of water.*
8. Sequencing			X	*Entire activity: toileting, cleaning self, undressing, filling tub with water. Putting toothpaste on brush before brushing.*
9. Categorization				*N/A*
10. Concept Formation	X			*Image of how one wants to look after bathing and dressing.*
11. Spatial Operations		X		*Line self up with toilet. Align body to get into tub. Turning dial on tub or top of toothpaste.*
12. Problem Solving		X		*Water is too hot or cold. Forget to close the drain. Forget to take medication.*
13. Learning	X			*One can learn in each step; depends on client.*
14. Generalization		X		*Previous bathing.*
C. Psychosocial Skills and Psychological Components 1. Psychological a. Self-Concept			X	*Attaining independence may affect one's value of the physical self.*
2. Social a. Social Conduct				*N/A*
b. Interpersonal Skills				*N/A*
c. Self-Expression	X			*Preferred clothing style. Hair style. Express the need for assistance.*

For each performance components, determine the level of challenge required to perform. (Min = minimum, Mod = moderate, Max = maximum).	Level of Challenge			Comments (Indicate N/A if Not Applicable)
	Min	Mod	Max	
3. Self-Management				
a. Coping Skills		X		*Solving any problems.*
b. Time Management		X		*Finishing entire activity to fit in the schedule of one's day.*
c. Self-Control				*N/A*

Performance Context	
	Comments
A. **Temporal Aspects** 1. Chronological	*Toilet training often begins around 1 1/2 years of age, and the self-care process continues to be elaborated upon throughout the life span.*
2. Developmental	*Anal stage (Freud). Autonomy vs. shame and doubt (Erikson).*
3. Life Cycle	*Acquiring independent self-care skills.*
4. Disability Status	*N/A*
B. **Environmental** 1. Physical	*Bathroom. Type of bathtub, toilet, towel rack, and sink influences performance.*
2. Social	*Availability of social support systems may affect whether a person must achieve independence in this area, or whether he or she can seek assistance.*
3. Cultural	*Different levels of independence may be expected from different cultures in regard to self-care activities. Additionally, there may be different styles for performing these activities.*

Adaptations, Grading, and Structuring:

Activity or Task

1. *Two-in-one shampoo*

2. *Large labels for hot and cold*

3. *Prepoured shampoo*

4. *Soap hung on a rope*

Environment

1. *Bedside routine*

2. *Contrasting colors for towel, wall, and soap*

3. *Walk-in shower*

4. *Personal care assistant*

Personal Approach

1. *Choice of shower or bath*

2. *Sit while brushing hair or teeth*

3. *Sponge bath*

Assistive and Adaptive Equipment:

1. *Buzzer to remind client to take medicine*

2. *Hand-held shower*

3. *Bars for balance around toilet and tub*

4. *Raised toilet seat*

5. *Toilet tissue holder*

6. *Velcro® strap to hold brush to hand*

7. *Shower seat*

8 *Pill box to allocate medication for each day*

9. *Long-handled comb*

10. *Toothpaste squeezer*

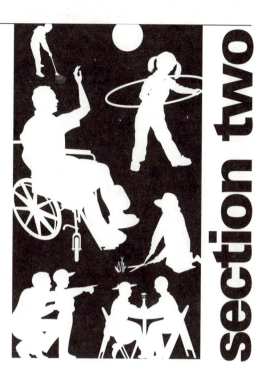

section two

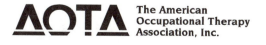

AOTA The American
Occupational Therapy
Association, Inc.

SECTION TWO: CHILDREN

"Childhood is hopeful and joyful and ever new. The spirit, the playfulness, and the joy of childhood creates the context for occupational therapy with children" (Case-Smith, 1996, p. 3).[1]

The role of pediatric practitioners is to enhance social role functioning and adaptation by facilitating occupational engagement in activities of daily living, productive and educational activities, and play and leisure pursuits. Occupational therapists evaluate children with disabilities to identify underlying performance components and contexts that support or constrain functional performance (Case-Smith, 1996). Intervention addresses performance components and contexts that limit or restrict current or expected future occupational performance. The American Occupational Therapy Association (1996) reported that 34% of registered occupational therapists and 20% of certified occupational therapy assistants worked primarily in pediatrics in 1995.

Section Two provides occupational therapy students with the opportunity to refine task analysis skills by applying this assessment and intervention tool to the occupational performance problems demonstrated by particular children. The meaning and purpose of pediatric play is reviewed in the chapter "Purposeful Play," while an overview of the therapeutic value of many different childhood activities is provided in the chapter "Children's Cultural Crafts and Games." Completing the Occupational Performance Analysis Form after engaging in a children's craft or game will require the student to integrate and apply knowledge acquired in Section One of this text. The hypothetical occupational therapy client cases titled **Bob, Tina, Sidney,** and **Miguel** provide realistic contexts for the use of task analysis as an assessment and intervention tool. These case vignettes demonstrate application of the Occupational Performance Practice Model for Service to Individuals, which was introduced in the chapter "Task Analysis: The Contribution of Occupational Therapy to Health."

Bob has difficulty engaging in educational, play, and leisure pursuits, and his parents are concerned about his confidence, self-esteem, lack of knowledge of academic concepts, and difficulty engaging in playground activities. Task analysis is used to identify performance components that affect specific play and leisure skills and to design a purposeful activity to challenge Bob's sensorimotor and cognitive skills, boost his confidence, and increase his self-esteem. Probe questions are provided to guide development of skills needed for task analysis. An obstacle course that was designed during a previous treatment session is used to demonstrate the therapeutic potential of play.

Tina has difficulty performing certain educational activities and learning some specific preacademic concepts. The kindergarten case manager is concerned about Tina's attention span and lack of interest in tabletop and quiet time activities. Task analysis is used to identify the performance components that limit Tina's success in specific educational activities, to design a purposeful activity to challenge her sensorimotor and cognitive skills, and to teach others how to structure therapeutic activities for use with this child. Completion of long-term and short-term goals that address performance components and contexts will be required. Probe questions are provided to guide task analysis skill development. Suggestions for therapeutic activity are included to facilitate the design of a purposeful activity.

[1]From "An Overview of Occupational Therapy with Children" (p. 3) by J. Case-Smith in *Occupational Therapy for Children* (3rd ed.) edited by J. Case-Smith, A. Allen, and P. Pratt, (1996), St. Louis, MO: Mosby. Copyright 1996 by Mosby. Reprinted with permission.

Sidney also has difficulty in engaging in educational tasks. Her parents would like a therapist to (a) use adaptive equipment to promote Sidney's engagement in meaningful and purposeful classroom activities and to enhance her peer interaction; and (b) adapt the performance context by educating others. This chapter includes information on the application of simple assistive technology and devices to promote engagement in educational activities. Task analysis is used to grade and adapt classroom activities.

Miguel has difficulty with a number of self-care, educational, play, and leisure activities that his parents and teachers would like addressed. Completion of the case will require greater independence in applying task analysis during assessment and intervention. Probe questions are provided to guide the process of client assessment and intervention.

The exercises throughout Section Two require the use of task analysis as an assessment and intervention tool to address pediatric activities of daily living, educational, play, and leisure performance areas. Task analysis is used to identify the performance components (sensorimotor, cognitive, psychosocial, and psychological) and performance contexts (social, cultural, and physical) that limit, restrict, or promote engagement. These pediatric client cases require occupational therapy students to develop and use task and activity analysis skills to (a) understand occupational performance profiles, (b) design and use purposeful activities to improve children's performance component skills and abilities, (c) structure practice opportunities for children to learn new methods, (d) teach others how to structure tasks for use with children with disabilities, and (e) alter environments and use adaptive equipment to facilitate role performance, boost confidence, and enhance self-esteem in children with disabilities. Completion of the client case assignments will require students to incorporate the remedial, functional, and preventative approaches to intervention.

References

American Occupational Therapy Association. (1996). OT practitioners work more with elderly patients. *OT Practice, 1*(3), 17.

Case-Smith, J. (1996). An overview of occupational therapy with children. In J. Case-Smith, A. Allen, & P. Pratt (Eds.), *Occupational therapy for children* (3rd ed., pp. 3–17). St. Louis, MO: Mosby.

PURPOSEFUL PLAY

"The purpose is the goal, the expected end result. The meaning is the value that accomplishment of the goal has for the person" (Trombly, 1995, p. 968).[1]

Chapter Objectives

1. Describe the characteristics of play.
2. Describe the features, characteristics, and utility of purposeful activity.
3. Compare the constructs of play and purposeful activity to determine why occupational therapy practitioners use play during evaluation and intervention.
4. Explain how play can be used as an assessment and treatment modality.
5. Engage in a group discussion about the use of play in practice.
6. Appraise the value of purposeful activities versus rote exercise.

Purposeful Activity and Play

Play is the primary occupation of children (Canadian Association of Occupational Therapists, 1996) and is a precursor to the productive work habits and roles of adulthood (Reilly, 1974). It is internally controlled and intrinsically motivating, focuses attention but suspends reality, simulates behavior, requires active participation, and allows freedom from externally imposed rules (Bundy, 1993; Rubin, Fein, & Vandenberg, 1983). It comprises both action and attitude and leads to the pleasure of doing (Ferland, 1992). Play promotes acquisition of skills and teaches symbolic learning and meaning (Reilly, 1974).

Occupational therapy practitioners use play as a therapeutic activity to assess function, promote skill development, and facilitate adaptation. Play activities may be used as a treatment modality to promote sensorimotor, cognitive, psychological, and psychosocial development. Physical and social environmental influences that support or hinder play are also of concern to the occupational therapist (Missiuna & Pollock, 1991).

When pediatric clients need to develop particular skills and abilities, therapists may select and design purposeful activities for use in intervention. Purposeful activities are therapeutic when they (a) are relevant, meaningful, and goal-directed; (b) elicit coordination among sensorimotor, cognitive, psychological, and psychosocial systems; and (c) promote mastery and feelings of self-competence (American Occupational Therapy Association, 1993; Fidler & Fidler, 1978; Trombly, 1995). Occupations that have "added purpose" are motivating and may be more effective for developing new motor skills than rote exercise alone (Van der Weel, Van der Meer, & Lee, 1991; Wu, Trombly, & Lin, 1994). Play is one occupation that is meaningful and has more added purpose for children than exercise does.

Assignment

1. Read the article *Position Paper: Purposeful Activity* (AOTA, 1993) (Appendix K).
2. What are the features or characteristics of a purposeful activity?
3. How are purposeful activities used by occupational therapy practitioners?
4. Separate into groups. Each member of the group should select, obtain, and review one of the articles in the Learning Resources section. Share with all group members what the journal article describes about the use of play as a therapeutic activity for children with disabilities.
5. Is play a purposeful activity? What is the potential therapeutic value of play?

---

[1]From "Occupation: Purposefulness and Meaningfulness As Therapeutic Mechanisms," by C. A. Trombly, 1995, *American Journal of Occupational Therapy, 49,* p. 968. Copyright 1995 by the American Occupational Therapy Association. Reprinted with permission.

6. Identify a rote exercise that could be used to improve muscle strength. Identify a purposeful activity that would increase muscle strength. Compare the two activities to determine how they are similar and different.

The information that follows will (a) provide students and instructors with resources to enhance the learning experience and (b) assist the student in completing the assignment.

Learning Resources

American Occupational Therapy Association. (1993). *Position paper: Purposeful activity.* Bethesda, MD: Author.

Bracegirdle, H. (1993). The use of play in occupational therapy for children: What is play? *British Journal of Occupational Therapy, 55,* 107–108.

Bundy, A. (1993). Assessment of play and leisure: Delineation of the problem. *American Journal of Occupational Therapy, 47,* 217–222.

Canadian Association of Occupational Therapists. (1996). Occupational therapy and children's play. *Canadian Journal of Occupational Therapy, 63*(2), Insert 1–9.

Fewell, R., & Glick, M. P. (1993). Observing play: An appropriate process for learning and assessment. *Infants and Young Children, 5,* 35–43.

Gunn, S. I. (1975). Play as occupation: Implications for the handicapped. *American Journal of Occupational Therapy, 29,* 222–225.

Missiuna, C., & Pollock, N. (1991). Play deprivation in children with physical disabilities: The role of the occupational therapist in preventing secondary disability. *American Journal of Occupational Therapy, 45,* 882–888.

Parham, D., & Fazio, L. (1997). *Play in occupational therapy for children.* St. Louis, MO: Mosby.

Schaaf, R. C. (1990). Play behavior and occupational therapy. *American Journal of Occupational Therapy, 44,* 68–75.

Vandenberg, B., & Kielhofner, G. (1982). Play in evolution, culture, and individual adaptation: Implications for therapy. *American Journal of Occupational Therapy, 36,* 20–28.

Study Questions

1. Identify five characteristics of play.
2. Identify five characteristics of a purposeful activity.
3. Is riding a tricycle a purposeful activity? Why or why not?
4. Identify a play activity that could be used to assess static balance.
5. Identify a play activity that could be used to treat an impairment in static balance.

References

American Occupational Therapy Association. (1993). *Position paper: Purposeful activity*. Bethesda, MD: Author.

Bundy, A. C. (1993). Assessment of play and leisure: Delineation of the problem. *American Journal of Occupational Therapy, 47*, 217–222.

Canadian Association of Occupational Therapists. (1996). Occupational therapy and children's play. *Canadian Journal of Occupational Therapy, 63*(2), Insert 1–9.

Ferland, F. (1992). Le jeu en ergothérapie: Reflexion préable à l'élaboration d'un noveau modèle de pratique. *Canadian Journal of Occupational Therapy, 59*, 95–101.

Fidler, G., & Fidler, J. (1978). Doing and becoming: Purposeful action and self-actualization. *American Journal of Occupational Therapy, 32*, 305–310.

Missiuna, C., & Pollock, N. (1991). Play deprivation in children with physical disabilities: The role of the occupational therapist in preventing secondary disability. *American Journal of Occupational Therapy, 45*, 882–888.

Reilly, M. (1974). *Play as exploratory learning: Studies in curiosity behavior*. Beverly Hills, CA: Sage.

Rubin, K., Fein, G. G., & Vandenberg, B. (1983). Play. In P. H. Mussen (Ed.), *Handbook of child psychology (4th ed.): Volume 4: Socialization, personality and social development* (pp. 693–774). New York: Wiley.

Trombly, C. A. (1995). Occupation: Purposefulness and meaningfulness as therapeutic mechanisms. *American Journal of Occupational Therapy, 49*, 960–972.

Van der Weel, F. R., Van der Meer, A. L., & Lee, D. N. (1991). Effect of task on movement control in cerebral palsy: Implications for assessment and therapy. *Developmental Medicine and Child Neurology, 33*, 419–426.

Wu, C-Y., Trombly, C. A., & Lin, K-C. (1994). The relationship between occupational form and occupational performance: A kinematic perspective. *American Journal of Occupational Therapy, 48*, 679–687.

CHILDREN'S CULTURAL CRAFTS AND GAMES

"Purposeful activities cannot be prescribed on the basis of analysis of their inherent characteristics alone; rather, by definition, prescription of purposeful activity is individual-specific" (AOTA), 1993, p. 1081).[1]

Chapter Objectives

1. Develop and refine skills in task and activity analysis by engaging in an activity, craft, or game and completing the Occupational Performance Analysis Form (Appendix A or C).
2. Identify many different activities, crafts, and games that may be of interest to children of different ethnic backgrounds.

Assignment

1. Select and perform one activity, craft, or game that may be of interest to children. Use the suggestions listed below if desired. The craft materials are commercially available through suppliers listed in Appendix M.
   Although the activities listed below are grouped by ethnicity, the prescriptive or therapeutic use of purposeful activity is individual-specific (AOTA, 1993). Children may enjoy participating in activities that have been popularized by their own ethnic culture or may not be familiar with or enjoy activities attributed to their ethnic heritage. They may also be interested in engaging in activities of other ethnic groups. The meaning and value attributed to different activities is individual-specific.
2. Complete the Occupational Performance Analysis Form on the selected activity, craft, or game.
3. Does this activity, craft, or game have potential therapeutic value for use with occupational therapy clients? Although the prescription or use of purposeful activity is individual-specific, what performance component deficits might be challenged or improved through engagement in this craft or game?

American Crafts and Games
Select any popular American craft or game.

African Crafts and Games
Sponge Art: Although the first wood block prints are credited to the Japanese, the Asante people of Ghana are also known for their Adinkra cloth stamped patterns (Gomez, 1992; Terzian, 1993). Today many children enjoy using sponge and rubber stamps to make patterns or pictures on both fabric (e.g., shirts, canvas totes) and paper (e.g., cards, wrapping paper).

Kente Cloth: The Asante people of Ghana weave rayon or silk threads into 3- to 6- inch strips. The strips are stitched together to form a Kente cloth (Terzian, 1993). After becoming familiar with the heritage and history of fabric, children may enjoy weaving tapestry or place mats by folding a piece of paper in half and making cut lines to create the warp. Use colored paper strips to weave the weft (see Figure 1). When weaving on a loom the warp threads extend lengthwise and the weft is woven crosswise.

Figure 1. Kente Cloth.

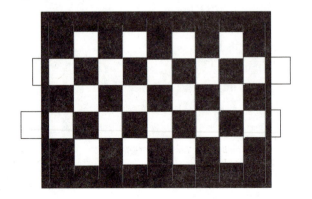

Asian Crafts and Games

Paper Making: Paper was invented by a Chinese government worker over 2 thousand years ago (Gomez, 1992). Pulp can be made with water, cotton fiber or newsprint, a wire mesh screen frame, and a food processor (Breines, 1995). Adding paint or fabric dyes, confetti, sequins, and flower fragments to wet pulp enhances the decorative appearance of the finished product. Pulp is drained over a wire mesh screen to produce paper. Many modern crafters use pulp molds to make paper sculptures. Paper-making kits and molds for paper sculptures are commercially available.

Origami: Paper folding, or origami, has a long Japanese tradition. Brightly colored, decorative origami paper is commercially available and kits usually include instructions for folding various projects (see Figure 2).

Uchiwa Paper Fans: Uchiwa or Japanese paper fans can be made by attaching folded paper (plain, origami, or decorated) to a piece of bamboo or wood (e.g., tongue depressor) (Terzian, 1993).

Paper Cutouts:
Chinese paper cutouts are used during festivals and celebrations as a sign of good luck. Chinese cutouts are made by folding a piece of paper in half and cutting out a figure. Once the paper is unfolded the figure is complete (see Figure 3).

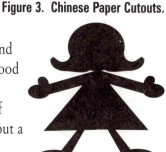

Figure 3. Chinese Paper Cutouts.

European Crafts

Wycinanki Paper Cutouts: Complex paper cutouts called **Wycinanki** are a traditional Polish craft (Gomez, 1992). Wycinanki cutouts are made by making one or two folds in paper and then making multiple scissor cutouts. When unfolded the project can be used for decorative purposes (see Figure 4). White paper cutouts look like snowflakes.

Figure 4. Wycinanki Paper Cutout.

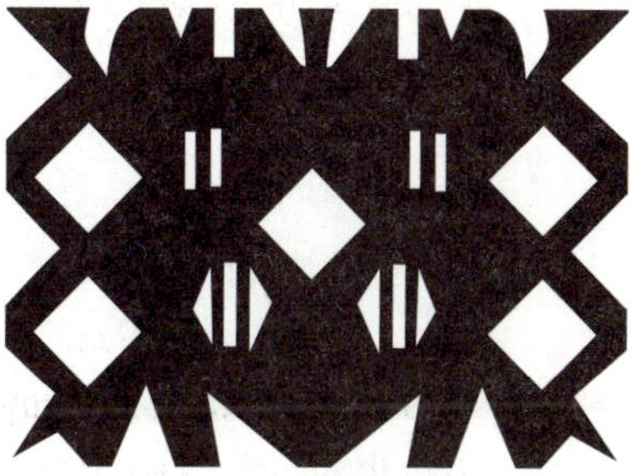

Figure 2. Japanese Origami.

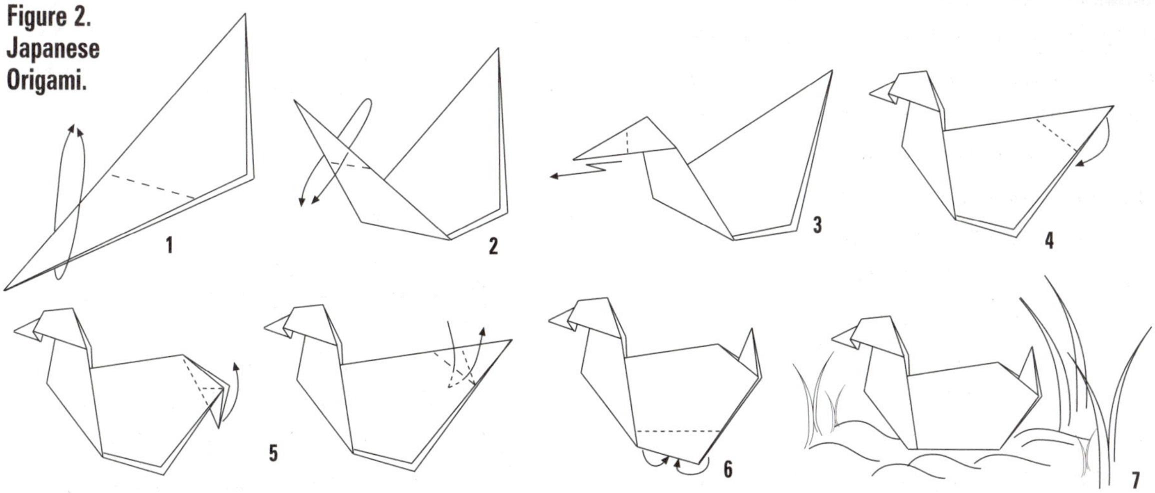

1
2
3
4
5
6
7

Origami Duck:
1 Fold a diamond shaped piece of paper as shown in illustration 1.
2 Outside reverse fold again.
3 Form the beak with a double reverse fold (2), as shown.

4 Reverse fold the tail down...
5 ...and reverse fold the tip up.
6 Fold inwards from front and back.
7 The duck completed.

Inside crimp:
The way of folding a bird's tail shown in steps 4 and 5 is called an "inside crimp". Usually the two folds are treated as a single move, and drawn as shown here.

151

Clay Vases: Ceramic clay vases, or Amphorae, are a Greek tradition with origins in the 11th and 6th centuries b.c. (Gomez, 1992). Amphora urns have a distinctive shape and can be made with a pinch pot technique or with the coil clay method (see Figure 5). Many Native American and Mexican ethnic groups are also known for their pottery and low-temperature clay firing methods. Self-hardening or nonhardening modeling clay that is nontoxic, colorful, pliable, and clean is commercially available.

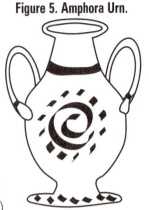

Figure 5. Amphora Urn.

Mexican Crafts and Games

Huichol Yarn Art: The Huichol Indians from the Pacific northwest of Mexico tell stories about their history and religion with paintings made of yarn and warm beeswax (Gomez, 1992; Terzian, 1993). Huichol yarn paintings can be made by applying glue and yarn to any picture (see Figure 6). Kits are also available from some craft supply catalogues and stores. Wax-coated, flexible, sticky string (i.e., Wax Works™ and Wikki Stix™) is also commercially available.

Figure 6. Huichol Yarn Art.

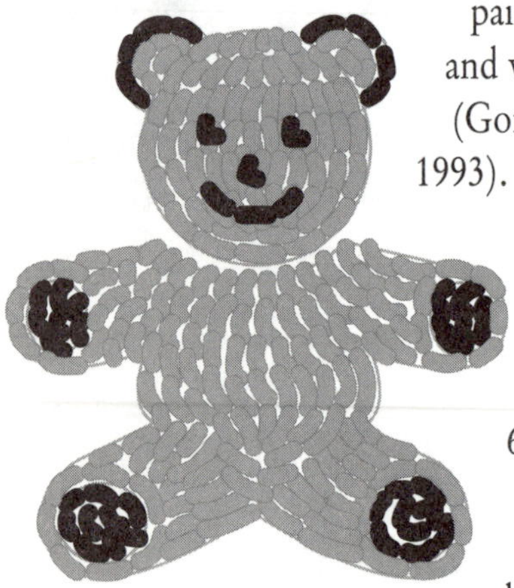

Papier-Mâché: The papier-mâché piñata is a popular Christmas or party treat for Mexican children. Piñatas are made by applying layer after layer of papier-mâché over an inflated balloon or paper bag (Drake, 1992). Once dry, the hollow structure is decorated and filled with children's treats. The piñata is suspended in the air while blindfolded children attempt to break it with a stick.

Native American Crafts and Games

Sand paintings are a medicinal tradition of the Navajo people, who live in the American Southwest. Traditional paintings are made with finely ground sand from different colored rocks such as coral, turquoise, lapis, and onyx. Trained "medicine people" create the paintings by letting sand slowly flow through their fingers onto the soil floor of a traditional home, or hogan. One painting will be completed over the course of a few days. At the end of the healing ceremony the sand painting is destroyed and buried because it has captured the spirit that caused sickness. Sand painting designs that hold these healing powers are not documented in books or shared with artists outside of the Navajo community. The artistic designs available for sale or shown in books are for decorative use only. Colored sand and sand painting kits are commercially available.

Native American Shields: The Plains Indians make rawhide shields with pictures of spirits to protect themselves (Terzian, 1993). Paper shields can be made with poster board with handles on the back. Shields can be hung up with sinew or laced with leather to make a small bolo tie. Attaching beads and feathers can create Native American designs.

Finger Puppets: While masks and puppets are used by many different cultures, Inuit women wear finger puppets during traditional dance ceremonies (Terzian, 1993). Finger puppets can be made with scrap materials or are commercially available in kits.

Learning Resources

Breines, E. B. (1995). *Occupational therapy: Activities from clay to computers.* Philadelphia: F. A. Davis.

Cook, D. (1995). *The kids' multicultural cookbook: Food & fun around the world.* Charlotte, VT: Williamson.

Drake, M. (1992). *Crafts in therapy and rehabilitation.* Thorofare, NJ: Slack.

Gomez, A. (1992). *Crafts of many cultures: 30 authentic craft projects from around the world.* New York: Scholastic.

Milord, S. (1992). *Hands around the world: 365 creative ways to build cultural awareness and global respect.* Charlotte, VT: Williamson.

S & S. (1996). *Arts, crafts, games and activities for healthcare.* Colchester, CT: Author.

S & S. (1996). *Developmentally appropriate crafts for children 6–12 years old.* Colchester, CT: Author.

S & S. (1996). 99 *Crafts for under 50¢.* Colchester, CT: Author.

References

American Occupational Therapy Association. (1993). Position paper: Purposeful activity. *American Journal of Occupational Therapy, 47,* 1081–1082.

Breines, E. B. (1995). *Occupational therapy: Activities from clay to computers.* Philadelphia: F. A. Davis.

Drake, M. (1992). *Crafts in therapy and rehabilitation.* Thorofare, NJ: Slack.

Gomez, A. (1992). *Crafts of many cultures: 30 authentic craft projects from around the world.* New York: Scholastic.

Terzian, A. M. (1993). *The kids' multicultural art book: Art and craft experiences from around the world.* Charlotte, VT: Williamson.

CHILDHOOD LEISURE ACTIVITIES: THE CASE OF BOB

"Play is viewed by occupational therapists as a need-fulfilling and important occupation in the life of every person" (Canadian Association of Occupational Therapists, 1996, p. 1).[1]

Chapter Objectives

1. Categorize case information into the domains of concern to the occupational therapy practitioner by completing the Occupational Performance Profile Form.
2. Identify the performance components that affect play and leisure performance of a young child.
3. Establish and delineate intervention priorities by completing the Client Goals Form.
4. Evaluate an activity to determine whether it addresses a particular client's needs.
5. Design a purposeful play and leisure activity that addresses a client's unique characteristics, skills, abilities, and needs.
6. Do role modeling of therapist-client interaction for developing therapeutic use of self.

Using Task Analysis and Purposeful Engagement to Develop Skills, Boost Confidence, and Increase Self-Esteem

Throughout our lives we engage in occupations that promote the development of performance capabilities in the sensorimotor, cognitive, psychological, and psychosocial domains. To encourage children to master new challenges, parents allow them to perform activities in adapted ways or alter the environment to enhance their chances for success. Repetition and practice foster confidence, self-esteem, and the development of intrinsic skills and abilities.

Consider the first time you tried to ride a two-wheeled bike. Initially, you may have been given training wheels. When you gained confidence, those extra wheels were removed. To compensate for the greater difficulty and extra balance challenge, you may have sat on the seat and propelled the bike with your feet on the ground. With practice you could lift your feet and coast without falling. As your confidence increased, so did your willingness to try pedal propulsion. As your balance, bilateral integration, and gross coordination improved, so did your chances for success. The self-confidence gained through riding a bike eventually allowed you to participate in the neighborhood bicycle races and to venture long distances on errands. Enhanced sensorimotor performance influenced your community mobility, social interaction, and self-concept.

Occupational therapists, who work with clients who want to improve their occupational performance, may design or adapt activities or alter environments to promote the development of specific abilities and functional skills. It is through the development of these abilities and skills that children achieve greater success in engaging in the activities, tasks, and roles that give meaning and purpose to their lives. Successful engagement, in turn, boosts self-concept and confidence. Although most pediatric occupational therapists and programs aim to improve self-esteem, little explicit measurement and evaluation of outcomes takes place in this domain (Mayberry, 1990; Willoughby, King, & Polatajko, 1996).

Assignment

1. Separate into groups of four. Read the Person-Activity-Environment Fit section of the document

Uniform Terminology for Occupational Therapy (American Occupational Therapy Association [AOTA], 1994a) (Appendix E) and *Uniform Terminology: Application to Practice* (AOTA, 1994b) (Appendix F).

2. Read the case about Bob. Use the Occupational Performance Profile Form (Table 1) to document information on the occupations that are important to Bob; his unique values, interests, goals, and performance components; and the contexts in which he performs. The Occupational Performance Profile Form has been started for you. This form will enable you to compile screening and evaluation information as recommended on the Occupational Performance Practice Model for Service to Individuals, which was introduced in the chapter "Task Analysis: The Contribution of Occupational Therapy to Health."

Case Study: Bob

Bob is a 4-year-old child who has just been assigned to your caseload following an evaluation by a registered occupational therapist at ABC Assessment Unit. Bob lives with his parents and sister in an apartment complex in a small town. He spends a lot of time at his grandparents' farm and helps to care for their animals. Bob's father indicates that Bob is interested in dinosaurs and enjoys horses and the Saturday morning cartoons.

Bob's parents are worried about his confidence and self-esteem and are concerned about his fear of playgrounds and lack of understanding of academic concepts. Bob cannot identify letters, basic shapes or colors, or sort objects into same and different categories. He is unable to put on or remove his overcoat or manage his zipper and often places his shoes on the wrong feet. Bob is so afraid of the slide, swing set, and merry-go-round that he refuses to play on his own at his day care. Bob rides a

tricycle short distances, but cannot ride with the speed, agility, and precision of his friends. Some of his older friends have graduated to two-wheel bikes. Unfortunately, a number of children tease him because of his "clumsiness."

The occupational therapy report indicates that Bob's self-care, academic, play, and leisure performance is delayed in comparison to his peers. He has poor postural control, gross and fine coordination, bilateral integration, visual motor integration, and spatial operations skills. Sensory testing is suggestive of poor proprioceptive, tactile, and vestibular processing (see Table 3, Developmental Coordination Disorder).

3. Why do you think Bob is fearful of the slide, swing, and merry-go-round? What sensorimotor performance components are required for success on all three pieces of equipment? Does the occupational therapy report indicate that Bob has difficulty in these areas?

4. Why do you think Bob has difficulty riding his tricycle with "speed, agility, and precision"? What sensorimotor performance components are required to complete this activity? Does the occupational therapy report indicate that Bob has difficulty in these areas?

5. Why do you think Bob is unable to put on or remove his overcoat or manage his zipper and places his shoes on the wrong feet? What performance components are required to complete this activity?

6. Use the information you have compiled to complete the Client Goals Form (Table 2). This table has been started for you. Ensure that your goals maintain or promote function and prevent dysfunction, and that they fit the concerns, priorities, and resources of this family. In the clinical setting these goals would be established in collab-

Table 1: Occupational Performance Profile Form

Occupations	Person	Contexts
Roles	**Values, Interests, and Goals**	**Temporal**
Son *Day-care student* *Brother*	*Interested in dinosaurs and enjoys horses and cartoons. Fear of playgrounds.*	*4-year-old boy*
Tasks and Activities	**Performance Components**	**Social**
Activities of Daily Living	Sensorimotor components	
Unable to manage overcoat.		*Parents and sister. Spends a lot of time at grandparents' farm.*
Work and Productive Activities	**Cognitive Integration and Cognitive Components**	**Cultural**
Cannot label letter/shapes/colors.		
Play or Leisure Activities	**Psychosocial and Psychological Components**	**Physical**
Unable to be alone on slide/swing/merry-go-round.	*Parents worry about self-concept and self-esteem.*	*Day care*

oration with Bob and his parents. Be prepared to modify these recommendations after discussing them with Bob's parents.

Long-term goals document expected functional outcomes in occupational performance areas that clients want addressed (AOTA, 1994c). Short-term objectives relate to the performance components or impairments that must be addressed or to the environmental parameters that must be altered in order to achieve the long-term goal. Goals must be as specific, objective, and as measurable as possible. Refer to Appendix H for more information.

7. During the last treatment session Bob participated in a therapeutic activity. An obstacle course (an imaginary farm) was designed to enhance Bob's skill and confidence on the playground by enhancing his sensorimotor, cognitive, and psychological performance components. Bob cut out a yellow paper star (sheriff's badge), wore a weighted vest (cowboy jacket) to walk across a balance beam (barnyard fence), threw red and blue beanbags (hay bales) into separate baskets, and bounced on a small trampoline (horse).

   Why was Bob asked to cut out a paper star? Why did Bob wear a weighted vest?

   What performance components were challenged to walk across the balance beam, sort and throw beanbags, and bounce on a trampoline? Did these task demands challenge the performance components with which Bob has difficulty?

   Why was an imaginary farm concept used during this activity?

8. Reconstruct and perform this obstacle course. Assume that Bob has mastered this activity. How could you increase the task demands to enhance the challenge and continue to develop Bob's skills?
   OR

   Design and construct an additional activity for Bob to do while engaging in this obstacle course.

The activity should challenge and promote the development of the performance components identified in the short-term objectives. Use balls, mats, balance beams, barrels, beanbags, hoops, foam blocks, swings, and so on. Be sure to create a meaningful context for this play and leisure activity. This could be accomplished through pretend play or by acting out a story line.

9. Bob has mastered this new activity. Continue to provide Bob with a challenge that is achievable by grading the activity to make it slightly more difficult. Explain why purposeful activities should balance achievement with challenge.

10. Take turns role playing as Bob and his therapist. This will increase the accuracy of your activity analysis and enable you to practice interacting with a toddler. The verbal and nonverbal interactive relationship between the therapist and client may provide a source of encouragement, motivation, and feedback to reinforce and facilitate learning.

Optional:

11. What gross motor play and leisure activities did you participate in and enjoy during early childhood? What are the characteristics and qualities of these activities that promoted your development?

12. Review the article *Position Paper: Purposeful Activity* (AOTA, 1993) (Appendix K). Does the imaginary farm obstacle course meet the criteria of a purposeful and therapeutic activity?

13. After designing and participating in the imaginary farm obstacle course, complete the Occupational Performance Analysis Form (Appendix A and C).

Table 2. Client Goals Form

Client Goals Form

Long-Term Goal #1

Bob will independently play on a swing for 3 minutes with confidence.

Short-Term Objective #1A

Improved vestibular and proprioceptive processing, postural control, and visual motor integration to walk across a balance beam without falling.

Short-Term Objective #1B

Improve vestibular and proprioceptive processing, and postural control to stand on one foot for 5 seconds.

Long-Term Goal #2

Bob's parents will be satisfied with his understanding of academic concepts.

Short-Term Objective #2A

Bob will separate red and blue objects into color categories.

Short-Term Objective #2B

Long-Term Goal #3

Bob will ride his tricycle through an obstacle course with improved speed and agility.

Short-Term Objective #3A

Short-Term Objective #3B

Table 3: Developmental Coordination Disorder

Clumsiness in children is associated with learning, communication, and attention deficit disorders (Kaplan & Sadock, 1996). Although the prevalence of developmental coordination disorder is not known, it has been estimated that 6 to 18% of general elementary school children have motor coordination problems (Cratty, 1986; Kaplan & Sadock, 1996). Risk factors include prematurity, low birth weight, and factors that result in central nervous system lesions (Kaplan & Sadock, 1996).

Occupational therapy practitioners frequently treat children with motor incoordination when their difficulties interfere with engagement in valued activities, tasks, and roles. Willoughby and Polatajko (1995) suggest that (a) the child will likely be the expert at determining which tasks are difficult and which portions of the activity cause the most problems, (b) there is no single effective and efficient treatment approach, and (c) the cause of the difficulty varies from child to child.

The information that follows will (a) provide students and instructors with resources to enhance the learning experience and (b) assist the student in completing the assignment.

Learning Resources

American Occupational Therapy Association (AOTA). (1993). Position paper: Purposeful activity. *American Journal of Occupational Therapy, 47,* 1081–1082.

AOTA. (1994a). *Uniform terminology for occupational therapy* (3rd ed.). Bethesda, MD: Author.

AOTA. (1994b). *Uniform terminology: Application to practice.* Bethesda, MD: Author.

Fink, B. E. (1989). *Sensory-motor integration activities.* Tucson, AZ: Therapy Skill Builders.

Haldy, M. (1995). *Making it easy: Sensorimotor activities for home and school.* San Antonio, TX: Therapy Skill Builders.

Orlick, T. (1982). *Cooperative sports and games book.* New York: Pantheon Books.

Sher, B. (1995). *Popular games for positive play.* San Antonio, TX: Therapy Skill Builders.

Witoski, M. L. (1992). *It's not just a parachute: Integrative activities for children of all abilities.* San Antonio, TX: Therapy Skill Builders.

Study Questions

1. Walking across a 4-inch-wide by 5-foot-long balance beam requires integration of which sensorimotor skills and abilities?

2. Maintaining balance while standing with eyes closed requires integration of which sensorimotor performance components?

3. Throwing beanbags toward a target while lying prone on a hammock swing requires integration of which sensory systems?

4. How can the social and physical environmental context of play be altered to reduce complexity?

5. Why are a client's values and interests important to designing purposeful activities?

6. Do long-term goals refer to expected outcomes in occupational performance areas, components, or contexts?

7. Define **person-activity-environment fit**. Why is this concept applicable to justifying and designing occupational therapy intervention?

8. What is **rapport** and why is it important in the therapy process?

References

American Occupational Therapy Association (AOTA). (1994a). *Uniform terminology for occupational therapy* (3rd ed.). Bethesda, MD: Author.

AOTA. (1994b). *Uniform terminology: Application to practice.* Bethesda, MD: Author.

AOTA. (1994c). *Elements of clinical documentation* (Rev. ed.). Bethesda, MD: Author.

Canadian Association of Occupational Therapists. (1996). Occupational therapy and children's play. *Canadian Journal of Occupational Therapy, 63*(2), Insert 1–9.

Cratty, B. J. (1986). *Perceptual and motor development in infants and children.* Englewood Cliffs, NJ: Prentice-Hall.

Kaplan, H. I., & Sadock, B. J. (1996). *Concise textbook of clinical psychiatry.* Baltimore: Williams & Wilkins.

Mayberry, W. (1990). Self-esteem in children: Considerations for measurement and intervention. *American Journal of Occupational Therapy, 44,* 729–734.

Willoughby, C., King, G., & Polatajko, H. J. (1996). A therapist's guide to children's self-esteem. *American Journal of Occupational Therapy, 50,* 124–132.

Willoughby, C., & Polatajko, H. J. (1995). Motor problems in children with developmental coordination disorder: Review of the literature. *American Journal of Occupational Therapy, 49,* 787–793.

CHILDHOOD EDUCATIONAL ACTIVITIES: THE CASE OF TINA

"Occupational therapists enable all people, regardless of ability, age or other characteristics, to choose and engage in occupations which give meaning and purpose to their lives"

(Canadian Association of Occupational Therapists, 1994, p 294).[1]

Chapter Objectives

1. Describe how occupational therapy practitioners use task analysis as an assessment and intervention tool to enhance role functioning of a young client.
2. Categorize case information into the domains of concern to the occupational therapy practitioner by completing the Occupational Performance Profile Form in Table 1.
3. Identify the performance components that affect engagement in educational tasks and activities of a young student.
4. Establish and delineate intervention priorities by completing the Client Goals Form in Table 2.
5. Evaluate an activity to determine whether it addresses a particular client's needs.
6. Develop and apply skills in creative analysis to select and design a purposeful activity to address a client's unique characteristics, skills, abilities, and needs.
7. Develop and refine skills in task analysis through personal engagement.

Using Task Analysis and Purposeful Engagement to Develop Skills and Enhance Role Functioning

Occupational therapists work with parents and teachers to enable children to assume student roles by promoting the child's development of academic skills and abilities or creating an optimal environment for learning. The American Occupational Therapy Association (1996) reports that 18.7% of registered occupational therapists and 14.8% of certified occupational therapy assistants worked within the school system in 1995.

Children perform a number of tasks each day while engaging in their student role. Traveling from home to school and moving around the classroom and playground requires community and functional mobility. Removing an overcoat in the morning, changing clothes for physical education, and visiting the bathroom requires skills in dressing and toilet hygiene. Snack or lunch time requires feeding and eating skills, and socialization occurs throughout the day. Recess and after-school activities provide many play and leisure opportunities, and academic educational activities challenge students to learn.

While 90% of children with learning difficulties demonstrate fine motor and handwriting difficulties, 85% of elementary school class time is spent on paper-and-pencil tasks, and 15% of class time is spent on manipulative tasks (McHale & Cermack, 1992; Tarnolpol & Tarnolpol, 1977). Therapists who work with preschoolers and young students who have motor delays or impairments frequently analyze the sensorimotor foundations that are required to perform functional classroom activities and then use strategies and techniques to improve these skills (Case-Smith, 1996). Therapists promote functional performance of students with these impairments by (a) developing in-hand manipulation, grasp patterns, visual motor integration, motor control, and strength; and (b) promoting skill

---

[1]From "Position Statement on Everyday Occupations and Health," by the Canadian Association of Occupational Therapists (CAOT), 1994, *Canadian Journal of Occupational Therapy 61*(5), p. 294. Copyright 1994 by CAOT Publications. Reproduced with permission.

generalization in varied classroom contexts (Case-Smith, 1995; Case-Smith, 1996; Cornhill & Case-Smith, 1996; McHale & Cermak, 1992).

While educational activities occupy many hours in the life of a child, the importance of the student role and academic achievement varies among different children and families. Occupational therapists and teachers collaborate with parents to identify educational goals that are important to individual students and their families. These educational goals are documented in an individualized education program (IEP). Intervention with students may be directed at restructuring tasks, providing purposeful activities to enhance performance components, providing opportunities for students to practice new methods, teaching and consulting with teachers and parents, altering the environment, and providing adapted equipment.

Assignment

1. Separate into groups of two. Read the case about Tina.
2. Use the Occupational Performance Profile Form in Table 1 to document information on the occupations that are important to Tina; her unique values, interests, goals, and performance components; and the contexts in which she performs. The Occupational Performance Profile Form has been started for you.
3. Why do you think Tina has difficulty completing puzzles, using scissors, and spelling her name? What skills and abilities or performance components are required for success in these activities? Will Tina need to be independent in these activities in her role as a student?
4. The case manager indicates that Tina is a very active child and there is concern about her attention span and interest in tabletop or quiet-time activities. How do temporal factors such as chronological and developmental age and the

social and cultural context of ABC Day Care and Kindergarten affect Tina and her role performance?

5. Complete the Client Goals Form in Table 2. Ensure that your goals maintain or promote function and prevent dysfunction, and that they fit the concerns, priorities, and resources of this family and day care. In the clinical setting these goals would be established in collaboration with Tina, her father, the teacher, and any other special education professionals at ABC Day Care and Kindergarten. Be prepared to modify these recommendations after discussing them with Tina's father and teacher. If you would like assistance defining goals and objectives refer to Appendix H.
6. Although ABC Day Care and Kindergarten has supplies for many different crafts, the tissue art project, Woodsies™ (Forster Inc.®), and Puzzle Power™ (S & S) catch your attention (see the following Therapeutic Activity Suggestions). From experience working with young children you recognize the potential for using these crafts to address some of Tina's goals. What features of these activities make them particularly attractive for use with children with perceptual and fine motor difficulties?

Theraputic Activity Suggestion: Tissue Art
Materials
    Colored paper
    Coloring book picture
    Glue
    Magnetic strip or gummed hanger (optional)
    Pencil or crayon
    Tissue paper
    Scissors
    Tissue-Paper-Collage project available from S & S craft suppliers (Appendix M). Nasco Arts & Crafts' Corrugated Paper Pegboard offers an alternative tissue art method that only provides a moderate level of fine motor coordination challenge.

Figure 1A. Sample Tissue Art Project.

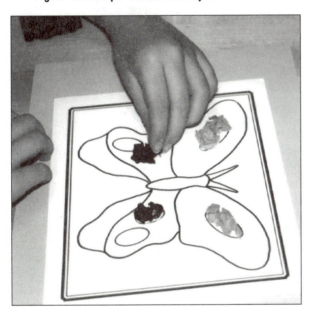

Figure 1B. Sample Tissue Art Project.

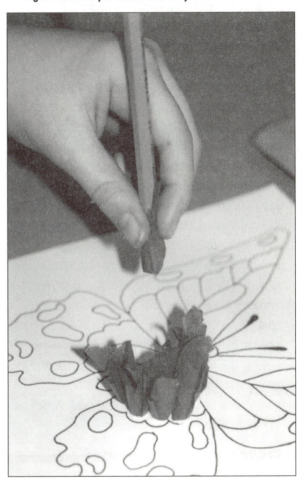

1. Select a picture from a coloring book and glue it onto colored paper.
2. Cut or rip the tissue paper into 1- or 2-inch squares.
3. Roll the tissue paper into tiny balls between your fingers, or wrap the tissue paper around the end of a pencil or crayon.
4. Apply glue to a small area of your picture, or if using a pencil or crayon, dip the tissue end of the pencil or crayon into white glue.
5. Fill in all of the picture spaces with your tissue paper.
6. Attach a magnetic strip or gummed hanger to the back of your picture to hang it up.
7. Select one of these projects or a craft from the chapter "Children's Cultural Crafts and Games." Design and structure this activity to maximize its therapeutic value with Tina. After analyzing an activity or task for its potential to address treatment goals, adaptations may be necessary to maximize its therapeutic value (Trombly, 1995).
8. Explain why purposeful activities should balance achievement with challenge.
9. After selecting, adapting, and fabricating this project, complete the Occupational Performance Analysis Form (Appendix A or C). Will you

recommend assistive and adaptive equipment, particularly crayons and scissors, for Tina? Review equipment supplier catalogues for ideas (Appendix M).

10. The purpose of using this therapeutic craft with Tina is to enhance her role functioning by promoting development of predetermined performance components. ABC's case manager, however, requested occupational therapy consultation rather than direct intervention. What therapeutic activities would you recommend that the staff at ABC Day Care and Kindergarten do with Tina? Occupational therapy intervention may be directed at teaching or consulting with others and altering sociocultural environments. What recommendations do you have regarding alterations to Tina's sociocultural environment?

Optional:

11. What activities did you participate in and enjoy when you were 5 years old? What are the characteristics and qualities of these activities that promoted your development in early childhood?

12. Review Cornhill and Case-Smith (1996) to become familiar with how research can be used to validate the relationship between performance components and task performance. Participate in a group discussion about this article's conclusions and relevance to the task analysis process.

13. Review Sooy Griswold (1994) to become familiar with methods of classroom environmental analysis. Participate in a group discussion about this article's conclusions and relevance to the task analysis process.

Therapeutic Activity Suggestion: Woodsies™

Materials

- Acrylic paints (optional)
- Colored paper
- Felt markers (optional)
- Glitter (optional)
- Glue
- Wiggly eyes (optional)
- Woodsies™

Figure 2. Woodsies™ Character Patterns.

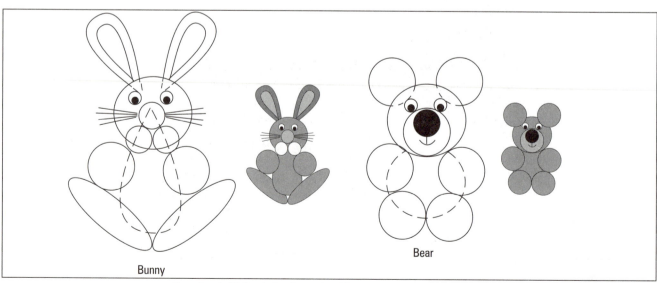

Bunny

Bear

Reproduced with Permission. Forster Inc., PO Box 657, Wilton, ME 04294.

Woodsies™ projects available from most craft suppliers, including S & S and Nasco Arts & Crafts (Appendix M).

1. Select a Woodsie™ character design.
2. Identify and locate the wooden shapes that are required for this character.
3. Assemble wood pieces.
4. Paint, color, and decorate before or after gluing project.
5. Create a background with paper, or attach a magnet, pin, or stick to use the character as an ornament, brooch, or puppet.

Therapeutic Activity Suggestion: Puzzle Power™

Materials
- Pencil and eraser
- Puzzle Power

- Watercolor or permanent marker
- Stencil (optional)

This creative craft project from S & S enables individuals to draw on blank cardboard puzzles. Information on arts and craft suppliers is available in Appendix M.

1. Select a picture or topic to illustrate on the blank Puzzle Power™ project.
2. Use a pencil to draw on the puzzle or use a stencil to assist in this process.
3. Use watercolor or permanent markers to color.
4. Deconstruct and then reassemble puzzle.

Figure 3. Sample Puzzle Power Project.

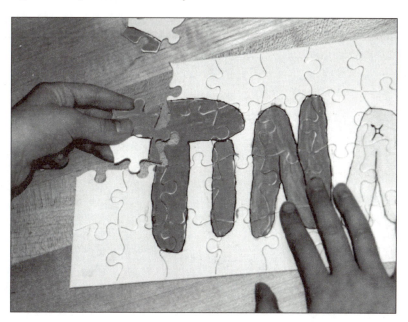

Case Study: Tina

Tina will be turning 6 years old next month and has already started to talk about her upcoming birthday party at ABC Day Care and Kindergarten. The child-care workers and teachers at ABC are very fond of Tina, as they have taken care of her on weekdays since she was 9 months old. Tina is an only child and lives with her father. ABC's case manager requests an occupational therapy consultation and explains Tina's situation.

According to her case manager, Tina has always been a very active child. "Although she is very weak for her age, she loves gross motor activities and is usually a daredevil on the playground. Her social skills have always been her greatest asset, and she has more friends than you could ever imagine." "Over the past year or so I have been concerned about her short attention span and lack of interest in tabletop or quiet-time activities. She has great difficulty completing puzzles, and becomes frustrated when trying to operate scissors. She can cut a straight line, but I have to explain how to turn the paper to cut around shapes." Tina likes to color, but is not very good at it. Although she puts great effort into printing, Tina cannot spell her name.

After spending a half hour interviewing some of the staff, you come to realize that ABC provides a very unstructured approach to learning. Children are encouraged to pursue activities of interest to themselves. Although the teachers offer projects that facilitate learning, the students can choose not to participate.

After Tina's evaluation is complete, it is determined that she has poor fine motor coordination, a very immature pencil grasp, and has not yet established a hand dominance. Her visual closure, spatial opera- tions, and sequencing skills are also below average. Tina appears to be very self-conscious about her performance when completing puzzles and during paper-pencil activities. She loves animals, the circus, and gymnastics.

Table 1: Occupational Performance Profile Form

Occupational Performance Profile		
Occupations	**Person**	**Contexts**
<u>Roles</u> *Kindergarten student.* *Daughter.*	<u>Values, Interests, and Goals</u> *Loves animals, the circus, gymnastics, and parties.*	<u>Temporal</u>
<u>Tasks and Activities</u> Activities of Daily Living	<u>Performance Components</u> Sensorimotor Components *Poor fine motor coordination.* *Immature pencil grasp.* *No hand dominance.*	Social *Lives with father.* *ABC staff very fond of Tina. Teachers provide group exercises.*
Work and Productive Activities *Difficulty completing puzzles.*	Cognitive Integration and Cognitive Components *Concern about attention span.*	<u>Cultural</u> *Unstructured approach to learning.* *Children choose educational activities.*
Play or Leisure Activities	Psychological and Psychosocial Components *Self-conscious.* *Values gross motor activities.* *Social skills greatest asset.*	<u>Physical</u>

Table 2: Client Goals Form

Client Goals

Long-Term Goal #1

Tina will print her name independently.

Short-Term Objective #1A

Tina will trace the letters in her name.

Short-Term Objective #1B

Tina will sequence the letters in her name.

Short-Term Objective #1C

Tina will establish a hand dominance and improve her fine motor coordination.

Short-Term Objective #1D

Long-Term Goal #2

Tina will color a picture of an animal and stay within the lines.

Short-Term Objective #2A

Short-Term Objective #2B

Long-Term Goal #3

Short-Term Objective #3A

Short-Term Objective #3B

The information that follows will (a) provide students and instructors with resources to enhance the learning experience and (b) assist the student in completing the assignment.

Learning Resources

Bal, D. (1996). OT in the public schools. *OT Week, 10*(30), 18–19.

Coling, M., & Carrett, J. (1995). *Activity-based intervention guide.* San Antonio, TX: Therapy Skill Builders.

Cornhill, H., & Case-Smith, J. (1996). Factors that relate to good and poor handwriting. *American Journal of Occupational Therapy, 50,* 732–739.

Klein, M. (1990a). *Pre-writing skills* (Rev. ed.). San Antonio, TX: Therapy Skill Builders.

Klein, M. (1990b). *Pre-scissor skills* (3rd ed.). San Antonio, TX: Therapy Skill Builders.

Loiselle, L., & Shea, S. (1995). *Curriculum based activities in occupational therapy: An inclusion resource.* Framingham, MA: Therapro.

Pascale, L. (1991). *Multi-arts resource guide.* Boston: Very Special Arts Massachusetts.

Press, J. (1994). *The little hands art book: Exploring arts and crafts with 2 to 6 year olds.* Charlotte, VT: Williamson.

Sher, B. (1992). *Extraordinary play with ordinary things.* Tucson, AZ: Therapy Skill Builders.

Sooy Griswold, L. (1994). Ethnographic analysis: A study of classroom environments. *American Journal of Occupational Therapy, 48,* 397–402.

Study Questions

1. Your 6-year-old client has great difficulty copying new spelling words from the board to his notebook. Completion of this activity requires integration of which sensorimotor, cognitive, psychosocial, and psychological performance components? How can the environment be restructured to facilitate completion of this activity?

2. Identify five self-care and educational activities in which students are expected to be independent upon entry into first grade?

3. What are the name and characteristics of the most mature pencil grasp pattern?

4. Your 7-year-old client is unable to use the zipper on his overcoat. Completion of this activity requires integration of which sensorimotor, cognitive, psychosocial, and psychological performance components? How can the task equipment be altered to facilitate completion of this activity?

5. Identify an activity that could be used to enhance a 5-year-old client's bilateral integration and fine motor coordination.

6. How can the activity of cutting with scissors be graded and adapted to increase or decrease the level of challenge to performance components?

7. Explain why purposeful activities are adapted to provide a challenge that is achievable.

References

American Occupational Therapy Association. (1996). Comparison of work settings 1990/95. *OT Practice, 1*(3), 14.

Case-Smith, J. (1995). The relationships among sensorimotor components, fine motor skill, and functional performance in preschool children. *American Journal of Occupational Therapy, 49,* 645–652.

Case-Smith, J. (1996). Fine motor outcomes in preschool children who receive occupational therapy services. *American Journal of Occupational Therapy, 50,* 52–60.

Cornhill, H., & Case-Smith, J. (1996). Factors that relate to good and poor handwriting. *American Journal of Occupational Therapy, 50,* 732–739.

McHale, K., & Cermak, S. A. (1992). Fine motor activities in elementary school: Preliminary findings and provisional implications for children with fine motor problems. *American Journal of Occupational Therapy, 46,* 898–903.

Sooy Griswold, L. (1994). Ethnographic analysis: A study of classroom environments. *American Journal of Occupational Therapy, 48,* 397–402.

Tarnolpol, L., & Tarnolpol, M. (1977). *Brain function and reading disabilities.* Baltimore: University Park Press.

Trombly, C. A. (1995). Purposeful activity. In C. A. Trombly (Ed.), *Occupational therapy for physical dysfunction* (pp. 237–253). Baltimore: Williams & Wilkins.

SWITCH ACCESS TO LEARNING: THE CASE OF SIDNEY

"It is doubtful that any child may reasonably be expected to succeed in life if he is denied the opportunity of an education. Such an opportunity, where the state has undertaken to provide it, is a right which must be made available to all on equal terms" (Brown v. Board of Education, 1954).

Chapter Objectives

1. Define the terms and give examples of **assistive technology devices** and **environmental control units.**
2. List a variety of different switches and describe how they can be used to operate a toy or appliance.
3. Operate a battery operated and electrical appliance with a switch.
4. Describe the relevance of assistive technology devices to special education.
5. Use task analysis skills to assess a child's Occupational Performance Profile and design intervention.
6. Apply the person-activity-environment fit concept described by the American Occupational Therapy Association (1994) to the selection and use of assistive technology devices.
7. Use logical thinking and creative analysis to restructure tasks and alter environmental context to enable a student to engage in a student role.

Using Assistive Technology to Enhance Role Functioning and Increase Self-Esteem

Assistive technology devices are an integral part of special education and the individualized education program (Individuals with Disabilities Education Act [IDEA], 1990; Shuster, 1993). An assistive technology device is "any item, piece of equipment, or product system, whether acquired commercially off the shelf, modified, or customized, that is used to increase, maintain, or improve functional capacities of individuals with disabilities" (IDEA, 1990; Technology-Related Assistance for Individuals with Disabilities Act, 1988).

Many individuals have disabilities that cannot be eliminated through the application or use of therapeutic modalities. "A disability is any restriction or lack (resulting from an impairment) of ability to perform an activity in the manner or within the range considered normal for a human being" (World Health Organization, 1980, p. 143). Disabilities may arise as a direct consequence of impairments at the organ level or as a response by an individual to an impairment. The role of the occupational therapy practitioner is to ensure that not all impairments cause disability. This may be accomplished through the use of assistive technology to compensate for impairments. Assistive technology, however, may be used to remediate or develop skills, particularly in the sensorimotor and cognitive domains.

By restructuring tasks and altering environments through the use of assistive technology devices, occupational therapy practitioners can enable people to control their patterns of occupation. During the evaluation process, therapists consider a person's sensorimotor, cognitive, psychological, and psychosocial skills and abilities, task demands, environmental constraints, and lifestyle to ensure useful and appropriate application of technology (AOTA, 1991b). The use of technology in treatment and intervention is guided by client and family values and needs, sociocultural and environmental factors, financial resources, and cost-effectiveness (AOTA, 1991b; Shuster, 1993; Swinth, 1996).

Occupational therapy practitioners use low-technology assistive devices (e.g., typing aides, reachers) and high-technology assistive devices (e.g., switches, computers, power wheelchairs, and environmental control units) to provide intervention services aimed at ensuring maximum independence of people of all ages (AOTA, 1991b). **Environmental control units** (ECUs) provide a means by which individuals can manage their environment by remote control (Lange, 1996). Controlling the environment through the use of assistive technology devices enables children with disabilities to maintain interest in interacting with their world and may prevent learned helplessness (Swinth, 1996).

Switch Access to Educational Experiences

Switches are used by people of all ages to activate battery operated or electrical appliances and devices including toys, fans, radios, computers, door openers, televisions, power wheelchairs, home appliances, and so on. Switch access to toys and computer cause-and-effect programs can be controlled by children as young as 6 to 9 months of age (Glickman, Deitz, Anson, & Stewart, 1996; Swinth, Anson, & Deitz, 1993). Switches that are connected to environmental control units enable individuals with disabilities to maintain a more independent level of activity and improve their relationships with family, personal assistants, and other people. Switches can also be used to provide access to computer programs and online services.

All battery operated toys and appliances require activation of an on/off switch. Movement of this lever completes an electrical circuit that supplies the motor with power. Typical on/off switches require fine motor coordination and strength. By changing this lever to a switch, the size and location of this lever can be modified to reduce the level of

challenge demanded of these sensorimotor performance components.

Switches function as alternative on/off control levers and are commercially available in many different shapes, colors, and sizes (see Figure 1 and Table 1). Several manufacturers make toys or other battery operated appliances with external switch jacks, while other devices have switches permanently attached. Some switches provide sensory feedback by vibrating, illuminating, and playing music or other auditory stimulation. The BIGmack™ (AbleNet® Inc.) single switch, for example, has 20 seconds of memory to record and play back audio messages.

Battery adapters are a very inexpensive means of enabling clients to activate or operate any battery operated appliance with a switch. Battery device adapters have a copper wafer at one end and a plug at the other as illustrated in Table 1. The copper wafer is placed between the battery and the lead on the appliance and the on/off lever is turned on. The appliance motor will not operate because the battery adapter has interrupted the electrical circuit. Once the switch is plugged into the battery adapter plug and pressed, the electrical circuit is complete and the motor will operate. On/off control has been transferred from the appliance to the switch.

Figure 1. A Variety of Switches.

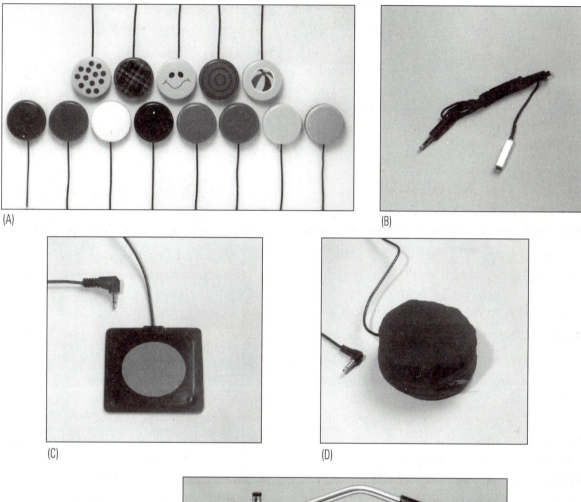

(A)

(B)

(C)

(D)

(A) Buddy Button Switches
(B) Tip or Mercury Switch
(C) Plate Switch
(D) Soft Switch
(E) Flex and leaf switches with
mount hardware

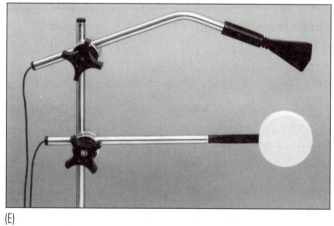

(E)

*Photographs courtesy of Tash International
Inc. 800-463-5685*

Table 1: Commonly Used Switches and Interfaces

Name/Example	Activation	Comments	Vendors
Flat Switch	Small low-force movement of arms, hands, legs, head, etc.	• flatness allows placement under many objects • notebook switch provides larger surfaces	Don Johnson TASH
Leaf Switch	Flexible switch that is activated when bent or pressed gently.	• requires mounting • can improve head control and fine motor skills	Don Johnson TASH Enabling Devices
Mercury (Tilt) Switch	Gravity sensitive switch activates when tilted beyond a certain point.	• can improve head or other posture control • attaches easily with Velcro® strap	HCTS TASH Enabling Devices
Plate Switch - Rectangular	Downward pressure on plate by hand, foot arm, leg or other reliable movement.	• most common • can be covered with various textures • some offer light, music, vibration, vertical position	Don Johnson TASH Enabling Devices
Plate Switch - Circular	Light touch anywhere on the top of surface.	• recommended for young children • click provides auditory feedback • 5" diameter and smaller size available	Ablenet TASH
Voice Activated	Significant vocalizations 1-2 seconds) required.	• can improve vocalizations • sound sensitivity control	Enabling Devices
Wobble Switch	Requires slight press to midline for activation; audible click.	• versatile and multi faceted • available with goose-neck positioner • sturdy	Prentke-romich Enabling Devices
Puzzle switch	Pieces must be properly inserted to activate toy.	• ideal for introducing children to basic cognitive concepts • can improve fine motor skills • complexity of task can be varied	Enabling Devices

Table 1: Commonly Used Switches and Interfaces, continued

Name/Example	Activation	Comments	Vendors
Battery Device Adapter	Allows a battery-operated device to be activated by a switch.	• nonpermanent • can be used with most on/off toys, radios, and tape recorders	Ablenet Don Johnson Enabling Devices
Computer Switch Interface	Allows single-switch access to an Apple computer.	• accepts one or two switches • subnstitute switches for joy sticks	Ablenet Don Johnson TASH
Control Unit	Enables electrical devices to be activated by a switch.	• allows children to participate with peers • used with continuous closure or on/off • timer can be set from 2-90 seconds	Ablenet Don Johnson TASH
Series Adapter	Connects two switches and one toy. Both switches must be activated at the same time.	• encourages bilateral movement • promotes cooperation between two children	Don Johnson HCTS Enabling Devices
Switch Latch Interface	Turns the device on and off with each switch activation.	• good for children who are unable to maintain switch closure for any length of time	Ablenet Don Johnson HCTS Enabling Devices
Timer Module	When switch is closed, a toy is activated for a preset time.	• the toy activates for 1-90 seconds, depending on the vendor	Ablenet HCTS Enabling Devices
Jack Adapter	Works to convert the size of the jack to the size required by the toy or device.	• must be mono to work with switches	Radio Shack

From "Using Assistive Technology for Play and Learning: Children, from Birth to 10 Years of Age" (pp. 131–163), by S. G. Mistrett and S. J. Lane, 1995, in *Assistive Technology for Persons with Disability* (4th ed.), edited by W. Mann and J. Lane, Bethesda, MD: American Occupational Therapy Association. Copyright 1995 by the American Occupational Therapy Association. Reproduced with permission.

Switches activate battery operated appliances only when they are depressed, unless a latch switch or a latch interface device is used. Activation of the latch switch will turn the appliance on, but a second activation will be required to turn the appliance off. A television remote control switch, for example, is a latch switch. An illustration of a switch latch interface is also found in Table 1.

Single, dual, and multiple switches enable clients to activate an assortment of appliances and devices. The ULTRA 4 Remote System (TASH International Inc.) is an environmental control unit that allows remote control of electrical appliances. The ULTRA 4 contains a transmitter box with four latch switches. Four receiver boxes are plugged into the electrical receptors on the wall between the electrical appliance and the outlet. The appliance is turned on but the motor will not operate until a switch on the transmitter box is pressed. The ULTRA 4 Remote System has transferred the appliance's on/off lever to the latch switch on the transmitter. Communication

between the transmitter and receivers occurs through ultrasound signals. Four different color transmitter switches operate four color-coded receivers. Figure 2 shows two different transmitters, and Figure 3 shows the Scanning ULTRA 4. This transmitter enables a person to use four single switches or one switch to scan and select signals.

The PowerLink 2® Control Unit (AbleNet) enables direct, latch, and timed switch control of any electrical appliance. The PowerLink 2 Control Unit is plugged into the wall, and an appliance is plugged into the unit. Although the appliance on/off lever must be in the on position, the appliance motor will not operate until the switch is plugged into the unit and pressed. Selection of direct, latch, and timed mode is made with a dial control, but this control requires fine motor coordination and strength. An illustration of a control unit is provided in Table 1.

Figure 2. Two Different Transmitters for the ULTRA 4 Remote System.

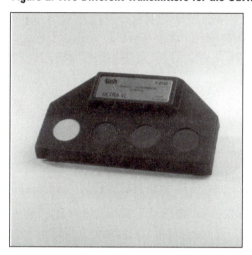 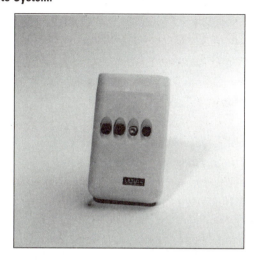

Figure 3. Scanning ULTRA 4 Transmitter with Four Buddy Button Switches.

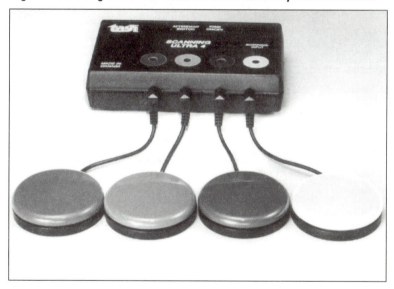

Photographs courtesy of Tash International Inc. 800-463-5685

Assignment

1. Read the documents *Broadening the Construct of Independence: A Position Paper* (AOTA, 1995) (Appendix L); *Evaluating Toddlers for Assistive Technology* (Swinth, 1996); or *Environmental Control Units 101* (Lange, 1996).

2. Review the different types of switches that are commercially available through supplier catalogues and the World Wide Web sites listed in the Learning Resource section of this chapter. Figure 1 and Table 1 provide examples.

   Set up a single switch to control a battery operated toy or electrical appliance. Use the information provided in the section Switch Access to Educational Experiences to assist you.

3. Separate into groups of three or four. Read the case about Sidney. Use the Occupational Performance Profile Form to document the information on the occupations that are important to Sidney, her parents, and teacher; Sidney's unique values, interests, goals, and performance components; and the contexts in which she performs. A copy of the Occupational Performance Profile Form is located in Appendix G.

4. What are your initial impressions about Sidney's neuromusculoskeletal and motor skills and abilities? Why do you think Sidney uses a wheelchair? Why does she have a special seating insert? Sidney's seating insert has a firm back and base, offers lateral support, and positions her hips, knees, and ankles in 90 degrees of flexion. Why was the insert designed with these features?

5. Sidney has a mental retardation diagnosis. What are your initial impressions about her cognitive skills and abilities? Is there evidence in the case that Sidney understands cause and effect? Do you believe that cause and effect is a prerequisite skill for the use of switches or is it a cognitive skill that can be taught through the use of a switch? What is the advantage of using a vibrating switch to teach cause and effect?

6. Do you have any initial impressions about Sidney's psychological performance components such as values, interests, and self-concept?

7. Do you have any initial impressions about Sidney's psychosocial performance components?

8. Do you have any initial impressions about Sidney's sociocultural environment at home and school?

9. Sidney's parents would like switch use to be incorporated into educational activities. This will be accomplished by identifying appropriate opportunities for switch use and consulting with the school teacher. Use Table 2 to list all of the battery operated or electrical appliances that may be available in Sidney's school, and to list the educational activities and tasks that occur within typical second-grade art, science, mathematics, music, and physical education classes. How could you incorporate the use of Sidney's switch using appliances within these classes?

   For example, if the students are painting pictures in art, Sidney could use Twirl-O-Paint® (The Ohio Art Company) for her project. During mathematics, when students are learning addition or multiplication, Sidney's classmates could place plastic pegs into group clusters on a Light Brite® (Milton Bradley) board while Sidney activates the light mechanism. Use the Canfield and Locke (1996) text to supplement your curriculum-based classroom activity ideas.

   It is possible to operate a computer with a switch when special hardware and software is installed. These assistive technology devices will be described in the chapter "Computer Access to Education: The Case of Greg."

Optional:

10. Read the chapter titled Real People and Their Success Stories in the book *Computer Resources for People with Disabilities: A Guide to Exploring Today's Assistive Technology.* (Alliance for Technology Access, 1994).

11. How does the Cordless Big Red® (AbleNet), mercury, grip, or puff switch operate?

Case Study: Sidney

Sidney was diagnosed with spastic cerebral palsy and mental retardation at a young age (see Table 3 for a discussion on cerebral palsy and mental retardation). Sidney is now a 7-year-old student who just moved to a new school district. She has a manual wheelchair for functional and community mobility but is unable to propel independently. Sidney's upper and lower limbs are very hypertonic but her trunk is hypotonic. She has poor postural control and is unable to sit independently. When her head and trunk are reclined toward supine, Sidney's arms extend and her lower extremities extend, abduct, and internally rotate. Her current wheelchair has a special seating insert that positions her hips, knees, and ankles at 90 degrees of flexion. The insert has lateral supports and the seat and back cushions are firm.

At the age of 4, Sidney began to learn to use a switch to control her environment and participate in new activities. She has progressed from using one vertical-toggle single switch to two single switches (2-inch diameter) that are attached to her wheelchair tray. She uses these switches to operate toys, a radio, and some kitchen appliances. Throughout the day, Sidney tends to rest her arms in a flexed position on her wheelchair tray. When she reaches for her switch, Sidney internally rotates and slightly flexes her shoulder and extends her elbow. She depresses the switch with a fisted grasp pattern.

Sidney remains nonverbal but uses a basic communication board that has slots for four 3-inch pictures. Sidney has a collection of approximately 15 pictures that represent people and activities that interest her, but only four pictures can be used on her board at one time. When provided with smaller pictures, Sidney's reach is occasionally inaccurate, making it difficult to determine which pictures she is selecting.

Sidney's parents are interested in incorporating switch use into Sidney's educational curriculum and ask you to provide some suggestions to the classroom teacher. One of the goals on Sidney's individualized educational program (IEP) is to maximize her participation in classroom learning experiences. The teacher at ABC Elementary has limited experience with assistive technology devices and would like you to provide specific activity recommendations. He also indicates a preference for switch activities that fit into regular weekly scheduled art, science, math, music, and physical education classes. Sidney is the only child with cerebral palsy in her school and she has not made any new friends.

Sidney's home life centers around sports and recreation. Her father is a baseball coach and her brother plays baseball and soccer. Sidney loves to attend the games and screams for her brother from the sidelines when he scores a goal. Her mother works full time at a local bakery and sends Sidney to school with freshly baked cookies every Monday. Sidney uses the PowerLink 2 Control Unit at home with kitchen appliances to bake with her mother. Her father has attached a switch to a red rotating light that Sidney activates during exciting moments at the baseball or soccer games.

Table 2: Battery Operated or Electrical Appliances Integrated in Classroom Educational Activities

Activities and Tasks	Lite Brite ™	Tape Recorder	Battery Operated or Electrical Appliances			
Art Activities						
Science Activities						
Mathematics *Learning addition and multiplication.*	*Classmates place pegs in groups while Sidney illuminates.*					
Music						
Physical Education						

Table 3: Cerebral Palsy and Mental Retardation

Cerebral palsy (CP) is a nonprogressive disorder of posture and movement that occurs following damage to the immature brain (Batshaw, Perret, & Kurtz, 1992). CP was the third most frequent health problem of occupational therapy clients in 1990, following cerebral vascular accident and developmental delay (AOTA, 1991a). Spastic CP occurs when the motor cortex or descending motor neurons in the central nervous system are damaged. Damage to these descending pathways causes hypertonia, hyperreflexia, and may cause clonus. Individuals with CP have varying degrees of involvement in sensorimotor, cognitive, psychological, and psychosocial performance components.

Approximately two-thirds of the children with CP have mental retardation (Eicher & Batshaw, 1993). A diagnosis of mental retardation requires evidence of significant subaverage intelligence quotient (IQ) scores, concurrent deficits in adaptive functioning, and an age of onset before 18 years (American Psychiatric Association, 1994). Adaptive functioning is an individual's degree of effectiveness in meeting the standards expected for his or her age, as defined by his or her cultural group in certain skill areas.

The information that follows will (a) provide students and instructors with resources to enhance the learning experience and (b) assist the student in completing the assignment.

Learning Resources

Books and Periodicals

Alliance for Technology Access. (1994). *Computer resources for people with disabilities: A guide to exploring today's assistive technology.* Alameda, CA: Hunter House.

American Occupational Therapy Association (AOTA). (1995). *Broadening the construct of independence: A position paper.* Bethesda, MD: Author.

Angelo, J. (1996). *Assistive technology for the rehabilitation therapist.* Philadelphia: F. A. Davis.

Canfield, H., & Locke, P. (1996). *A book of possibilities: Activities using simple technology.* Minneapolis, MN: AbleNet.

Denziloe, J. (1994). *Fun & games: Practical leisure ideas for people with profound disabilities.* Boston: Butterworth Heinemann.

Hammel, J. (Ed.). (1996). *Occupational therapy and assistive technology: A link to function. AOTA Self Study.* Bethesda, MD: American Occupational Therapy Association.

Lange, M. L. (1996). Environmental control units 101. *OT Practice, 1*(12), 27–31.

Lear, R. (1993). *Play helps: Toys and activities for children with special needs.* Boston: Butterworth Heinemann.

Levin, J., & Enselein, K. (1990). *Fun for everyone: A guide to adapted leisure activities for children with disabilities.* Minneapolis, MN: AbleNet.

Levin, J., & Scherfenberg, L. (1990). *Selection and use of simple technology in home, school, work, and community settings.* Minneapolis, MN: AbleNet.

Mistrett, S. G., & Lane, S. J. (1995). Using assistive technology for play and learning: Children, from birth to 10 years of age. In W. Mann & J. Lane (Eds.), *Assistive technology for persons with disability* (4th ed., pp. 131–163). Bethesda, MD: American Occupational Therapy Association.

Morris, L., & Schultz, L. (1989). *Creative play activities for children with disabilities.* (2nd ed.). Champaign, IL: Human Kinetics Books.

Pellicciotto, N. A. (1995). Incorporating technology into activity-based intervention. In M. Coling & J. Garrett (Eds.), *Activity-based intervention guide* (pp. 59–69). San Antonio, TX: Therapy Skill Builders.

Shuster, N. (1993). Addressing assistive technology needs in special education. *American Journal of Occupational Therapy, 47,* 993–997.

Swinth, Y. (1996). Evaluating toddlers for assistive technology. *OT Practice, 1*(3), 32–41.

Wright, C., & Nomura, M. (1985). *From toys to computers: Access for the physically disabled child.* San Jose, CA: Authors.

Supplier Catalogues

AbleNet. 1081 Tenth Avenue SE, Minneapolis, MN 55414. 612-379-0956. 800-322-0956.

Don Johnston Developmental Equipment, Inc. PO Box 639, 1000 North Rand Road, Building 115, Wauconda, IL 60084-0639. 708-526-2682. 800-999-4660. http://www.donjohnston.com

Flaghouse - Special Populations Catalogue. 150 North MacQuesten Parkway, Mount Vernon, NY 10550. 914-699-1900. 800-793-7900.

Jesana, Ltd. 979 Saw Mill River Road, Yonkers, NY 10710. 800-443-4728.

The Ohio Art Co., Bryan, OH 43506.

Sammons, Inc. PO Box 32, Brookfield, IL 60513. 708-325-1700. 800-323-5547.

TASH International Inc. Unit #1, 91 Station Street, Ajax, ON, Canada LS H2. 905-686-4129. 800-463-5685.

Toys for Special Children, Inc. 385 War burton Avenue, Hastings-On-Hudson, NY 10706. 800-832-8697.

This list of suppliers is not exhaustive, nor does it represent endorsements by the author or AOTA.

Web Sites

ABLEDATA. The National Institute on Disability and Rehabilitation Research—U.S. Department of Education, http://abledata.com

Assist-TECH, http://www.assis-tech.com

RESNA. Rehabilitation Engineering and Assistive Technology Society of North America, http://www.resna.com

Technology Assistive Resource Program (TARP), http://members.gnn.com/tarp/tarp.htm

Study Questions

1. Define or describe the terms **assistive technology device, environmental control unit, switch, and latched switch.**

2. List four examples of a low-technology device.

3. List two examples of a high-technology device.

4. Give two examples of environmental control units.

5. List four types of commonly used switches. How are the switches activated?

6. Describe how a switch can be used to turn a lamp on and off.

7. Your client has severe physical limitations and enjoys music. Describe how a switch could be used to turn a battery operated radio on and off.

8. Identify a switch and toy that could be used together to teach the concept of cause and effect to a severely disabled individual.

9. Explain how the concept of person-activity-environment fit applies to the selection and use of appropriate assistive technology devices.

References

American Occupational Therapy Association (AOTA). (1991a). *1990 membership data survey.* Bethesda, MD: Author.

AOTA. (1991b). *Position paper: Occupational therapy and assistive technology.* Bethesda, MD: Author.

AOTA. (1994). *Uniform terminology for occupational therapy* (3rd ed.). Bethesda, MD: Author.

American Psychiatric Association. (1994). *Diagnostic and statistical manual of mental disorders* (4th ed.). Washington, DC: Author.

Batshaw, M. L., Perret, Y. M., & Kurtz, L. (1992). Cerebral palsy. In M. L. Batshaw & Y. M. Perret (Eds.), *Children with disabilities: A medical primer* (pp. 441–470). Baltimore: Paul H. Brookes.

Brown v. Board of Educ., 347 U.S. 483 (1954).

Canfield, H., & Locke, P. (1996). *A book of possibilities: Activities using simple technology.* Minneapolis, MN: AbleNet.

Eicher, P. S., & Batshaw, M. L. (1993). Cerebral palsy. *Pediatric Clinics of North America, 40,* 537–551.

Glickman, L., Deitz, J., Anson, D., & Stewart, K. (1996). The effect of switch control site on computer skills of infants and toddlers. *American Journal of Occupational Therapy, 50,* 545–553.

Individuals With Disabilities Education Act of 1990, Pub. L. No. 101-476, §101, 104 Stat. 1103 (1990).

Lange, M. L. (1996). Environmental control units 101. *OT Practice, 1*(12), 27–31.

Shuster, N. (1993). Addressing assistive technology needs in special education. *American Journal of Occupational Therapy, 47,* 993–997.

Swinth, Y. (1996). Evaluating toddlers for assistive technology. *OT Practice, 1*(3), 32–41.

Swinth, Y., Anson, D., & Deitz, J. (1993). Single-switch computer access for infants and toddlers. *American Journal of Occupational Therapy, 47,* 1031–1038.

Technology-Related Assistance for Individuals With Disabilities Act of 1988, Pub. L. No. 100-407, 29 U.S.C. §2202.

World Health Organization. (1980). *International classification of impairments, disabilities, and handicaps: A manual of classification relating to the consequences of disease.* Geneva: Author.

CHILDHOOD OCCUPATIONS: THE CASE OF MIGUEL

"Although functional performance can be analyzed into specific skills and skill components, it is the spirit of a child that holds those components together. The maturation of a child and the complexity of the interrelationships between mind and body and between physical and social development are beyond human analytic ability" (Case-Smith, 1996, p. 3).[1]

Chapter Objectives

1. Categorize case information into the domains of concern of the occupational therapy practitioner as delineated on the Occupational Performance Profile Form.

2. Independently identify and document client goals.

3. Synthesize knowledge of the use of task analysis in pediatrics to independently select and design a purposeful activity for intervention.

4. Determine whether a remedial or functional intervention approach is appropriate.

5. Justify the use of a specific intervention activity or plan according to the criteria established in the document Position Paper: *Purposeful Activity* (American Occupational Therapy Association, 1993).

Assignment

1. Read the case about Miguel. Use the Occupational Performance Profile Form to document the information on the occupations that are important to Miguel, his family, and the teacher; Miguel's unique values, interests, goals, and performance components; and the contexts within which he performs. A copy of the Occupational Performance Profile Form is located in Appendix G.

2. In which occupational performance areas does Miguel's impairment (Down's syndrome) cause disability or handicap? Table 1 describes developmental expectations for children. Refer to Erhardt (1994) and Parks (1992) if more developmental information is desired. Table 2 describes Down's syndrome.

3. Why do you think that Miguel avoids fine motor challenges such as drawing, cutting, and printing his name? Why might he have difficulty learning to print his name?

   Why do you think Miguel requires a moderate amount of assistance getting dressed at home and at his preschool? Why might he have difficulty learning to (a) orient his shoes and clothing garments, (b) manage his clothing fasteners, and (c) tie his shoes? Why do you think Miguel needs close supervision on the playground?

4. What are the goals and priorities of this family and teacher? How do they compare with Miguel's values, interests, goals, and priorities? Use this information to identify the occupational performance areas, components, and contexts requiring intervention. Define your intervention goals using the Client Goals Form located in Appendix H. In practice these goals would be established in collaboration with Miguel's family and teacher.

5. Work individually or in small groups. Design a therapeutic activity for Miguel to do during one 30-minute direct treatment session. This purposeful activity should (a) address the concerns and priorities of this family and teacher, (b) meet the developmental needs of this child, and (c) satisfy the criteria for a purposeful activity as delineated by the American Occupational Therapy Association (1993). This document is located in Appendix K.

---

[1]From "An Overview of Occupational Therapy with Children" (p. 3) by J. Case-Smith in *Occupational Therapy for Children* (3rd ed.), 1996, edited by J. Case-Smith, A. Allen, and P. Pratt, St. Louis, MO: Mosby. Copyright 1996 by Mosby. Reproduced with permission.

OR

Work individually or in small groups. Assume that Miguel is expected to learn to dress himself. Complete the Occupational Performance Analysis Form on the task of dressing, in particular the activities of putting on underpants, socks, shirt, pants, and shoes. The Occupational Performance Analysis Form is located in Appendix A and C. Design an intervention plan to increase Miguel's independence in dressing. Consider using the strategies identified in the Occupational Performance Practice Model for Service to Individuals provided in the chapter "Task Analysis: The Contribution of Occupational Therapy to Health."

6. Does the intervention activity or plan used in Question 5 reflect a remedial or functional approach?

7. Present your intervention activity or plan to your class and explain why it meets the criteria of a purposeful activity.

Case Study: Miguel

Sue Ann is an occupational therapy student who is completing her clinical fieldwork at an agency that provides evaluation and intervention services to children with disabilities. During the first week of December, Sue Ann's clinical supervisor initiated an evaluation of Miguel at his preschool. Miguel is a 5-year-old Hispanic child with Down's syndrome who lives with his mother and grandparents. His mother works full time during the week at a coffee kiosk from 6:00 a.m. to 2:00 p.m. Miguel's father is a construction worker and both grandparents are retired. Miguel spends the first hour of each day eating breakfast and watching television with his grandfather. By 7:30 a.m. Miguel's grandmother gets him groomed and dressed for preschool.

Sue Ann participates in an interview with Miguel's mother, teacher, and both grandparents. During the interview process the family and teacher indicate that Miguel avoids all fine motor activities, cannot print his name, requires a moderate amount of assistance getting dressed, and is very clumsy on the playground. Miguel's mother expresses pride in her son and speaks highly of his accomplishments. Mother and teacher request assistance to "help Miguel academically and socially" and "improve his independence at preschool." Both grandparents suggest that Miguel should be more independent in getting dressed in the morning.

Books, constructional games, and gross motor play are Miguel's favorite activities. He spends hours looking at books and enjoys identifying different animal pictures. He likes trucks, motorcycles, baseball, and airplanes. He enjoys creating imaginary buildings with large foam blocks but his structures are not well designed or constructed. Miguel indicates that "Dad builds houses too" and that he wants to be a construction worker or a fireman when he grows up. Miguel appears to be one of the most active children at the school, is described as one of the most clumsy, and needs very close supervision on the playground equipment. He can throw a large ball with some accuracy but cannot catch. Sue Ann notices that Miguel's muscle tone is very low and his joints are hypermobile.

Miguel frequently attempts to direct other children's play and his behavior is described as destructive by the teacher. He is adamant and refuses to share. Despite these interactions, Miguel has not learned the names of his playmates. He is able to put on his shoes but occasionally has them on the wrong feet and cannot tie his laces. Miguel occasionally puts his own jacket on, but will often wear it backwards or inside out. He appears frustrated that he is unable to manage buttons, zippers, or snaps.

Miguel is able to cut out simple shapes with scissors within 1/2 inch from the outline. He is able to correctly identify the color green, can count to two, and is beginning to recognize the letter M in his name. When given a crayon, Miguel makes pictures with random squiggle lines using a palmar grasp pattern. He is able to draw a circle but is not able to draw a face.

Occupational therapy assessment of performance components indicates that Miguel has poor fine motor dexterity, postural control, bilateral integration, gross motor coordination, and visual motor integration. Visual memory, spatial relations, and position in space perceptual skills are delayed. He has difficulty with sequencing and spatial operations.

Table 1: Developmental Expectations for Children

Dressing	Puts on socks, shoes, and shorts (2 years); ties laces (5 to 6 years). Needs help with buttons and right or left shoe (3 years). Knows front and back of clothing (4 years). Buttons (4.5 years) and unbuttons (4 years) front-opening garments. Zips up front-opening clothing (5 years).
Socialization	Tells names of friends, relatives (4 years). Adamant about making own decisions (2 to 3 years). Parallel play (1.5 to 2 years); cooperative play (> 2 years); interactive play (> 3 years). Behaves according to peer group norm (4 to 5 years).
Educational Activities	Cuts paper with scissors (3 years); curved lines/simple shapes (5 years). Draws recognizable face (4 to 5 years). Palmar pencil grasp (1 to 2 years); static tripod (3 to 4 years); dynamic tripod (4 to 6 years) with pencil to draw circles (3 years), squares (4.5 years), and triangles (5 years). Matches objects (3 years); primary colors (3 years); 6 colors (5 years). Counts to three (4 years).
Play or Leisure Performance	Catches large ball from 5 feet (2.5 to 3 years). Catch small ball (>3 years). Throws overhand method 3 feet (1.5 to 2 years). Kicks a stationary ball (3 years). Rides tricycle without pedals (1.5 to 2 years); uses pedals (2.5 to 3 years).

Table 2: Down's Syndrome

Down's syndrome is the most common form of mental retardation and occurs in approximately 1 in 700 births (Kaplan & Sadock, 1996; Batshaw & Perret, 1992). Individuals with Down's syndrome often have a short and stocky stature, a small flattened skull, excessive neck skin, obliquely placed eyes, cardiac malformations, and hypotonia. The majority of individuals with Down's syndrome are moderately to severely mentally retarded (Kaplan & Sadock, 1996). The chromosomal abnormality that leads to the musculoskeletal structural malformations and immature neurons and synaptic connections that cause the syndrome are likely related to incomplete embryogenesis rather than deviant development (Batshaw & Perret, 1992).

Individuals with Down's syndrome generally perform at near-normal levels of intellectual functioning throughout the first year of life, but cognitive development slows thereafter. To receive a mental retardation diagnosis, the Diagnostic and Statistical Manual of Mental Disorders (DSM IV) requires evidence of significantly subaverage intelligence quotient (IQ) scores, concurrent deficits in adaptive functioning, and an age of onset before 18 years (American Psychiatric Association, 1994). Adaptive functioning is an individual's degree of effectiveness in meeting the standards expected for his or her age, as defined by his or her cultural group, in certain skill areas.

The information that follows will (a) provide students and instructors with resources to enhance the learning experience and (b) assist the student in completing the assignment.

Study Questions

1. How do occupational therapists judge the value of an activity for a given purpose?
2. Which activity(ies) would be appropriate to recommend that Miguel do during his leisure time: build plastic truck models, complete a coloring book of animal pictures, ride a tricycle, or dress up in costumes? Why?
3. Recommending that Miguel use sweat pants instead of jeans with a zipper front at school is an example of a remedial or functional intervention approach?

References

American Occupational Therapy Association. (1993). *Position paper: Purposeful activity.* Bethesda, MD: Author.

American Psychiatric Association. (1994). *Diagnostic and statistical manual of mental disorders* (4th ed.). Washington, DC: Author.

Batshaw, M. L., & Perret, Y. M. (1992). *Children with disabilities: A medical primer.* Baltimore: Paul H. Brookes.

Case-Smith, J. (1996). An overview of occupational therapy with children. In J. Case-Smith, A. Allen, & P. Pratt. (Eds.), *Occupational therapy for children* (3rd ed., pp. 3–17). St. Louis, MO: Mosby.

Erhardt, R. P. (1994). *Developmental hand dysfunction: Theory, assessment, and treatment* (2nd ed.). Tucson, AZ: Therapy Skill Builders.

Kaplan, H. I., & Sadock, B. J. (1996). *Clinical textbook of clinical psychiatry.* Baltimore: Williams & Wilkins.

Parks, S. (1992). *Inside HELP: Administration and reference manual for the Hawaii Early Learning Profile (HELP).* Palo Alto, CA: Vort.

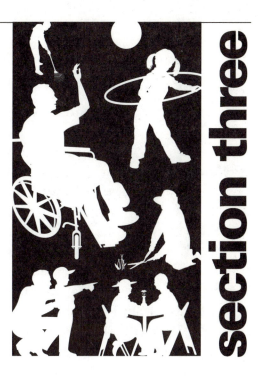

section three

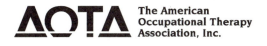

AOTA The American
Occupational Therapy
Association, Inc.

SECTION THREE: ADOLESCENTS

"Understanding the interplay of development and contextual factors is important to assessing risk and opportunity in adolescent development and in planning appropriate intervention" (Kenny, 1996, p. 476).[1]

The adolescent decade marks a transition from childhood roles, dependency, and reliance on others, to adult roles, personal directedness, and self-sufficiency. To make a successful transition to adulthood, an individual must internalize societal norms that will enable him or her to develop economic independence, form viable family units, and accept responsibility for self and others (Zahn-Waxler, 1996). Positive changes occur in the direction of increased competence and maturity. Adolescents gain reproductive potential, enhance their levels of self-esteem, and develop their capacity to establish and maintain social relationships (Peterson, 1993). Research suggests that individuals vary in their adolescent adaptation and adjustment (Hauser, Borman, Powers, Jacobson, & Noam, 1990) and the effects of change during the developmental transition of adolescence can be long-lasting (Peterson, 1993).

Adolescents must assume a variety of adult roles, perform new tasks and activities, and participate in new environments. When individuals have difficulty engaging in these new roles, tasks, and activities, occupational therapy practitioners begin to address the difficulty by first analyzing the dynamic relationship between the individuals and their occupations and environments. Intervention is then directed at reestablishing a fit among these three variables. Professions other than occupational therapy also emphasize a transactional approach to understanding the dynamic and interactive relationship between adolescents and their environments (Peterson, 1993; Zahn-Waxler, 1996).

Section Three provides occupational therapy students with the opportunity to refine their skills in task analysis by applying this assessment and intervention tool to resolve the occupational performance problems demonstrated by individual adolescents. An overview of the therapeutic value of different activities of interest to adolescents is provided in the chapter "Adolescent Activities, Crafts, and Games." The Occupational Performance Analysis—Short Form is introduced. Its use in completing assignments in this section will streamline the task analysis process.

The hypothetical occupational therapy client cases in Section Three provide realistic contexts for students to apply task analysis as an assessment and intervention tool. Occupational therapy students are required to independently evaluate client occupational performance profiles, determine appropriate outcome goals and objectives, and target intervention according to client priorities and needs.

Ali, Barb, Carl, and Dana all have psychological and psychosocial needs that must be addressed in individual and group therapy sessions. In this chapter, after evaluating client occupational performance profiles and specifying outcome goals and objectives for these four adolescents, students are asked to design a purposeful activity for one client or plan a group therapy session. Students will complete the therapeutic project or will role-model the therapy session to increase the accuracy of their analysis, develop skill in individual and group interaction, and acquire insight into the therapeutic value of group dynamics and client rapport.

Sylvie and Laureal will be attending a therapy cooking group. After evaluating both clients' occupational performance profiles, students must plan interventions. Students will use creative analysis to design and structure a purposeful activity for use during a group therapy session to address the sensorimotor, cognitive, psychological, and psychosocial needs of these adolescents. Students may find it helpful to participate in meal preparation to increase the accuracy of their analysis and acquire insight into the potential therapeutic value of social groups. Both Sylvie and Laureal have traumatic brain injuries and Sylvie is taking medication for depression.

Greg is having more and more difficulty accessing and operating his computer for educational and leisure pursuits. After evaluating Greg's occupational performance profile, students will use task analysis to assess the task and contextual demands of accessing a traditional computer keyboard and to identify the potential assistive technology devices and alternative input methods most appropriate for Greg. Logical thinking and creative analysis will be used to restructure tasks and alter environmental context to minimize disability, promote independence, enhance role performance, and maintain self-esteem. Students will also evaluate low- and high-technology assistive devices for computer access.

Daniel will be making the transition from a student role to participating in vocational activities and would like to work at a local grocery store. Although his mother is proud of his social skills and keen sense of responsibility, Daniel currently has difficulty performing many of the physical and cognitive tasks required by his

desired vocation. After evaluating Daniel's occupational performance profile, students are asked to use task analysis to conduct a job analysis to identify the performance components and contexts that would limit Daniel's employment success. Students are required to complete a consultation report to document their intervention strategies.

Completion of the assignments in Section Three requires students to use task analysis as an assessment and intervention tool to address adolescent activities of daily living, educational, play, and leisure performance areas. Task analysis is used to identify intervention strategies and target the performance components (sensorimotor, cognitive, psychosocial, and psychological) and performance contexts (temporal and environmental) that limit or restrict engagement. Completion of the case assignments will require students to incorporate remedial, functional, and preventative intervention strategies with clients whose occupational performance is impaired by physical disability, mental illness, or developmental disorder.

References

Hauser, S. T., Borman, E. H., Powers, S. I., Jacobson, A. M., & Noam, G. G. (1990). Paths of adolescent ego development: Links with family life and individual adjustment. *Psychiatric Clinics of North America, 13*, 489–510.

Peterson, A. C. (1993). Presidential address: Creating adolescents: The role of context and process in developmental trajectories. *Journal of Research on Adolescence, 3*(1), 1–18.

Zahn-Waxler, C. (1996). Environment, biology, and culture: Implications for adolescent development. *Developmental Psychology, 32*(4), 571–573.

ADOLESCENT ACTIVITIES, CRAFTS, AND GAMES

"The use of tasks and activities within a therapeutic relationship is a hallmark of the practice of occupational therapy. As occupational therapists, we select particular activities for the properties they possess that are most applicable to the treatment of the condition of concern. These properties are discovered through the process of activity or task analysis" (Llorens, 1973, p. 453).[1]

Chapter Objectives

1. Identify many different activities, crafts, and games that may be of interest to adolescents.

2. Develop and refine skills in task analysis by using personal engagement in an activity, craft, or game and completing the Occupational Performance Analysis–Short Form.

Using Activity Analysis to Design Purposeful Activities

Activity analysis refers to the process of analyzing an activity, craft, or game to determine whether its inherent properties motivate and fulfill a client's needs in areas of occupational performance or performance components (Llorens, 1993). This chapter contains a number of adolescent activities, crafts, and games. Although these activities may be of interest to some adolescents, the prescriptive or therapeutic use of purposeful activity is individual-specific because the meaning and value attributed to different activities is dependent on the client and his or her performance contexts (AOTA, 1993). In addition, "we [occupational therapists] select particular activities for the properties they possess that are most applicable to the treatment of the condition of concern" (Llorens, 1973, p. 453).

Assignment

1. Select and perform one activity, craft, or game that may be of interest to adolescents. Use the suggestions listed below if desired. Craft suppliers are listed in Appendix M.

2. Complete the Occupational Performance Analysis–Short Form (Appendix B) on the selected activity, craft, or game. This short form will streamline the analysis process by requiring documentation of only those performance components that are required to a moderate or maximum degree. Examples of completed Occupational Performance Analysis–Short Forms are located in Section Six.

3. Does this activity, craft, or game have potential therapeutic value for use with occupational therapy clients? Although the prescription or use of purposeful activity is individual-specific, what performance component deficits might be challenged or remedied through engagement in this craft or game?

The information that follows will (a) provide students and instructors with resources to enhance the learning experience and (b) assist the students in completing the assignment.

Bead Jewelry
Karin Sandstrom, Occupational Therapy Student, Class of 1998

Bead jewelry is believed to have been worn in prehistoric times by both men and women from around the world (Erickson, 1969). While men wore beads as a sign of their manliness, women wore them for decoration. Beads adorned the dead, which demonstrates their importance and value. Beads were also bartered in the early trade routes to and from the Mediterranean. Throughout time beads

---

[1]From "Activity Analysis for Cognitive-Perceptual-Motor Dysfunction," by L. A. Llorens, *American Journal of Occupational Therapy, 27,* p. 453. Copyright 1973 by the American Occupational Therapy Association. Reprinted with permission.

have had many different names including "trinket," "joyas," "bijou," and "bauble." Beads are still popular today and are worn by people around the world. A large selection of bead jewelry can be mail-ordered through Fire Mountain Gems (Appendix M).

Materials

- Beads (any size, shape, or color)
- Fishing line (heavy weight) or elastic cords
- Necklace clasps

1. Cut a piece of fishing line longer than needed to fit around your neck.
2. Tie the clasp to one end of the fishing line.
3. Place beads onto the fishing line in the sequence that you want by putting the fishing line through the center of the beads.
4. Once all of the beads are on, tie the other part of the clasp to the other end of the fishing line and then screw the clasps together.

Dream Catchers
Karin Sandstrom, Occupational Therapy Student, Class of 1998

The use of Dream Catchers has been credited to the Chippewa and Cherokee tribes. Dream Catchers are hung over beds and cradles to protect their sleepers from evil dreams. When dreams come at night, the pleasant dreams pass through the web to the sleeper while the evil dreams get caught in the web to perish with the morning sun. Beads and feathers are hung from the Dream Catchers, as demonstrated in Figure 1, to store the bad dreams and let the good dreams float free (Terzian, 1993).

Figure 2. Threading a Dream Catcher.

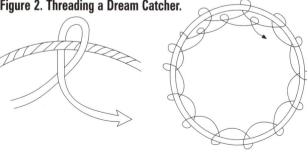

Figure 1. Dream Catcher.

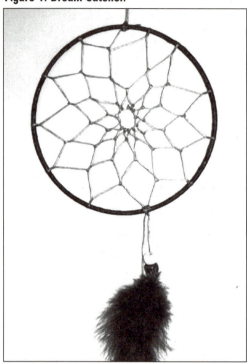

Materials

- Metal hoop
- Brown tape (yarn or suede can be substituted)
- Artificial sinew (or embroidery floss)
- Assorted feathers
- Beads

1. Wrap brown tape around the entire wire hoop.
2. Cut 6 to 10 feet of sinew and tie it securely to the hoop.
3. Wrap the sinew around the hoop about every 2 inches using half-hitch knots (Figure 2).
4. Once the wire hoop is covered use the loops already created for the base of the next set of hoops. Beads can be placed anywhere throughout the sinew.
5. Continue until you determine that tension on the sinew will produce a taut web. Pull the sinew to create tension and knot it in the middle.
6. Tie a loop of sinew to the top of the hoop so it can be hung.
7. Feathers and beads can be attached to the wire hoop for added effect.

Friendship Bracelet
Carolyn Silva and Susan Finora, Occupational Therapy Students, Class of 1998

Materials
- Embroidery floss (different colors)
- Scissors
- Safety pin

1. Choose four different colors of embroidery floss and cut two 3-foot strands from each color.
2. Tie the eight strands together in one knot approximately 1 inch from the end. Stick a safety pin through center of knot and secure to stable object as demonstrated in Figure 3A.
3. Take the first strand (A1) and wrap it over then under the second strand (A2) as demonstrated in Figure 3B.
4. Hold firmly onto the second strand (A2) while pulling up on the first strand (A1). Pull toward the large knot you made in Step 1.
5. Repeat Steps 3 and 4 to make a second small knot. You have now completed a double knot

around (A2). Leave the second strand (A2).
6. Take the first strand (A1) and make a similar knot around the third strand (B1), wrapping (A1) over then under (B1). Make a second knot around (B1) to complete a double knot.
7. Continue making double knots across the row around remaining strands. Strand (A1) will be at far right side of this row of strands when all double knots are complete.
8. Use A2 to complete a second row of double knots.
9. Continue making knots on the bracelet until desired length is reached. Alternate colors as desired.
10. When finished, tie a knot at the end of the bracelet. Cut string, leaving 1 inch of excess at both ends for tying around wrist.

Figure 3A & 3B. Tying a Friendship Bracelet.

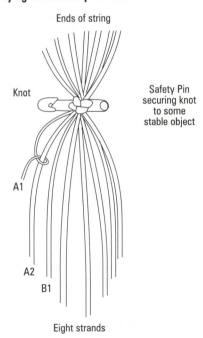

Ends of string

Knot

Safety Pin securing knot to some stable object

A1

A2

B1

Eight strands

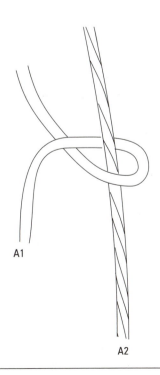

A1

A2

Ojo de Dios
Carolyn Silva, Occupational Therapy Student, Class of 1998

Materials

- Two wooden dowels (3 to 10 inches in length)
- Yarn
- Scissors
- Pencil
- Ruler

1. Measure and mark the center of two dowels.
2. Measure and cut a 5-inch piece of string (any color). Cross the dowels where they are marked and tie them together with the 5-inch piece of cut yarn.
3. Decide what color of yarn you would like to use for your project.
4. Secure one end of the yarn to the string that was used to tie the two dowels together.

5. Bring the yarn around one of the dowels as shown in Figure 4, Step 1.
   Bring the yarn under the next dowel and twist it around as shown in Figure 4, Step 2.
   Bring the yarn under the next dowel and repeat the twist as shown in Figure 4, Step 2.
6. Wrap the yarn around each dowel, moving clockwise until the dowels are covered within 1 inch of the ends. Hold the yarn taut when wrapping.
7. Cut the end of the yarn and push the end underneath the yarn at the back of the nearest dowel.

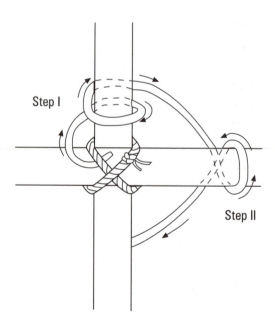

Step I

Step II

Figure 4. Tying an Ojo de Dios.

String Art
Rachel Budney, Occupational Therapy Student, Class of 1998

In the United States, the art of string pictures came to the foreground in the late 1960s and '70s. The acceptance of string design has been slow even though several outstanding string compositions are on exhibit in well-known museums around the world. Teachers of the arts or mathematics may use string pictures as a medium to bridge the gap between art and math (Sharpton, 1975).

Materials
- Six-strand embroidery thread
- Patterns
- Hammer and nails
- Scissors
- Pliers
- Wood block
- Tape
- Colored paints and brushes (optional)

1. Paint one side of wood block (optional).
2. Cut out paper pattern and tape it, centrally, onto the wood block.
3. Hammer nails into corresponding dots on pattern until about 1/4 inch sticks out. Pliers may be used to steady nails while hammering.
4. Straighten all nails using pliers.
5. Cut string into three 4-foot lengths and separate six-stranded thread into three sets of two strands each.
6. Knot string around starting-point nail.
7. Follow pattern on instruction sheet and tie off knots when thread runs short.
8. Upon completion of pattern, cut any remaining long pieces of string and push string down to the bottom of the nails.

The information that follows will (a) provide students and instructors with resources to enhance the learning experience and (b) assist the student in completing the assignment.

Learning Resources

Breines, E. B. (1995). *Occupational therapy activities from clay to computers: Theory and practice.* Philadelphia: F. A. Davis.

Drake, M. (1992). *Crafts in therapy and rehabilitation.* Thorofare, NJ: Slack.

Johnson, C., Lobdell, K., Nesbitt, J., & Clare, M. (1996). *Therapeutic crafts: A practical approach.* Thorofare, NJ: Slack.

S & S. (1996). S & S Catalogue: *Arts, crafts, games and activities for health care.* Colchester, CT: Author.

References

American Occupational Therapy Association. (1993). Position paper: Purposeful activity. *American Journal of Occupational Therapy, 47,* 1081–1082.

Erickson, J. M. (1969). *The universal bead.* New York: W. W. Norton.

Llorens, L. A. (1973). Activity analysis for cognitive-perceptual-motor dysfunction. *American Journal of Occupational Therapy, 27,* 453–456.

Llorens, L. A. (1993). Activity analysis: Agreement between participants and observers on perceived factors in occupation components. *Occupational Therapy Journal of Research, 13,* 198–211.

S & S. (1996). S & S Catalogue: *Arts, crafts, games and activities for health care.* Colchester, CT: Author.

Sharpton, R. (1975). *String art: Step-by-step.* Radnor, PA: Chilton.

Terzian, A. M. (1993). *The kids' multicultural art book: Arts & craft experience from around the world.* Charlotte, VT: Williamson.

IN SEARCH OF SELF AND OTHERS: THE CASE OF ALI, BARB, CARL, AND DANA

"Causal intent is a direct precipitant of action; purpose, action, and occupation are inextricable. The will to 'make a difference' pervades human beings. People feel that they must influence their world. This compelling feature of human behavior permeates human occupation" (Breines, 1989, p. 51).[1]

Chapter Objectives

1. Evaluate the occupational performance profiles of adolescent clients to identify the psychological and psychosocial performance components and environmental contexts that affect adaptation.
2. Identify and document appropriate therapy outcome goals and objectives.
3. Use creative analysis to design a purposeful activity to address a particular client's needs or plan a group therapy session to address mutual needs.
4. Describe the role of occupational therapy practitioners in promoting adolescent mental health.
5. Describe how occupational therapy differs from other therapies in its approach to mental health.
6. Role model therapist–client and therapist–group interaction.

Using Task Analysis and Activity Engagement to Develop Personal and Social Identity

The adolescent decade marks a transition from childhood roles, dependency, and reliance on others to adult roles, personal directedness, and self-sufficiency. The components of a successful transition include completing one's education, living independently, achieving economic self-sufficiency, and developing personal autonomy and a social lifestyle (Gorski & Miyake, 1985). Adolescents clarify their roles and career aspirations by defining a personal ideology through identification and confirmation of beliefs, values, and ideals (Erikson, 1964). The development of a personal identity occurs throughout childhood, adolescence, and adulthood.

Parents and peer groups provide the necessary social environment and support system for this transition.

Research has revealed a substantial increase in criminal activity, antisocial patterns, suicidal behavior, alcohol and drug abuse, low achievement, eating disorders, and depression among adolescents (Rutters, 1995; Zahn-Waxler, 1996). Adolescence is not a time of normative pathology and emotional turmoil, but is an age of vulnerability resulting from the developmental transition from childhood to adulthood (Carnegie Council on Adolescent Development, 1995). "It is important to recognize the coherence or continuity in development across life stages as well as the factors that contribute to discontinuity.... Understanding the interplay of developmental and contextual factors is important to assessing risk and opportunity in adolescent development and in planning appropriate interventions" (Kenny, 1996, p. 476).

Occupational therapy practitioners work with adolescents who have difficulty engaging in the new roles, tasks, and activities that characterize this developmental stage. Intervention is directed at achieving clients' goals in these occupational performance areas, and services may be provided through schools, community agencies, and hospitals. Task analysis is used to analyze the dynamic relationship between adolescents and their occupations and environments and to conduct evaluations and target intervention strategies. Occupational therapy is concerned with the consequences of adjustment problems that affect daily living roles, activities, and

[1]From "Making a Difference: A Premise of Occupation and Health," by E. B. Breines, 1989, *American Journal of Occupational Therapy, 43*, p. 51. Copyright 1989 by the American Occupational Therapy Association. Reprinted with permission.

socialization. Socialization refers to one's ability to respond to opportunities and interact with other people in appropriate contextual and cultural ways to meet one's emotional and physical needs (AOTA, 1994).

Occupational therapy practitioners use a number of intervention strategies to address the needs of clients with psychosocial and psychological difficulties, including (a) purposeful activity, (b) interpersonal relationships, and (c) activity groups.

Use of **purposeful activities** is what separates occupational therapy from the verbal therapies (CAOT, 1993). Active engagement in purposeful activity is a catalyst in the development of self and in the fulfillment of social membership and can be "understood as motivation toward achieving a sense of competence, self-reliance, social role learning, and societal contribution" (AOTA, 1995, p. 1021). A purposeful activity is selected for use in intervention by determining whether an individual or group project, craft, or game motivates and fulfills a client's psychosocial and psychological needs. "Congruence between the characteristics of an activity and the biopsychosocial characteristics of the person" qualify an activity as purposeful (AOTA, 1995, p. 1021; Fidler, 1981).

Interpersonal relationships that involve therapeutic use of self, interpersonal rapport, and collaboration characterize the helping relationship and are an essential feature of practice (AOTA, 1995; Mosey, 1986). This therapeutic relationship is "one of the most important and powerful tools in client-centered intervention" because the emotional atmosphere of therapy influences client expectations, attitude, and trust. This relationship transforms the adolescent's behavior from "constructive dependency" to "functional autonomy" (CAOT, 1991, p. 61).

Activity groups that provide both a therapeutic activity and a social context are designed to induce changes in individual members. The activity, social milieu, and group dynamics are all structured to replicate the daily living challenges encountered by individuals in their natural social environments (Davidson, 1991). The verbal and nonverbal interactive group process may provide a source of motivation, support, and feedback to reinforce learning and promote adaptation. Therapists who lead adolescent groups must be flexible, offer appropriate and sincere encouragement, possess interpersonal sensitivity, teach new skills, share information, and provide guidance (Gorski & Miyake, 1985).

Assignment

1. What individual activities did you participate in and enjoy when you were an adolescent? What were the activities' characteristics and qualities that promoted your personal and social development during adolescence?
2. What group activities did you participate in and enjoy when you were an adolescent? What were the activities' characteristics and qualities that promoted your personal and social development during adolescence?
3. Read the document *Position Paper: The Psychosocial Core of Occupational Therapy* (AOTA, 1995) and describe AOTA's perspective on the role of occupational therapy in addressing the psychosocial needs of clients.
4. Read the case profiles of Ali, Barb, Carl, and Dana, four adolescents who are being followed by your outpatient psychiatric clinic. Complete Project A to design a therapeutic activity for one client or complete Project B to plan a group therapy session.

Project A

1. Work with a partner to select one client. Evaluate the adolescent client's occupational performance profile and identify and document therapeutic outcome goals and objectives. If you would like assistance with this challenge, use the Occupational Performance Profile Form (Appendix G) and the Client Goals Form (Appendix H). Within the clinical context these outcome goals and objectives would be made collaboratively with your client and intervention team.

2. Select and design a purposeful activity for use with this adolescent. Individual treatment sessions in your facility are 20 minutes in length. Purposeful activities are therapeutic when they (a) are relevant, meaningful, and goal-directed; (b) elicit coordination among sensorimotor, cognitive, psychological, and psychosocial systems; and (c) promote mastery and feelings of competence (AOTA, 1993; Fidler & Fidler, 1978; Trombly, 1995). Ensure that the selected therapeutic activity addresses the client's goals, interests, values, and needs.

3. Determine how you will structure the activity and the engagement process. After analyzing an activity for its potential to address client goals, you may decide that adaptations may be necessary to maximize therapeutic value. Therapists who are skilled at analysis are able to select the most appropriate activity from among those of interest to a particular client (Trombly, 1995) or to adapt an activity that a client has selected to optimize its therapeutic value.

4. Engage in the activity you have selected and structured for this client. Take turns with your partner role-playing the client and therapist. This will provide insight into the therapeutic value of rapport and enable students to increase the accuracy of analysis and develop skill in client interaction.

5. How might occupational therapy practitioners work with other professionals to address contextual factors that influence this client's adaptation?

Project B

1. Divide into groups of five to design a therapy session for Ali, Barb, Carl, and Dana. Group therapy sessions last 30 minutes.

2. Evaluate the occupational performance profiles of these adolescents. If you would like assistance with this challenge, use multiple copies of the Occupational Performance Profile Form (Appendix G) to document information on the occupations that are relevant to each adolescent; their respective values, interests, goals, and performance components; and the contexts in which they perform.

3. Identify and document mutual client interests, values, needs, and therapy goals. If you would like some assistance with this challenge, use the Client Goals Form (Appendix H).

4. Select and design a purposeful group activity for use with all or some of these adolescents. Ensure that the therapy session addresses mutual goals and the interests, values, and performance component and context profiles of these adolescents. Purposeful activities are therapeutic when they (a) are relevant, meaningful, and goal-directed; (b) elicit coordination among sensorimotor, cognitive, psychological, and psychosocial systems; and (c) promote mastery and feelings of competence (AOTA, 1993; Fidler & Fidler, 1978; Trombly, 1995). If you would like some assistance in this area, review the Gorski and Miyake (1985) article listed in the Learning Resources section.

5. Determine how you will structure the group activity and engagement process. After analyzing an activity for its potential to address client goals, you may decide adaptations may be necessary to

maximize therapeutic value. Therapists who are skilled at analysis are able to select the most appropriate activity from among those of interest to a particular client (Trombly, 1995) or to adapt an activity that a client has selected to optimize its therapeutic value.

6. Participate in the selected group activity. Take turns with your group members role-playing each adolescent and the occupational therapist. This will increase the accuracy of analysis, develop skill in facilitating client interaction and managing group dynamics, and provide insight into the therapeutic value of rapport.

Case Study: Ali

Ali is a 14-year-old adolescent who lives with his father and brother in a small town. Six months ago, both parents agreed to a marital separation. Ali's mother and two sisters now live with his maternal grandparents approximately 500 miles away. Ali's mother has not called her sons since the separation and his father indicates that she apparently had been hospitalized a few months ago for a major depressive episode.

Prior to the family's separation, Ali was academically an above-average student who enjoyed race cars, reading, martial arts, and acting. One month after his mother's departure, Ali's father received a telephone call informing him that Ali had missed 3 days of school. When discussing this unexplained absence with his son, Ali's father received only a vague explanation. Although Ali returned to class, he failed to complete homework assignments or participate in class discussions. After 3 months of Ali's aggressive verbal outbursts at teachers and other students and a large backlog of incomplete course work, Ali's father removed him from school for the remainder of the academic year. Ali has stopped going to karate practice and recently canceled his engagement to play a part in the drama

club's year-end production. Ali's teacher and father jointly initiated behavioral health services.

During your initial interview with Ali, he complains that his father is "useless." Ali is disappointed that his father does not cook or clean their home as well as his mother did. He repeatedly describes his brother as "lazy." Ali dislikes performing the chores he has been assigned and indicates that he does not have time for school or karate. He is not aware of his mother's hospitalization and is upset that she has not called. Ali tends to focus on hypothesizing about and evaluating the potential reasons his family has been separated. Ali's father suggests that Ali is so preoccupied with his thoughts, distress, and desires that he is unable to concentrate on academics, acting, or karate. Ali's brother suggests that his reminiscing and rationalizing must be very tiring, because Ali spends 4 to 5 hours a day sleeping on the couch.

Case Study: Barb[2]

Barb is a 16-year-old who lives at home with her parents. She is the oldest of four children. Barb's mother is a recovering alcoholic who has been sober for 5 years. Her father uses alcohol occasionally but drinks excessively when unemployed. During several of these binges, her mother has taken the children to a shelter for battered women. A restraining order against Barb's father has been obtained on two occasions. Once Barb's father is reemployed and stops binge drinking, the family returns home.

Barb is an average student who has never excelled in any subject or sport. She was hospitalized at age 13 with a diagnosis of depression with suicidal behavior. Her mother indicates that Barb will turn on the television when she comes home from school and watch movies until three in the morning. Barb shows poor problem-solving skills, and her mother indicates that she takes little responsibility for her

[2]By Neil Penny, MS, OTR/L. Printed with permission.

actions. Barb has lost interest in spending time at the theater or in the shopping mall with her friends. Her boyfriend discontinued their relationship recently and has started dating Barb's girl-friend. Barb indicates that she feels "rejected" by both her boyfriend and girlfriend and admits feeling "worthless."

Barb's father has recently lost his job and tension has increased in the family. Her mother has threatened to leave if he starts to drink heavily. Barb appears to lack the coping skills to deal with the stress of recurrent family problems and has become more irritable with her parents and brothers.

Case Study: Carl

Carl has always been an above-average student. He is interested in the arts and has a number of artistic talents including painting, sculpting, and poetry writing. Carl plays football and tennis although he does not practice these activities regularly. Although Carl is a high achiever in many domains, he has anxiety and panic attacks that occasionally limit his ability to function in social and stress-provoking situations. These episodes are characterized by intense anxiety, palpitations, sweating, and sensations of shortness of breath and choking.

Over the past 2 months Carl has had a number of panic attacks that have caused him to avoid social outings. He has missed 3 weeks of school and high-school graduation is approaching. He has not decided whether to attend his graduation ceremony nor has he determined who he will invite to this momentous occasion. Carl expresses feelings of resentment toward a boyfriend who ended their homosexual relationship 2 months ago.

Carl uses alcohol and marijuana on a regular basis and indicates that he has been experimenting with cocaine and "other stuff" for approximately 1 year.

Three months ago Carl found out that he was HIV positive. At the request of his family physician, Carl sought behavioral health services. His family is not aware of his homosexuality or that he is attending therapy.

Case Study: Dana

Dana graduated from high school 2 years ago. She expresses disappointment with the completion of her academic studies and misses her position as a cheerleader. Shortly after graduation Dana was hired as a cashier at a retail clothing store. Although she makes very little money, she spends many hours shopping with her girlfriends. Dana has a large wardrobe of recent purchases that she uses for work and to go dancing every Friday and Saturday night. Dana attends aerobics three times a week and is considering taking courses to be a certified instructor. She is also considering an evening position as a disc jockey to supplement her income and support herself. Dana's mother is not supportive of this initiative.

Dana is interested in music and can identify an artist or song title after listening to only a few verses. Between the ages of 2 and 7 she traveled between pubs and taverns around the country listening to her father play in a band. Dana has not seen her father in years and lives with her mother. Dana does not speak highly of her mother and her mother's mental health problems, nor does she have positive memories of her abusive, alcoholic father. She has had a number of boyfriends over the past few years, but these relationships do not last more than 1 to 2 months. Dana indicates that she wants a relationship that is nurturing and satisfying.

Dana's binge-eating behavior began close to 1 year ago, but she was able to control weight gain by using laxatives. The frequency of Dana's binge episodes has increased and she is now purge vomiting to limit her weight gain. However, she is gaining weight. Dana has sought therapy services to deal with her anger toward her mother and feelings of guilt about binge eating and purging. Table 1 describes the disorders of these four adolescents.

The information that follows will (a) provide students and instructors with resources to enhance the learning experience and (b) assist the student in completing the assignment.

Learning Resources

Brollier, C., Hamrick, N., & Jacobson, B. (1994). Aerobic exercise: A potential occupational therapy modality for adolescents with depression. *Occupational Therapy in Mental Health, 12(4),* 19–29.

Gorski, G., & Miyake, S. (1985). The adolescent life/work planning group: A prevention model. *Occupational Therapy in Health Care, 2(3),* 139–150.

Study Questions

1. Your adolescent client drinks alcohol throughout the day to avoid unwanted responsibilities. This characteristic would be considered under which psychosocial or psychological performance component in *Uniform Terminology for Occupational Therapy* (AOTA, 1994)?

2. Your client's father is a binge drinker when unemployed. This observation is considered under which performance context area?

3. Which of the following activities would be most appropriate to increase social interaction between three depressed adolescents: checkers, bingo, or charades?

4. Which of the following activities would be most appropriate to assess self-concept: play a competitive game, draw a self portrait, or complete a 500-piece puzzle?

5. Describe four ways a therapist could provide positive reinforcement to a client in a group session.

6. Describe two ways a therapist could provide negative reinforcement to a client who behaves inappropriately in a group session.

7. What qualities distinguish occupational therapy's approach to mental health from the other therapies?

Table 1: Adjustment Disorder, Bulimia, Depression, and Suicide

Adjustment disorders are characterized by emotional and behavioral symptoms; marked distress; and significant impairment in social, vocational, and academic functioning that occurs in response to an identifiable stressor(s) (American Psychiatric Association [APA], 1994). Although adjustment disorders are most common in adolescents, they may occur at any age. Common precipitating stressors include school problems, parental rejection, parental divorce, and substance abuse (Kaplan & Sadock, 1996).

Bulimia nervosa is characterized by recurrent episodes of binge eating with inappropriate compensatory behavior in order to prevent weight gain (APA, 1994). Binge eating often occurs in private, and individuals frequently feel guilt, depression, or self-disgust after the episode terminates. Bulimia occurs much more often in females than in males and estimates of prevalence range from 1% to 3% of young women (Kaplan & Sadock, 1996). Individuals with bulimia are often of average weight, tend to be high achievers, and many are depressed. Their families tend to be conflictual, neglectful, and rejecting (Kaplan & Sadock, 1996). Self-evaluation is unduly influenced by body shape and weight (APA, 1994).

Major depressive disorder is characterized by sustained internal emotional state of depressed mood or loss of interest or pleasure that is a change from previous functioning, causing distress or disability in social and occupational functioning. The lifetime prevalence of major depressive disorder is 15% for the general population and 25% for women (APA, 1994). Dysthymic disorder is characterized by the chronic presence of these symptoms to a less severe degree. Individuals with dysthymic disorder commonly have substance-abuse-related disorders (Kaplan & Sadock, 1996).

Each year 30,000 deaths are attributed to **suicide** in the United States; however, the estimates of attempted suicide are 8 to 10 times that number (Kaplan & Sadock, 1996). The rate of attempted and completed suicide among young people is rising. Suicide is now the third leading cause of death in 15- to 24-year-olds after accidents and homicide. One to 2 million young adults in this age group attempt suicide annually. Almost 95% of all individuals who attempt or commit suicide have a diagnosed mental disorder, and highly significant psychiatric factors include depressive disorders, substance abuse, and schizophrenia.

References

American Occupational Therapy Association (AOTA). (1993). *Position paper: Purposeful activity.* Bethesda, MD: Author.

AOTA. (1994). *Uniform terminology for occupational therapy* (3rd ed.). Bethesda, MD: Author.

AOTA. (1995). Position paper: The psychosocial core of occupational therapy. *American Journal of Occupational Therapy, 49* 1021–1022.

American Psychiatric Association. (1994). *Diagnostic and statistical manual of mental disorders* (4th ed.). Washington, DC: Author.

Breines, E. B. (1989). Making a difference: A premise of occupation and health. *American Journal of Occupational Therapy, 43,* 51–52.

Canadian Association of Occupational Therapists (CAOT) & Health Services Directorate, Health Services and Promotion Branch, Health and Welfare Canada. (1991). *Occupational therapy guidelines for client-centred practice.* Toronto, ON: Author.

CAOT. (1993). *Occupational therapy guidelines for client-centred mental health practice.* Ottawa, ON: Minister of Supply and Services Canada.

Carnegie Council on Adolescent Development. (1995). *Great transitions: Preparing adolescents for a new century.* New York: Carnegie Corporation.

Davidson, H. (1991). Performance and the social environment. In C. Christiansen & C. Baum (Eds.), *Occupational therapy: Overcoming human performance deficits* (pp. 144–177). Thorofare, NJ: Slack.

Erikson, E. H. (1964). *Insight and responsibility.* New York: W. W. Norton.

Fidler, G. (1981). From crafts to competence. *American Journal of Occupational Therapy, 35,* 567–573.

Fidler, G., & Fidler, J. (1978). Doing and becoming: Purposeful action and self-actualization. *American Journal of Occupational Therapy, 32,* 305–310.

Gorski, G., & Miyake, S. (1985). The adolescent life/work planning group: A prevention model. *Occupational Therapy in Health Care, 2*(3), 139–150.

Kaplan, H. I., & Sadock, B. J. (1996). *Concise textbook of clinical psychiatry.* Baltimore: Williams & Wilkins.

Kenny, M. E. (1996). Promoting optimal adolescent development from a developmental and contextual framework. *The Counseling Psychologist, 24,* 475–481.

Mosey, A. (1986). *Psychosocial components of occupational therapy.* New York: Raven Press.

Rutters, M. (1995). *Psychosocial disturbances in young people: Challenges for prevention.* Cambridge, MA: Cambridge University Press.

Trombly, C. A. (1995). Occupation: Purposefulness and meaningfulness as therapeutic mechanisms. *American Journal of Occupational Therapy, 49,* 960–972.

Zahn-Waxler, C. (1996). Environment, biology, and culture: Implications for adolescent development. *Developmental Psychology, 32,* 571–573.

ADOLESCENT ACTIVITIES OF DAILY LIVING: THE CASE OF SYLVIE AND LAUREAL

"Occupational therapists feel that everyday activities are significant and meaningful. They have a firm belief that it is important to be able to perform everyday activities and that those activities are essential to one's sense of self-worth" (Fleming, 1994, p. 104).[1]

Chapter Objectives

1. Evaluate the occupational performance profiles of two adolescents and determine the task demands and contextual variables that influence independence in meal preparation.

2. Use creative analysis to design a cooking group therapy session to individualize intervention.

3. Describe why cooking might be considered an instrumental activity of daily living, a work or productive activity, or a leisure pursuit.

4. Explain the difference between basic and instrumental activities of daily living.

5. Describe the use of cooking as a purposeful activity to increase independence in meal preparation or to challenge and develop interpersonal skills and social conduct.

Using Task Analysis to Promote Independence in Activities of Daily Living

According to the Bureau of the Census, 44 million people over the age of 15 in the United States in 1991 and 1992 had difficulty with or were unable to perform one or more functional activities. Of these individuals, 11.7 million had some difficulty with one or more instrumental activities of daily living (IADL) and 7.9 million had difficulty with activities of daily living (ADL). Four and one-half million individuals have difficulty with or need personal assistance preparing meals, which represents 2.5 percent of people over the age of 15 and 9.3 percent of those over the age of 65 (McNeil, 1993).

Basic **activities of daily living** (ADL) include self-care tasks, and **instrumental activities of daily living** (IADL) are the more complex tasks that are necessary to maintain independence in the home and community (Lawton & Brody, 1969). IADL are more complex because (a) they contain a number of subtasks and activities, (b) they require a high level of proficiency in performance components in comparison to basic ADL, (c) each client has a unique approach to task performance, (d) client and therapist perceptions about successful performance vary, and (e) the therapist's background and familiarity with these tasks may vary substantially (Culler, 1993). Foti and Pedretti (1996) include mobility, self-care, and communication as ADL and home management, community living tasks, health management, and safety management as IADL.

Meal preparation and cleanup is a home management task that encompasses planning nutritious meals; preparing and serving food; opening and closing containers, cabinets, and drawers; using kitchen utensils and appliances; and cleaning up and storing food safely (AOTA, 1994). Occupational therapy practitioners work with clients to improve functional performance in this area when a greater degree of independence in meal preparation is desired. Cooking is also used in therapy as a purposeful activity to develop specific sensorimotor, cognitive, psychological, and psychosocial performance components. Cooking groups are often used as a context for developing and practicing interpersonal skills and social conduct.

---

[1]From "A Common Sense Practice in an Uncommon World" (p. 104) by M. H. Fleming, 1994, in *Clinical Reasoning: Forms of Inquiry in a Therapeutic Practice,* edited by C. Mattingly and M. H. Fleming, Philadelphia: F. A. Davis. Copyright 1994 by F. A. Davis. Reproduced with permission.

Assignment

1. Read the case about Sylvie and Laureal.

2. Evaluate the occupational performance profiles of both adolescents. If you would like some assistance with this challenge, use two copies of the Occupational Performance Profile Form (Appendix G) to document information on the occupations that are relevant to each adolescent; their respective values, interests, goals, and performance components; and the contexts in which they perform.

3. Make a breakfast, lunch, or dinner or bake a dessert and complete the Occupational Performance Analysis—Short Form (Appendix B) to define the task and contextual demands placed on a cook. Define the task as Meal Preparation and Cleanup according to the term suggested in *Uniform Terminology for Occupational Therapy* (AOTA, 1994).

   When completing the physical environmental section of the Occupational Performance Analysis—Short Form, assume that Sylvie or Laureal's home has the same layout (e.g., shelf organization and utensils) as the kitchen you used to make a meal or bake a dessert. Within the clinical context you will be able to interview clients or conduct home evaluations to obtain this important information.

4. Meal preparation or baking requires the performance of a number of activities. After evaluating the client profiles and completing the Occupational Performance Analysis—Short Form, identify which activities you would expect Sylvie to have most difficulty performing. Which activities would you expect Laureal to have difficulty performing? What skills and abilities might you address in therapy to increase Sylvie's independence in these activities? How might you adapt or modify the task or environment to promote Sylvie's independence? Review ADL supplier catalogues if you would like some assistance selecting appropriate adaptive cooking equipment (Appendix M). What skills and abilities might you address in therapy to increase Laureal's independence in meal preparation? How might you adapt or modify the task or environment to promote Laureal's independence in this task? Would basic meal preparation be an appropriate vocational option for Laureal? Review ADL supplier catalogues if you would like some assistance selecting appropriate adaptive cooking equipment (Appendix M).

5. Plan a 45-minute cooking group therapy session. Specify what the group will cook, how the task and environment (social and physical) will be structured, and what each client is expected to contribute. This purposeful activity can be structured to address multiple client goals. Therapists always try to engage clients in selected activities for multiple reasons and to address simultaneous goals, and these choices are based on knowledge of the client's interests, motives, and the impact of the clinical condition on performance (Fleming, 1994).

   How could you structure peer interaction to optimize the social benefits of this purposeful activity?

   How could you structure the group cooking session to incorporate some of Sylvie's physical and speech therapy goals?

Case Study: Sylvie and Laureal

Ron is a certified occupational therapy assistant who works with the interdisciplinary, outpatient rehabilitation team at ABC Regional Outreach Center. Ron has read the occupational therapy evaluation reports for two new clients, Sylvie and Laurel, and is in the process of planning intervention for them. He wonders about the possibility of arranging for these two adolescents to work together during a cooking therapy group.

Sylvie was in a motor vehicle accident 4 months ago and sustained a traumatic brain injury. She was discharged from the hospital 2 weeks ago and will resume occupational, physical, and speech therapy services as an outpatient. Her current therapy goals center around reestablishing self-concept, improving social conduct, and achieving more independence in toilet hygiene, functional transfers, and meal preparation.

Sylvie is 17 years old and lives in a small suburban home with her father and 10-year-old sister. Their father's work day is very long, so Sylvie has traditionally been responsible for all of the homemaking chores. Prior to her accident Sylvie had applied for admission to a computer science program at a local college. She has a very large circle of friends but is particularly fond of four girlfriends. One girlfriend visited Sylvie daily during her inpatient hospitalization and Sylvie apparently had plans to live with this woman during college.

Sylvie is independent in feeding and eating but requires minimal assistance (Sylvie performs 75 to 100% of the task) with dressing, toilet hygiene, and functional transfers, and moderate assistance (Sylvie performs 50 to 75% of the task) with grooming, showering, meal preparation, and her medication routine. Assistance with these activities is primarily provided by Sylvie's younger sister. Sylvie mobilizes with a standard walker but spends most of her day in a lightweight wheelchair. Sylvie must use both hands to operate her walker due to her poor balance and lower limb spasticity. Physical therapy goals center around increased balance and coordination, use of a walker, and independence ascending and descending stairs. Sylvie's functional communication is influenced by articulation problems. Her fine motor dexterity is affected by a mild tremor, and performance during functional activities is affected by generalized upper limb weakness. Testing and

behavior during performance of activities of daily living suggests difficulty with short-term memory, problem solving, and speeded motor response. Her father is concerned about how introverted Sylvie has become and comments about her "limited verbal interaction," "impulsive behaviors," and "inappropriate comments." Sylvie is currently taking antidepressant medication. (Table 1 provides an overview of traumatic brain injury and depression in adolescents.)

Laureal was hit by a car while riding her bicycle 8 months ago and sustained a traumatic brain injury. Laureal received extensive inpatient rehabilitation and outpatient services for 3 months after her accident. The family is now concerned about her apparent lack of progress in the social and cognitive domains and Laureal's family physician requested that occupational therapy continue to provide intervention in these domains. The evaluation report indicates that Laureal is a 16-year-old adolescent who lives with both parents and a 19-year-old brother. Prior to her accident Laureal spent most of her time at school or working out with the high-school gymnastics team. She had been a gymnast for 5 years prior to her accident. Laureal also enjoys reading and collects cookbooks with her mother. Her father is a full-time chef, her mother is a part-time librarian, and her brother works full-time at a delicatessen. Her mother and father both express concerns about Laureal's poor grooming habits, interpersonal skills, and future employment prospects. Laureal indicates that she is interested in pursuing a career in coaching, cooking, or hairdressing.

Although Laureal was very active with her peer group prior to her accident and shortly after discharge, her brother reports that these relationships have been deteriorating. He indicates that she appears to be "insensitive" to the needs of her girlfriends and her behavior is "too aggressive." It has been 3 weeks since any of Laureal's friends have called her at home. Laureal demonstrates little insight into her poor social conduct.

Laureal has gained independence in basic self-care tasks but relies on verbal cues and written reminders from her family. Laureal has difficulty performing many instrumental activities of daily living and apparently did not participate in any home management activities prior to her accident. Her motor performance is negatively influenced by generalized hypotonia and incoordination. Formal evaluation of visual perception indicates that Laureal's performance in this area is much below average and that

she has most difficulty with figure-ground. She has difficulty sequencing instructions or following multistep directions during complex, novel tasks. Laureal is able to remember information from long-term memory but her short-term memory is very poor. Her therapy goals center around improving social and cognitive skills to enable her to reestablish positive social relationships with peers, gain independence in instrumental activities of daily living, and explore possible future vocations.

Table 1: Traumatic Brain Injuries and Depression in Adolescents

Traumatic brain injury (TBI) is the most common cause of traumatic death and acquired disability in children and young adults (Ghajar & Harari, 1992). Motor vehicle accidents are the most common cause of TBI in adolescents, followed by assault, sports and recreational accidents, and falls (Centers for Disease Control, 1990). The sequelae of head trauma is broad and ranges from mild (82%), moderate or severe (14%), to fatal (5%) (Kraus, Rock, & Hemyari, 1990). Deficits in behavior, cognition, sensation, perception, or motor function are common. Ninety percent of the long-term neurological outcome is generally achieved within 6 months to 1 year postinjury (Ghajar & Harari, 1992). Increases in intelligence quotients continue throughout the first year of recovery with slow improvements thereafter (Molnar & Perrin, 1992).

Parents report that 10 to 20% of adolescents experience depressed mood, while 20 to 35% of male adolescents and 25 to 40% of female adolescents report that they experience depressed mood. Approximately 3 to 8% of adolescents are clinically diagnosed with major depressive disorder. Depressive disorders are more common in female than male youth, and Native Americans and homosexual adolescents are at increased risk (Peterson et al., 1993).

The information that follows will (a) provide students and instructors with resources to enhance the learning experience and (b) assist the student in completing the assignment.

Learning Resources

Books and Periodicals

Culler, K. H. (1993). Home and family management. In H. L. Hopkins & H. D. Smith (Eds.), *Willard & Spackman's occupational therapy* (8th ed., pp. 207–226). Philadelphia: Lippincott.

Foti, D., & Pedretti, L. W. (1996). Activities of daily living: Self-care/home management. In L. W. Pedretti (Ed.), *Occupational therapy: Practice skills for physical dysfunction* (4th ed., pp. 463–499). St. Louis, MO: Mosby.

Neistadt, M. E. (1994). A meal preparation treatment protocol for adults with brain injury. *American Journal of Occupational Therapy, 48,* 431–438.

Steward, C. (1995). Retraining housekeeping and child care skills. In C. A. Trombly (Ed.), *Occupational therapy for physical dysfunction* (4th ed., pp. 319–328). Baltimore: Williams & Wilkins.

Supplier Catalogues

North Coast Medical, Inc. 187 Stauffer Boulevard, San Jose, CA 95125-1042. 800-821-9319.

Sammons, Inc. PO Box 32, Brookfield, IL 60513. 708-325-1700. 800-323-5547.

Smith & Nephew Rolyan Inc. One Quality Drive, Germantown, WI 53022. 800-228-3693.

This list of suppliers is not intended to be exhaustive, nor does it represent endorsements by the author or AOTA.

Study Questions

1. Your client has difficulty with short-term memory. Which cooking activities might be difficult for this individual to perform? How could these activities be modified to ensure independence?

2. Define and give three examples of **instrumental activities of daily living.**

3. List four reasons why instrumental activities of daily living are complex.

4. Describe the contexts in which cooking might be considered an activity of daily living, a work or productive activity, or a leisure pursuit.

5. Which of the following cooking activities would be most appropriate to challenge and develop interpersonal skills and social conduct in a group of three adolescent clients: making pizza, eating pizza, or washing dishes?

6. Identify the perceptual and cognitive skills that are required to visually locate a particular food item in a cluttered cupboard.

7. Identify the neuromusculoskeletal skills required to operate a hand-held mixer.

8. Determine whether the following tasks are basic or instrumental activities of daily living: balancing a checkbook, taking a bath, dusting, giving yourself a manicure.

References

American Occupational Therapy Association (AOTA). (1994). *Uniform terminology for occupational therapy.* Bethesda, MD: Author.

Centers for Disease Control. (1990). Childhood injuries in the United States. *American Journal of Diseases of Children, 144,* 627–646.

Culler, K. H. (1993). Home and family management. In H. L. Hopkins & H. D. Smith (Eds.), *Willard & Spackman's occupational therapy* (8th ed., pp. 207–226). Philadelphia: Lippincott.

Fleming, M. H. (1994). Conditional reasoning: Creating meaningful experiences. In C. Mattingly & M. H. Fleming (Eds.), *Clinical reasoning: Forms of inquiry in a therapeutic practice* (pp. 197–235). Philadelphia: F. A. Davis.

Foti, D., & Pedretti, L. W. (1996). Activities of daily living: Self-care/home management. In L. W. Pedretti (Ed.), *Occupational therapy: Practice skills for physical dysfunction* (4th ed., pp. 463–499). St. Louis, MO: Mosby.

Ghajar, J., & Hariri, R. J. (1992). Management of pediatric head injury. *Pediatric Clinics of North America, 39,* 1093–1125.

Kraus, J. F., Rock, A., & Hemyari, P. (1990). Brain injuries among infants, children, adolescents, and young adults. *American Journal of Diseases of Children, 144,* 684–691.

Lawton, M. P., & Brody, E. (1969). Assessment of older people: Self-maintaining and instrumental activities of daily living. *Gerontologist, 9,* 179–186.

McNeil, J. M. (1993). *Americans with disabilities: 1991–1992. U.S. Bureau of the Census. Current Population Reports P70-33.* Washington, DC: Government Printing Office.

Molnar, G. E., & Perrin, J. C. (1992). Head injury. In G. E. Molnar (Ed.), *Pediatric rehabilitation* (pp. 254–283). Baltimore: Williams & Wilkins.

Peterson, A. C., Compas, B. E., Brooks-Gunn, J., Stemmler, M., Ey, S., & Grant, K. E. (1993). Depression in adolescents. *American Psychologist, 48,* 155–168.

COMPUTER ACCESS TO EDUCATION: THE CASE OF GREG

"Many people like me who cannot speak also have other disabilities. They cannot use a keyboard. Instead, they can use one or more switches, operated by a head or hand movement.... I hope that others find in this book [Computer Resources for People with Disabilities: A Guide to Exploring Today's Assistive Technology] the inspiration and the technology, hardware and software, that can help them to communicate better—to express their human-ness" (Stephen Hawking & Alliance for Technology Access, 1996, vii–viii).[1]

Chapter Objectives

1. Evaluate the occupational performance profile of an adolescent and identify the task demands and contextual variables required for independence in computer use.
2. Apply the person-activity-environment fit concept (AOTA, 1994) to the selection and use of assistive technology devices.
3. Use logical thinking and creative analysis to restructure tasks and alter environmental context to enable an adolescent to independently access a computer.
4. List examples of low-technology assistive devices and high-technology assistive devices.
5. Attach and use an alternative input device to operate a computer.
6. List different types of alternative computer input devices.
7. Describe AOTA's (1995) perspective on the definition of independence.

Using Task Analysis to Identify Assistive Technology Devices to Maintain Independence

Many individuals have impairments that cannot be eliminated through the application or use of therapeutic modalities. For example, Alzheimer's disease, Duchenne muscular dystrophy, multiple sclerosis, and Parkinson's disease cause progressive deterioration in cognitive and motor performance over time. To assist individuals in compensating for their impairments, occupational therapy practitioners restructure tasks and alter environments through the use of assistive technology devices. By teaching clients how to use these devices and providing practice opportunities, therapists enable individuals with disabilities to control their patterns of occupation. "The [occupational therapy] profession recognizes independence as a state of self-determination.... Individuals are independent when they perform tasks themselves, when they perform tasks in an adapted environment, and when they appropriately oversee task completion by others on their own behalf" (AOTA, 1995, p. 1014).

Assistive technology devices are used in practice as an adjunctive modality to enable clients to overcome disability (Dow & Rees, 1995). The term **assistive technology device** refers to "any item, piece of equipment, or product system, whether acquired commercially off the shelf, modified, or customized, that is used to increase, maintain, or improve functional capacities of individuals with disabilities" (Technology-Related Assistance for Individuals With Disabilities Act [1988]). More than 13.1 million Americans used assistive technology devices in 1990 (U.S. Census Bureau, 1990).

---

[1]From *Computer Resources for People with Disabilities: A Guide to Exploring Today's Assistive Technology* (2nd ed.) (Foreword by Stephen Hawking, pp. vii–viii), by Alliance for Technology Access, 1996, Alameda, CA: Hunter House. Copyright 1996 by Hunter House. Permission granted by Alliance for Technology Access and Hunter House, Inc. To order please call 800-266-5592.

Occupational therapy practitioners use low-technology assistive devices (e.g., typing aids) and high-technology assistive devices (e.g., switches, computers, power wheelchairs, and environmental control units) to provide evaluation and intervention services aimed at ensuring maximum independence (AOTA, 1991a). Computers have been used as adjunctive modalities to enable performance or as purposeful activities to treat a client condition. In 1990 approximately 40% of registered occupational therapists and 30% of certified occupational therapy assistants used computers for treatment (AOTA, 1991b).

The use of assistive technology with individuals with disabilities requires a team of professionals. The occupational therapy practitioner contributes to the team's evaluation and intervention process by identifying the input and display methods most appropriate for a client's sensorimotor and cognitive skills and abilities (Smith, 1991). This process includes (a) assessing client priorities, needs, and skills, and device characteristics; (b) matching client and device characteristics; (c) trailing equipment and systems; (d) recommending equipment and systems; and (e) training in the use of personalized systems (Dow & Rees, 1995). Therapists must consider a person's lifestyle, performance component capabilities, and environmental constraints to ensure useful and appropriate application of technology (AOTA, 1991a).

Occupational therapy practitioners require skill in task analysis to complete the initial evaluation and to create the best fit between client and device characteristics. Many assistive technology device specialists propose evaluation and intervention models that require the establishment of a fit between the person, environment, and technology (Cook & Hussey, 1995; Smith, 1991). This approach to evaluation and intervention parallels the occupational performance approach to task analysis.

Computer Input Devices

When impairments affect an individual's ability to operate a traditional computer keyboard or mouse, an alternative input device is required. **Peripheral devices** or **peripherals** refer to equipment that is used to input and receive information from a computer. The keyboard and mouse are examples of peripheral input devices. Head sticks, mouth sticks, key guards, and typing aide orthoses are low-technology alternatives that can be used to assist clients in accessing conventional keyboards.

Keyboards that offer alternatives to the conventional shape, size, and key location are commercially available. Miniature and expanded keyboards are **alternative input devices** that offer smaller- or larger-than-normal letter, numeric, and function keys. The standard key location is called QWERTY after the letter sequence on the top left row of a traditional keyboard (Figure 1). Some alternative keyboards offer a frequency-of-use layout to

Figure 1. WinMini with QWERTY layout.

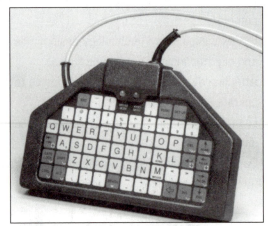

Photograph courtesy of TASH International, Inc. 800-463-5685.

enhance efficiency of movement (Figure 2A). The WinMini (TASH International Inc.) is a 7- by 4-inch keyboard that plugs directly into a personal computer (PC-compatible) keyboard port. This small keyboard is available in QWERTY or frequency-of-use key layouts. Figure 1 shows the WinMini with the QWERTY key layout. The MacMini (TASH International Inc.) is the Macintosh® version of the WinMini.

The WinKing (TASH International Inc.), MacKing (TASH International Inc.), Big Keys™ (Greystone Digital), Discover:Board™ (Don Johnston), and IntelliKeys® (IntelliTools, Inc.) are all large alternative keyboards that plug directly into a computer's keyboard port. Figure 2A shows the WinKing (21

by 11 inches) with a frequency-of-use key layout. Big Keys is a color-coded, alphabetized keyboard with extra-large numeric, letter, return key and space bar. Discover:Board (Figure 2B) is a large, colorful, programmable keyboard with speech output and overlay options. IntelliKeys (Figure 2C) is a large, touch-sensitive, programmable keyboard with overlay options and a port for switch access.

Figure 2. Various alternative large keyboards.

(A) WinKing Keyboard with frequency-of-use layout.
Photograph courtesy of TASH International Inc.
(B) Discover:Board. *Photograph courtesy of Don Johnston Inc.*
(C) IntelliKeys with standard overlays.
Photograph courtesy of IntelliTools, Inc. All rights reserved.

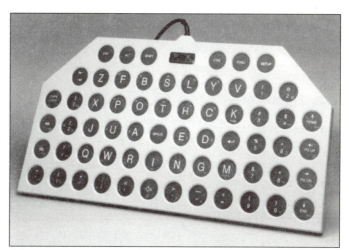

(A)

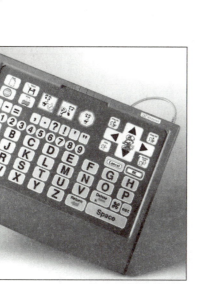

(B)

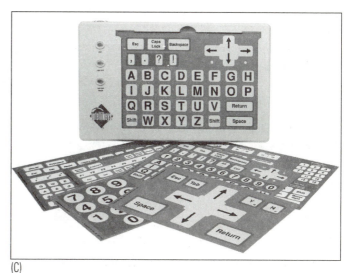

(C)

Switch Interface Systems

Alternative input computer devices include expanded or miniature keyboards, ultrasonic and infrared head pointers, voice controls, and switches. Indirect-control switch interface systems enable users to use switches to access a computer. These systems also allow users to (a) create and print custom overlays for programmable keyboards; (b) use on-screen keyboard displays, scanning, and Morse code to operate software programs; and (c) produce speech output. Indirect-control switch interface systems that are commercially available include the Adaptive Firmware Card™ (Don Johnston), DATAEntry (TASH), and Ke:nx® (Don Johnston) (pronounced "connects") systems (see Figure 3).

Assignment

1. Read the document *Broadening the Construct of Independence: A Position Paper* (AOTA, 1995) (Appendix L) and describe AOTA's perspective on the definition of independence.

2. Separate into groups of three or four. Read the case about Greg and evaluate his occupational performance profile. If you would like assistance with this challenge, use the form in Appendix G to document the information on the occupations that are relevant to Greg; his unique values, interests, goals, and performance components; and the contexts within which he performs.

   Why does Greg use a power wheelchair for functional and community mobility? Why does he need a special seating system? Why do you think that the upright position (90 degrees of hip flexion) is Greg's most functional sitting position?

   Why does Greg use his left hand to push his right arm toward the numeric or function keys or lean his entire trunk to the right in an effort to reach the keys at the outer borders of the keyboard? Why is he unable to return to a vertical position if he leans too far to the right or left?

Figure 3. The Ke:nx System.

Ke:nx is the key component for alternate access to the Macintosh. All of these input devices can be used with Ke:nx, an all-inclusive access package. In this photo, clockwise from the computer: keyguard, BASS switch, Ke:nx box, Mini keyboard, single switches, Rollerball, TouchWindow, Key Largo, and Ke:nx Easy Overlays. *Photograph courtesy of Don Johnston Inc.*

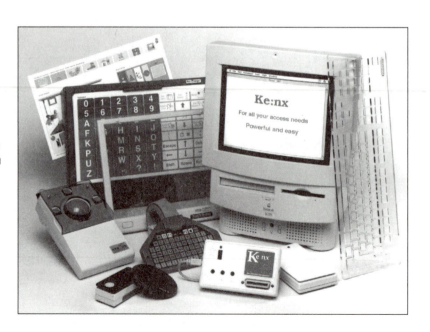

Why is Greg still able to control the joystick on his powered wheelchair?

3. Identify the task demands and contextual variables that currently challenge Greg beyond his capabilities?

4. You have collaborated with Greg and determined that the goal of intervention is to assist him in determining a method to independently access and operate his computer.

   Would repositioning the keyboard position on the table or a lap tray affect Greg's independence and success in accessing the function and numeric keys? How could you reposition the keyboard?

5. You have repositioned the keyboard so that it is closer to Greg. He smiles. He tried that trick already and it doesn't work. Greg is still unable to reach all of the function and numeric keys.

   What low-technology assistive device(s) would you consider trying with Greg?

   What high-technology assistive device(s) would you consider trying with Greg?

   Review the different low- and high-technology assistive devices that are commercially available through supplier catalogues and the World Wide Web sites listed in the Learning Resources section.

Optional:

6. Read the chapter titled "Real People and Their Success Stories" in *Computer Resources for People with Disabilities: A Guide to Exploring Today's Assistive Technology* by Alliance for Technology Access (1996).

7. Set up and operate the computer with a miniature and/or expanded keyboard.

8. Set up and operate the computer using a single switch using an interface device such as the Adaptive Firmware Card, DATAEntry, and Ke:nx systems. Practice using the scanning and Morse code access methods.

9. Use a mounting system such as the Mighty Mount (TASH), Universal Table Mount (TASH), Slim Armstrong™ (AbleNet), or Universal Mount (AbleNet) to set up a switch so that it can be controlled by a client's chin.

Case Study: Greg

Greg is a 15-year-old adolescent who was diagnosed with Duchenne muscular dystrophy as a boy (see Table 1). He drives his powered wheelchair to school every day using a joystick that is positioned just in front of his trunk at midline. He uses his right and left hand together to operate the joystick. Greg has a special seating system that tilts in space. When engaging in certain activities such as computer work, Greg prefers to have his trunk in an upright position with his hips at 90 degrees of flexion. This position is more functional for Greg than a reclined sitting position.

Greg has his own computer at home and school but he is having more difficulty reaching all of the keys on both keyboards. He spends many hours throughout the week typing his school work, playing computer games, and talking with friends using electronic mail. During a recent occupational therapy school visit, Greg indicates that the function keys at the top of the keyboard are "impossible to reach" and the numeric keys to the far right of his keyboard are "useless." Greg uses his left hand to push his right arm toward the function or numeric keys or leans his entire trunk to the right in an effort to reach the numeric keys. Both tasks require great effort and when Greg leans any distance he is unable to return to an upright trunk position. When this happens Greg laughs and calls for help. When working on a lengthy project, Greg eventually becomes very frustrated with the amount of assistance required. Evaluation of his bilateral muscle strength indicates that Greg has "poor minus" (i.e., poor –) shoulder flexion, abduction, and external rotation. His wrist strength is poor and his hand strength is poor minus.

Table 1: Duchenne Muscular Dystrophy

> Duchenne muscular dystrophy is a disease of muscle tissue that causes progressive weakness. Proximal muscles are most affected, but gradually all muscle groups become weak. Therapy is directed toward minimizing contractures, maximizing muscle strength, and compensating for weakness (Batshaw & Perret, 1992). Although occupational therapy practitioners may use purposeful activities to minimize contractures and maximize muscle strength, tasks also can be restructured and environments can be altered to compensate for weakness and promote independence and engagement in meaningful activities, task, and roles. This intervention strategy minimizes the disabling effects of muscular impairments.
>
> Occupational and physical therapists perform manual muscle testing to assess strength. When assigning a muscle grade, therapists consider the client's ability to complete a full range of motion with and without gravity and to hold a position. The degree of muscle strength ranges from zero (also referred to as 0/5), trace (1/5), poor (2/5), fair (3/5), good (4/5), to normal (5/5). The grade of "poor" is obtained when full range of motion occurs in a gravity-eliminated position only, while "poor minus" is obtained when only partial range of motion occurs in a gravity eliminated position (Hislop & Montgomery, 1995).

The information that follows will (a) provide students and instructors with resources to enhance the learning experience and (b) assist the student in completing the assignment.

Learning Resources

Books and Periodicals

Alliance for Technology Access. (1996). *Computer resources for people with disabilities: A guide to exploring today's assistive technology* (2nd ed.). Alameda, CA: Hunter House.

American Occupational Therapy Association (AOTA). (1991). *Position paper: Occupational therapy and assistive technology.* Bethesda, MD: Author.

AOTA. (1995). *Broadening the construct of independence: A position paper.* Bethesda, MD: Author.

Hammel, J. (Ed.) (1996). *Occupational therapy and assistive technology: A link to function.* Bethesda, MD: American Occupational Therapy Association.

Community Resources

ABLEDATA: The National Database of Assistive Technology Information, 8455 Colesville Road, Suite 935, Silver Spring, MD 20910-3319. 800-227-0216. 301-588-9284.

Alliance for Technology Access, 2175 East Francisco Blvd., Suite L, San Rafael, CA 94901. 415-455-4575.

Supplier Catalogues

Don Johnston Developmental Equipment, Inc.
PO Box 639, 1000 North Rand Road, Building 115, Wauconda, IL 60084-0639. 708-526-2682. 800-999-4660. http://www.donjohnston.com

Greystone Digital, Inc. PO Box 1888, Huntersville, NC 29078. 800-249-5397. http://www.caro.net.gdi

IntelliTools, Inc. 55 Leveroni Court, Suite 9, Novato, CA 94949. 800-899-6687.

Sammons, Inc. PO Box 32, Brookfield, IL 60513. 708-325-1700. 800-323-5547.

TASH International Inc. Unit #1, 91 Station Street, Ajax, ON Canada L1S 3H2. 905-686-4129. 800-463-5685.

This list of suppliers is not intended to be exhaustive, nor does it represent endorsements by the author or AOTA.

Videos

Child Development Media, Inc. (1994).
Adapting the computer: An overview. Van Nuys, CA: Author.

Center for Assistive Technology. (1995).
Applications for technology for persons with disabilities. Buffalo, NY: State University of New York. (Available from AOTA.)

Don Johnston Developmental Equipment, Inc. (1993). *Ke:nx basic training video.* Wauconda, IL: Author.

Web Sites

ABLEDATA. The National Institute on Disability and Rehabilitation Research—U.S. Department of Education. http://abledata.com

Assist-TECH. http://www.assis-tech.com

RESNA. Rehabilitation Engineering and Assistive Technology Society of North America. http://www.resna.com

Technology Assistive Resource Program (TARP). http://members.gnn.com/tarp/tarp.htm

Study Questions

1. Define the terms **assistive technology device** and **independence.**
2. Identify three low-technology assistive devices that can be used to assist clients in accessing conventional computer keyboards.
3. Identify two examples of high-technology assistive devices.
4. What three domains does a registered occupational therapist evaluate to ensure useful and appropriate application of assistive technology?
5. Identify two alternative keyboards and describe their distinctive features.
6. Describe how a single switch can be used to operate a computer.

References

American Occupational Therapy Association (AOTA). (1991a). *Position paper: Occupational therapy and assistive technology.* Bethesda, MD: Author.

AOTA. (1991b). *1990 Membership data survey.* Bethesda, MD: Author.

AOTA. (1994). *Uniform terminology for occupational therapy (3rd ed.).* Bethesda, MD: Author.

AOTA. (1995). Broadening the construct of independence: A position paper. *American Journal of Occupational Therapy, 49,* 1014.

Batshaw, M. L., & Perret, Y. M. (1992). *Children with disabilities: A medical primer* (3rd ed.). Baltimore: Paul H. Brookes.

Cook, A. M., & Hussey, S. M. (1995). *Assistive technologies: Principles and practice.* St. Louis, MO: Mosby.

Dow, P. W., & Rees, N. P. (1995). High-technology adaptations to overcome disability. In C. A. Trombly (Ed.), *Occupational therapy for physical dysfunction* (4th ed., pp. 611–643). Baltimore: Williams & Wilkins.

Hawking, S. (1994). Foreword. In Alliance for Technology Access. (1994). *Computer resources for people with disabilities: A guide to exploring today's assistive technology* (pp. vii–viii). Alameda, CA: Hunter House.

Hislop, H. J., & Montgomery, J. (1995). *Daniels and Worthingham's muscle testing: Techniques of manual examination* (6th ed.). Philadelphia: W. B. Saunders.

Smith, R. O. (1991). Technological approaches to performance enhancement. In C. Christiansen & C. Baum (Eds.), *Occupational therapy: Overcoming human performance deficits* (pp. 747–788). Thorofare, NJ: Slack.

Technology-Related Assistance for Individuals With Disabilities Act of 1988, Pub. L. No. 100-407, 29 U.S.C. §2202.

U.S. Census Bureau. (1990). *National health insurance interview survey on assistive devices.* Washington, DC: Author.

ADOLESCENT OCCUPATIONS: THE CASE OF DANIEL

"Roles for occupational therapy in transition programming are multifaceted. Occupational therapists not only teach functional daily living skills, they also help structure the physical, temporal, and social environments"
(Brollier, Shepherd, & Markley, 1994, p. 351).[1]

Chapter Objectives

1. Evaluate the occupational performance profile of an adolescent.
2. Evaluate the task demands and workplace contextual variables required for successful employment in a specific vocation.
3. Evaluate whether there is a fit between an individual, his or her employment tasks, and workplace contextual demands.
4. Use client goals and evaluation results to independently identify and document objectives.
5. Use logical thinking and creative analysis to develop an individualized intervention strategy.
6. Write an occupational therapy consultation report that demonstrates application of information compiled through task analysis.
7. Define the role of occupational therapy practitioners in transition services.

Using Task Analysis to Enable an Adolescent to Transition into the Workplace

Occupational therapists provide valuable assistance to adolescents with disabilities making the transition from school to adult roles, activities, and environments (Spencer, 1996). Transition services are mandated by federal law, which requires the provision of a

> *... coordinated set of activities for a student, designed within an outcome-oriented process, which promotes movement from school to post-school activities.... The coordinated set of activities shall be based upon the individual student's needs, taking into account the student's preferences and interests,*

> *and shall include instruction, community experiences, the development of employment and other post-adult living objectives, and, when appropriate, acquisition of daily living skills and functional vocational evaluation (Individuals with Disabilities Education Act, 1990, pp. 1103–1104).*

Occupational therapy practitioners use task analysis as an assessment and intervention tool during vocational evaluations to analyze the dynamic relationship between an adolescent, his or her anticipated job tasks, and expected work environments, targeting intervention to promote person-activity-environment fit. "Task analysis identifies not only all the steps necessary for successful performance of a task, but also the intellectual, psychosocial, perceptual, and motor skills required. Information gained from the analysis of a task is placed into a step-by-step learning sequence" (Brollier, Shepherd, & Markley, 1994, p. 351).

Within the school system, transition services require (a) collaboration among clients, families, professionals, service agencies, and members of the community; (b) curriculum models that promote performance in domestic, vocational, community, and leisure environments; and (c) the establishment and use of linkages among community service agencies (Spencer, 1996). Occupational therapy services could include any combination of direct service, consultation, monitoring, or referral to other agencies. Therapists assist in developing a client's functional skills and structuring the physical, temporal, and social environment to promote learning and independence (Brollier, Shepherd, & Markley, 1994).

---

[1]From "Transition from School to Community Living," by C. Brollier, J. Shepherd, and K. F. Markley, 1994, *American Journal of Occupational Therapy, 48*, p. 351. Copyright 1994 by the American Occupational Therapy Association. Reprinted with permission.

Assignment

1. Read the case about Daniel. Work individually or in small groups to (a) evaluate the fit between Daniel and his desired job tasks and workplace contextual demands, (b) delineate outcome-oriented goals and objectives, and (c) plan and document intervention recommendations.

2. Evaluate Daniel's occupational performance profile. If you would like some assistance with this challenge, use the form in Appendix G to document information on the occupations that are relevant to Daniel; his unique values, interests, goals, and performance components; and the contexts in which he performs.

   Use the case information to hypothesize about Daniel's current performance component skills and abilities. For example, what skills must he possess to independently complete bank transaction slips to deposit earnings? Why might Daniel's room always look like a "mess" with his "belongings all over the floor"?

3. Complete the Occupational Performance Analysis - Short Form (Appendix B) to define the task and workplace contextual requirements of an inventory clerk at Catriona's grocery store. Define the task as Work or Job Performance according to the term suggested in *Uniform Terminology for Occupational Therapy.* This term refers to the performance of job tasks in a timely and effective manner including necessary work behaviors (American Occupational Therapy Association, 1994).

   Consider the information you have been provided to form some hypotheses about the activities that Daniel will be required to perform. For example, Daniel may (a) work with the inventory manager to open boxes, count, and catalogue new inventory; (b) transport boxes of merchandise to appropriate shelf space; (c) put merchandise on appropriate shelves.

   Spend some time hypothesizing about all of the temporal, social, and physical environmental variables that would influence this inventory clerk job. For example, what temporal cues are available to assist Daniel in identifying when to begin or end a task? How high are most grocery store shelves? Use this information to complete the Occupational Performance Analysis–Short Form. In clinical practice you may be able to visit Catriona's grocery store to complete a more detailed job site analysis.

4. In an attempt to understand current function and imagine future potential, therapists think about the person, the disability, the meaning the illness or disease has for the client, and the performance contexts in which the client lives (Fleming, 1994). After evaluating Daniel's occupational performance profile, the job tasks of an inventory clerk, and the workplace contextual requirements at Catriona's grocery store, identify which activities would challenge Daniel beyond his current capabilities?

5. Use the information compiled in Question 4 to make a list of specific, measurable, outcome-oriented objectives for Daniel's goal of earning a living by working at Catriona's grocery store. In clinical practice these goals and objectives would be established in collaboration with Daniel, his family, the teacher, and Catriona. The Client Goals Form is located in Appendix H.

6. Use the information collected in Question 5 to identify intervention recommendations. If you would like some assistance with this challenge, consider using the various intervention strategies identified in the Occupational Performance Practice Model for Service to Individuals outlined in the chapter "Task Analysis: The Contribution of Occupational Therapy to Health."

7. Write an occupational therapy consultation report to document your recommendations. A sample documentation format is provided on the form Occupational Therapy Consultation Report: Transition Services that follows. The categories listed on the form under Recommendations for Educational Programming are selected from the Occupational Performance Practice Model for Service to Individuals.

Case Study: Daniel

Daniel is a 14-year-old adolescent who lives with his parents and 16-year-old sister. He expects to graduate from high school within the next few years, and his teachers and parents have requested special-education transition services. During recent discussions with these individuals about his future, Daniel has indicated that he would like to find a girlfriend, earn a living, and live in an apartment with his sister.

Daniel is a very social adolescent who is friendly with other students and all of his neighbors. His mother indicates that she is particularly proud of Daniel's social skills and keen sense of responsibility. Daniel's sister, however, remarks sarcastically that he "talks to everyone whether they want to talk to him or not" and "is excessively preoccupied being responsible for his stuff." Daniel was diagnosed with spastic quadriplegia and mental retardation at a very young age. Today he ambulates short distances around his community with a rolling walker. He avoids uneven terrain and must use curb cuts to cross the street. Although Daniel has a number of friends at school, he is disappointed that he doesn't have a "real girlfriend." His performance in mathematics is particularly poor and is a source of frustration. Daniel can count objects but has difficulty remembering or mentally manipulating numbers. He must use paper and pencil to add or subtract numbers greater than 10 and he requires a calculator for multiplication or division. He has great difficulty conceptualizing fractions and negative values, but understands the decimal system of currency. Daniel uses a digital watch to tell time, but has difficulty adding values of time or projecting the amount of time he will take to complete a project.

Daniel has his own bank account and independently completes a transaction slip to deposit any earnings from performing extra domestic chores. He collects the family's mail each day but requires assistance to reach envelopes he drops on the floor. His sister collects the newspaper or any parcel deliveries when they are either too heavy or bulky for Daniel to carry while manipulating his walker. Daniel is responsible for purchasing the familys bread and milk, which he carries home in his backpack. Although Daniel has been saving money to move out with his sister, she plans to live with a girlfriend when she starts college. Daniel continues to hope that his sister will change her mind. When asked why she wouldn't consider living with her brother, his sister responds, "I couldn't take care of him…. He can't cook anything, his room is always a mess, his belongings are all over the floor, and he couldn't afford the rent."

Daniel's family has lived in a condominium complex in a large metropolitan area for over a decade. Over the years Daniel has befriended a local grocery store owner, Catriona, who operates her business adjacent to the family's condominium complex. Daniel has spent many hours doing odd jobs to help Catriona's workers and he speaks admirably about their employment opportunities. Two months ago Daniel's parents approached Catriona about possible future employment for their son. Catriona responded positively but indicated that Daniel would have to be able to work independently for 3 to 4 hours at one time. She recommended that he work toward a position as an inventory control clerk.

Catriona's grocery store employs approximately 10 people who work either full or part time. Two inventory control clerks are responsible for collaborating with the inventory manager to catalogue new merchandise on arrival, transporting new merchandise from the receiving office to the store shelves, and modifying produce price signs during store sales. All employees are responsible for assisting customers, minimizing theft, and performing odd jobs as business requires them.

Laurie is an occupational therapist who works as a consultant to ABC School District; she provides school-based transition services to individuals with disabilities. Laurie participates in screening and evaluation and provides intervention services directed at adapting tasks and materials, altering performance component requirements, and modifying environmental constraints. Laurie returns to her office to write a consultation report to assist the educational team in compiling a coordinated set of activities to facilitate Daniel's successful future employment.

The information that follows will (a) provide students and instructors with resources to enhance the learning experience and (b) assist the student in completing the assignment.

Learning Resources

Brollier, C., Shepherd, J., & Markley, K. F. (1994). Transition from school to community living. *American Journal of Occupational Therapy, 48,* 346–353.

Spencer, K., & Sample, P. (1993). Transition planning and services. In C. Royeen (Ed.), *Classroom applications for school-based practice* (pp. 6–48). Rockville, MD: American Occupational Therapy Association.

Study Questions

1. List five activities required to complete the transport of new merchandise from a receiving office to a store shelf. List the physical environmental constraints that influence each of these activities.

2. Your client is unable to pick up objects from the floor. How might you restructure the task using adapted equipment? What performance components within the individual could be addressed to increase skill in this movement?

3. Your client's goal is to be able to operate a motorized scooter to carry large parcels. Define three specific, measurable, outcome-oriented objectives.

4. What is the role of the occupational therapy practitioner in providing transition services to adolescents with disabilities?

Occupational Therapy Consultation Report:
Transition Services

Outcome-Oriented Vocational Exploration Goals and Objectives:

Recommendations for Educational Programming:

• **Restructure the Following Tasks:**

• **Enhance Daniel's Ability to Perform the Following Activities:**

Occupational Therapy Consultation Report, page 2

• **Provide Practice Opportunities for the Following Skills:**

• **Collaborate with the Grocery Store Employees to:**

• **Alter the Workplace Environment by:**

• **Use the Following Adapted Equipment or Assistive Technology Devices:**

_____   _____

Occupational Therapist   **Date**

Note: The categories listed under "Recommendations for Educational Programming" are selected from the Occupational Performance Practice Model for Service to Individuals outlined in the chapter "Task Analysis: The Contribution of Occupational Therapy to Health."

References

American Occupational Therapy Association. (1994). *Uniform terminology for occupational therapy* (3rd ed.). Bethesda, MD: Author.

Brollier, C., Shepherd, J., & Markley, K. F. (1994). Transition from school to community living. *American Journal of Occupational Therapy, 48,* 346–353.

Fleming, M. H. (1994). A common sense practice in an uncommon world. In C. Mattingly & M. H. Fleming (Eds.), *Clinical reasoning: Forms of inquiry in a therapeutic practice* (pp. 94–116). Philadelphia: F. A. Davis.

Individuals with Disabilities Education Act of 1990, Pub. L. No. 101-476, §101, 104, Stat. 1103 (1990).

Spencer, K. C. (1996). Transition services: From school to adult life. In J. Case-Smith, A. S. Allen, & P. N. Pratt (Eds), *Occupational therapy for children* (3rd ed., pp. 808–822). St. Louis, MO: Mosby.

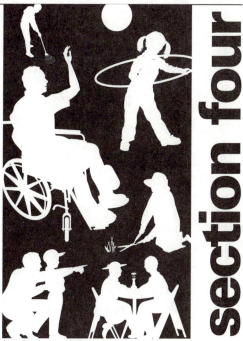

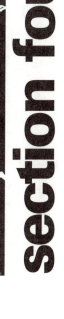

AOTA The American
Occupational Therapy
Association, Inc.

SECTION FOUR: ADULTS

"Human life includes a process of continuous adaptation. Adaptation is a change in function that promotes survival and self-actualization. Biological, psychological, and environmental factors may interrupt the adaptation process at any time throughout the life cycle. Dysfunction may occur when adaptation is impaired. Purposeful activity facilitates the adaptive process" (American Occupational Therapy Association, 1995, p. 1026).[1]

The American Occupational Therapy Association (1996) reports that 28% of registered occupational therapists and 18% of certified occupational therapy assistants provided services to adults between 19 and 64 years of age in 1995. Occupational therapy practitioners contribute to the health and wellness of individuals by working with clients to enable, maintain, or restore their occupational performance to enhance function, self-esteem, self-efficacy, and well-being (AOTA, 1994; CAOT, 1990; Trombly, 1995). This vision is accomplished in practice through the use of task analysis as a key process skill for assessment and intervention (Mosey, 1981; Trombly, 1995).

Section Four provides the opportunity for occupational therapy students to refine task analysis skills by applying this assessment and intervention tool to resolve the occupational performance problems demonstrated by adults between 28 and 52 years of age with acute or chronic disabilities. Students will review the literature and prepare a presentation on the therapeutic value of a selected activity, craft, or game appropriate for use with adult clients in the chapter "Adult Activities, Crafts, and Games." The hypothetical occupational therapy client cases in Section Four provide realistic contexts for the application of task analysis as an assessment and intervention tool. These clinical vignettes provide students with the opportunity to practice applying the Occupational Performance Practice Model for Services to Individuals, which was introduced in the chapter "Task Analysis: The Contribution of Occupational Therapy to Health."

Laurie is a 40-year-old wife, mother, and chief executive officer. She was in a motor vehicle accident 1 year ago and received rehabilitation services to recover from a left-upper-limb above-elbow amputation, extensive internal injuries, and multiple abrasions to her face and upper body. Despite achieving independence in self-care tasks, Laurie did not return to work following her injury. Laurie eventually sought medical services for depression at the request of her husband and attempted suicide 2 weeks later. Occupational therapy students are required to (a) evaluate this client's occupational performance profile and the apparent discrepancy between skill attainment and actual performance, and (b) design intervention to address client needs. The influence of personal causation, self-efficacy, and self-concept on adaptation is discussed.

Dawn is a 52-year-old woman who recently had a hip replacement. The surgeon's postsurgical restrictions for hip range of movement limit Dawn's ability to engage in basic activities of daily living. Dawn will be discharged from a rehabilitation hospital and must become independent in dressing and bathing. After evaluating this client's occupational performance profile, students will be required to

[1]From "The Philosophical Base of Occupational Therapy," by the American Occupational Therapy Association, 1995, *American Journal of Occupational Therapy, 49*, p. 1026. Reprinted with permission.

assess the task and contextual demands of dressing and bathing and determine the performance capabilities required to meet those demands. Logical thinking and creative analysis will be used to select appropriate adaptive equipment to alter task demands and environmental contexts. Students must also practice teaching a client new techniques for performing these activities of daily living.

Rick is a 28-year-old rehabilitation engineer who sustained a recent lower back and wrist injury. He would like to return to his job as a designer and fabricator of adapted equipment for children with disabilities. Students will complete an Occupational Performance/ Biomechanical Analysis Form by applying the biomechanical frame of reference to worker rehabilitation. Task analysis will be required to (a) identify performance components and contexts that affect work performance; (b) design a purposeful activity to build strength, endurance, and range of joint motion; and (c) recommend adapted equipment or alterations in the physical environmental context. By engaging in a woodworking or sewing project themselves, students will gain insight into Rick's job demands and have the opportunity to design and fabricate adapted equipment or sew. Completion of an optional neuromusculoskeletal assessment enables students in registered occupational therapy educational programs to apply knowledge from anatomy and kinesiology course work.

Jeff is a 32-year-old sports commentator who sustained a mild traumatic brain injury and a midthoracic, complete spinal cord injury during a recent motor vehicle accident. He would like to learn how to drive using assistive technology devices and participate in wheelchair sports. After evaluating Jeff's occupational performance profile, students will complete the Occupational Performance Analysis–Short Form to evaluate the task and contextual demands of driving a vehicle or participating in a sport that interests Jeff. Logical thinking and creative analysis are used to design intervention strategies that will enable Jeff to return to a meaningful and healthy lifestyle.

Rena is a 40-year-old, single mother who had a cerebral vascular accident. Rena must return to her role as a mother, primary caregiver, homemaker, and librarian. Students will be required to analyze the impact of this neurological condition on Rena's occupational performance profile and predict potential future performance. Task analysis is used to evaluate the fit between Rena and her desired roles, tasks, and activities. Creative analysis is used to design individualized intervention using a remedial or functional approach. The availability of community resource agencies and social support systems is reviewed.

Completion of the assignments in Section Four requires the use of task analysis as an assessment and intervention tool to address adult activities of daily living, work and productive activities, and play and leisure performance areas. Task analysis is used to identify and direct intervention strategies at the performance components (sensorimotor, cognitive, psychosocial, and psychological) and performance contexts (temporal and environmental) that limit or restrict engagement. Completion of the case assignments will require students to incorporate remedial, functional, and preventative intervention strategies with adults whose occupational performance is impaired by acute or chronic disabilities.

References

American Occupational Therapy Association (AOTA). (1994). *Uniform terminology for occupational therapy* (3rd ed.). Bethesda, MD: Author.

AOTA. (1995). The philosophical base of occupational therapy. *American Journal of Occupational Therapy, 49,* 1026.

AOTA. (1996). OT practitioners work more with elderly patients. *OT Practice, 1*(3), 17.

Canadian Association of Occupational Therapists (CAOT). (1990). *Position statement: Occupational therapy: Core identity.* Toronto, ON: Author.

Mosey, A. C. (1981). *Occupational therapy: Configuration of a profession.* New York: Raven Press.

Trombly, C. A. (1995). Purposeful activity. In C. A. Trombly (Ed.), *Occupational therapy for physical dysfunction* (4th ed., pp. 237–253). Baltimore: Williams & Wilkins.

ADULT ACTIVITIES, CRAFTS, AND GAMES

"Emerging occupational theory holds that there are inherent factors within tasks, activities, and occupation components that satisfy needs; engage intrinsic motivation; and facilitate growth, development, and adaptation to life roles and performance expectation" (Llorens, 1986, p. 104).[1]

Chapter Objectives

1. Become familiar with the range of purposeful activities used by occupational therapy practitioners with adults and seniors.
2. Access the professional literature.
3. Evaluate a purposeful activity for its potential therapeutic value.
4. Describe the appropriate use of physical agent modalities in clinical practice.
5. Compare the use of activity in occupational therapy to other professions.
6. Prepare and give a presentation on a selected purposeful activity.

Selecting and Researching Purposeful Activities

Countless examples of the different activities used by occupational therapy practitioners can be cited. All purposeful activities, however, have inherent properties that make them appropriate tools for use in therapy. In addition, the prescriptive use of purposeful activity is individual-specific because the meaning and value attributed to different activities is dependent on the client and his or her performance contexts (AOTA, 1993). "As occupational therapists, we select particular activities for the properties they possess that are most applicable to the treatment of the condition of concern. These properties are discovered through the process of activity or task analysis" (Llorens, 1973, p. 453).

Assignment

1. Select an activity, craft, or game that may be of interest and therapeutic value to adults and seniors.
2. Evaluate the therapeutic value of engagement in this activity by (a) analyzing the task demands and contextual variables, and (b) reviewing any relevant literature regarding the clinical use of this activity and its effectiveness in therapy. If you would like assistance with this challenge, use the Occupational Performance Analysis—Short Form (Appendix B) or the Learning Resources listed below.
3. Prepare and provide a presentation on the therapeutic potential, clinical use, and effectiveness of this purposeful activity.

Optional:

4. Read the document *Position Paper: Physical Agent Modalities* (AOTA, 1992). When is it appropriate for occupational therapy practitioners to use physical agent modalities? Compare the use of physical agent modalities to purposeful activity in clinical practice.
5. Engage in a discussion to compare and contrast the role of art therapists, music therapists, occupational therapists, physical therapists, and recreational therapists.

The information that follows will (a) provide students and instructors with resources to enhance the learning experience and (b) assist students in completing the assignment.

1From "Activity Analysis: Agreement Among Factors in a Sensory Processing Model," by L. A. Llorens, 1986, *American Journal of Occupational Therapy, 40,* p. 104. Copyright 1986 by the American Occupational Therapy Association. Reprinted with permission.

Learning Resources

Bernard, A. (1992). The use of music as purposeful activity: A preliminary investigation. *Physical and Occupational Therapy in Geriatrics, 10*(3), 35–45.

Boren, H. A., & Meell, H. (1985). Adolescent amputee ski rehabilitation program. *Journal of the Association of Pediatric Oncology Nurses, 2*(1), 16–23.

Breines, E. B. (1995). *Occupational therapy: Activities from clay to computers.* Philadelphia: F. A. Davis.

Brollier, C., Hamrick, N., & Jacobson, B. (1994). Aerobic exercise: A potential occupational therapy modality for adolescents with depression. *Occupational Therapy in Mental Health, 12*(4), 19–29.

Busuttil, J. (1990). An art therapy exhibition: A retrospective view. *British Journal of Occupational Therapy, 53*, 501–503.

Casby, J. A., & Holmes, M. B. (1994). Effect of music on repetitive disruptive vocalizations of persons with dementia. *American Journal of Occupational Therapy, 48*, 883–889.

Centoni, M., & Tallant, B. (1986). The projective use of drawings as a treatment technique with the depressed unemployed male. *Canadian Journal of Occupational Therapy, 53*(2), 81–87.

Curley, J. S. (1982). Leading poetry writing groups in a nursing home activities program. *Physical and Occupational Therapy in Geriatrics, 1*(4), 23–34.

Drake, M. (1992). *Crafts in therapy and rehabilitation.* Thorofare, NJ: Slack.

Fine, L., & Nichols, D. (1994). An evaluation of a twelve week recreational kayaking program: Effects on self-concept, leisure satisfaction and leisure attitudes of adults with traumatic brain injuries. *Journal of Cognitive Rehabilitation, 12*(5), 10–15.

Frye, B. (1990). Art and multiple personality disorder: An expressive framework for occupational therapy. *American Journal of Occupational Therapy, 44*, 1013–1022.

Garrett, G. (1994). A stroke of genius … The aquatic environment offers a range of opportunities for expanding practice. *Rehab Management, 7*(3), 56–59.

Grogan, G. (1994). The personal computer: A treatment tool for increasing sense of competence. *Occupational Therapy in Mental Health, 12*(4), 47–70.

Hamel, R. (1992). Getting into the game: New opportunities for athletes with disabilities. *Physician and Sports Medicine, 20*(11), 128–129.

Holtzinger, L. J. (1994). Vets join gingerbread house construction crew. *OT Week, 8*(40), 20.

Jamison, L., & Ogden, D. (1996). Aquatic therapy: Enhancing rehabilitation through teamwork. *OT Practice, 1*(5), 26–31.

Javernick, A. (1994). Renowned pianist thrives on limitations. *OT Week, 8*(10), 16–17.

Joe, E. (1996). Expressive therapy helps adults cope with past abuse. *OT Week, 10*(3), 17.

Kaplan, K., Mendelson, L., & Dubroff, M. (1983). The effect of a jogging program on psychiatric inpatients with symptoms of depression. *Occupational Therapy Journal of Research, 3*(3), 173–175.

King, T. I. (1992). The use of electromyographic biofeedback in treating patients with tension headaches. *American Journal of Occupational Therapy, 46*, 839–842.

Kirsteins, A., Dietz, F., Hwang, S. (1991). Evaluating the safety and potential use of a weight-bearing exercise, T'ai Chi Chuan, for rheumatoid arthritis patients. *American Journal of Physical Medicine and Rehabilitation, 70*(3), 136–141.

Krag, M. H., & Messner, D. G. (1982). Skiing for the physically handicapped. *Clinics in Sports Medicine, 1* (2), 319–332.

Langer, L. (1995). Tai Chi: Grasp the sparrow's tail. *OT Week, 1,* 22–23.

Lee, B., & Nantais, T. (1996). Use of electronic music as an occupational therapy modality in spinal cord injury rehabilitation: An occupational performance model. *American Journal of Occupational Therapy, 50,* 362–369.

MacKinnon, J., Noh, S., Laliberte, D., Lariviere, J., Allen, D. (1995). Therapeutic horseback riding: A review of the literature. *Physical and Occupational Therapy in Pediatrics, 15*(1), 1–15.

MacRae, A. (1992). Should music be used therapeutically in occupational therapy? *American Journal of Occupational Therapy, 46,* 275–277.

Madorsky, J. G. B., & Kiley, D. P. (1984). Wheelchair mountaineering. *Archives of Physical Medicine and Rehabilitation, 65,* 490–492.

Madorsky, J. G. B., & Madorsky, A. G. (1988). Scuba diving: Taking the wheelchair out of wheelchair sports. *Archives of Physical Medicine and Rehabilitation, 69*(3), 215–219.

Mathis, T. K. (1996). The MAGIC in a pecan pie. *OT Week, 10*(25), 16.

McBey, M. A. (1985). The therapeutic aspects of gardens and gardening: An aspect of total patient care. *Journal of Advanced Nursing, 10,* 591–595.

McCormick, G. (1991). *Therapeutic use of touch for the health professional.* Tucson, AZ: Therapy Skill Builders.

McCormick, G. L., & Galantino, M. L. (1997). Non-contact therapeutic touch. In C. M. Davis (Ed.), *Complementary therapies in rehabilitation* (pp. 83–100). Thorofare, NJ: Slack.

Neistadt, M.E. (1994). A meal preparation treatment protocol for adults with brain injury. *American Journal of Occupational Therapy, 48,* 431–438.

Nolinske, T. (1987). Patients find greener pastures in rehabilitation through horticulture therapy. *OT Week, 1*(41), 12–15.

Pasek, P. B., & Schkade, J. K. (1996). Effects of skiing experiences on adolescents with limb deficiencies: An occupational adaptation perspective. *American Journal of Occupational Therapy, 50,* 24–31.

Peloquin, S. M. (1996). Art: An occupation with promise for developing empathy. *American Journal of Occupational Therapy, 50,* 655–661.

Phillips, M. E. (1996). Looking back: The use of drama and puppetry in occupational therapy during the 1920s and 1930s. *American Journal of Occupational Therapy, 50,* 229–33.

Price-Lackey, P., & Cashman, J. (1996). Jenny's story: Reinventing oneself through occupation and narrative configuration. *American Journal of Occupational Therapy, 50,* 306–314.

Raible, R. (1995). Skiing: A therapeutic lift. *OT Week, 9*(14), 16–19.

Renner, A. L. (1994). Reclaiming lives with song and dance. *OT Week, 8*(21), 16–17.

Rubin, G., & Fleiss, D. (1983). Devices to enable persons with amputation to participate in sports. *Archives of Physical Medicine and Rehabilitation, 64*(1), 37–40.

Sanford, S. L., Cash, S. H., & Nelson, C. E. (1995). The use of arts and crafts in the rehabilitation of the adult burn patient. *Occupational Therapy in Health Care, 9*(4), 53–58.

Sayre-Adams, J. (1995). *The theory and practice of therapeutic touch.* New York: Churchill Livingstone.

Spink, J. (1993). *Developmental riding therapy: A team approach to assessment treatment.* Tucson, AZ: Therapy Skill Builders.

Stancliff, B. L. (1996). OTs recognize animals in therapy. *OT Practice, 1*(2), 12–13.

Standley, J. M. (1994). A case for music therapy. *OT Week, 8*(31), 54.

Taylor, L. P. S., & McGruder, J. E. (1996). The meaning of sea kayaking for persons with spinal cord injuries. *American Journal of Occupational Therapy, 50,* 39–46.

Tse, S., & Bailey, D. (1992). T'ai chi and postural control in the well elderly. *American Journal of Occupational Therapy, 46,* 295–300.

Webre, A. W., & Zeller, J. (1990).*Canoeing and kayaking for persons with physical disabilities.* Springfield, VA: American Canoe Association.

Zisselman, R. D., Rovner, B. W., Schmuely, Y., & Ferrie, P. (1996). Pet therapy intervention with geriatric psychiatric patients. *American Journal of Occupational Therapy, 50,* 47–51.

References

American Occupational Therapy Association (AOTA). Position paper: Physical agent modalities. *American Journal of Occupational Therapy, 16,* 1090–1091.

AOTA. (1993). *Position paper: Purposeful activity.* Bethesda, MD: Author.

Llorens, L. A. (1973). Activity analysis for cognitive-perceptual-motor dysfunction. *American Journal of Occupational Therapy, 27,* 453–456.

ARTS AND LITERATURE: THE CASE OF LAURIE

"Occupation that is relevant and appropriate to a given person's capacities and needs may also serve to alter his or her mood by capturing interest, focusing attention, creating a meaningful time structure, diminishing helplessness, establishing a sense of effectiveness and personal control, and meeting a range of cultural and social-interpersonal needs"

(Devereaux & Carlson, 1992, p. 175).[1]

Chapter Objectives

1. Use evaluation results and client goals to identify and document outcome-oriented objectives.
2. Define the terms **self-concept**, **perceived self-efficacy**, and **personal causation** and describe their effect on adaptation.
3. Use creative analysis to select and design a purposeful activity to address client needs.
4. Use the professional literature.

Using Purposeful Activity to Facilitate Adaptation

Adaptation refers to the adjustments made by individuals to enhance their ability to survive, contribute to the actualization of their potential, and master occupational challenges (King, 1978; AOTA, 1993). Adaptation requires individuals to take an active role in responding to specific environmental demands (King, 1978). Adaptation, then, requires, and is the result of, changes in individuals, their desired tasks, or their environment (AOTA, 1993; Mosey, 1986).

An individual's identity, self-concept, and life plans evolve and are influenced by life events (Polkinghorne, 1991). When an individual's ability to perform meaningful activities is impaired, life plans must undergo transformation (Frank, 1996; Polkinghorne, 1996). People are holistic entities, and injury or underdevelopment in one area may affect a person's entire identity; conversely, changes in a person's identity can influence the level of dysfunction caused by impairments (Polkinghorne, 1996). Occupational therapy practitioners facilitate adapta-

tion by evaluating and directing intervention toward individuals' desired tasks and performance contexts. "On the basis of evaluation, the occupational therapy practitioner, in collaboration with the individual, designs activity experiences that offer the individual opportunities for effective action" (AOTA, 1993, p. 1081). Therapists direct intervention toward (a) developing client skill in performing desired tasks, (b) ensuring that these skills transfer to performance outside of the clinical environment, and (c) enhancing the client's ability to cope with life stresses associated with their disability (Gage & Polatajko, 1994).

Assignment

1. Read the case of Laurie.
2. Work in groups of two to evaluate Laurie's past and present occupational performance profile. If you would like assistance with this challenge, use the form in Appendix G to document information on the occupations that are meaningful to Laurie; her unique values, goals, and performance component capabilities; and the contexts in which she performs.

Discuss your perceptions of Laurie's personal causation, perceived self-efficacy, and self-concept. **Personal causation** refers to an individual's belief in his or her abilities, perception of control over behavior and outcomes, and expectation of success in future endeavors (Kielhofner, 1985). **Perceived self-efficacy** refers to an individual's judgment of his or her capacity to use

[1]From "The Role of Occupational Therapy in the Management of Depression," by E. Devereaux and M. Carlson, 1992, *American Journal of Occupational Therapy, 46,* p. 175. Copyright by the American Occupational Therapy Association. Reprinted with permission.

existing skills to attain certain levels of performance (Bandura, 1986). **Self-concept** refers to the value that the individual places on the physical, emotional, and sexual self (AOTA, 1994). Consider the long-term potential, in terms of physical capacity and motor performance, for an individual with an above-elbow amputation. Has Laurie lived up to this potential? If not, what might be the reason(s)? Do you think Laurie's depression might be caused by or related to the accident? How might you determine the answers to these important questions?

3. Identify, prioritize, and document some specific, measurable, outcome-oriented goals and objectives for Laurie. If you would like some assistance with this challenge, use the Client Goals Form (Appendix H). Within clinical practice these goals and objectives would be modified when Laurie is prepared to work more collaboratively with the intervention team.

4. Select and design a purposeful activity for use with Laurie during treatment. It is possible to treat Laurie individually or within a group context. Ensure that the selected therapeutic activity addresses your perceptions of Laurie's needs, interests, and values.

    The activity could be directed toward having Laurie be more active in the construction of a life plan and therefore in the identification of her therapy goals and objectives. If you would like some assistance with this challenge, review some of the articles identified in the Learning Resources section.

5. Determine how you will structure the activity and engagement process. After analyzing an activity for its potential to address client goals, you may decide adaptations may be necessary to maximize therapeutic value. Therapists who are skilled at analysis are able to select the most appropriate

activity from among those of interest to a particular client (Trombly, 1995) or to adapt an activity that a client has selected to optimize its therapeutic value.

6. Engage in the activity you have selected and structured for this client. Take turns with your partner role-playing the client and therapist. This will provide insight into the therapeutic value of rapport and enable students to increase the accuracy of analysis and develop skill in client interaction.

7. What strategies might Laurie's prior occupational therapy practitioner have used with her or other individuals with traumatic and permanent disabilities to enhance adaptation over the long term? These strategies will enhance the quality of service provision and may minimize the likelihood of readmission.

Case Study: Laurie

Laurie is a 40-year-old, married woman who was the sole occupant in a single-vehicle automobile accident. She was driving home from a Christmas party where she had been drinking wine all evening. Laurie was always busy throughout the month of December with promotional parties and obligatory engagements. The business of marketing and advertising in the fashion industry is very competitive; and visibility, reputation, and consistency in performance were Laurie's secrets to success.

Laurie began her career as a fashion model at the age of 14. By the time she was in her early 20s she had posed on the cover of a number of national women's magazines. In her teens and early 20s she worked freelance selling fashion illustrations but never made enough money to support her desired lifestyle. She was married at the age of 25 to a successful interior designer and began a college program in journalism and photography shortly thereafter. It was during school that she decided to minor in art history. Immediately after graduation Laurie worked as a freelance journalist writing articles on women's apparel and accessories. As she gained more experience, she began publishing photographs to accompany her articles. Three years after graduation Laurie became the owner and chief executive officer of ABC Marketing, combining her knowledge of fashion and skills as a writer and photographer. The firm has three employees, profits have soared, and Laurie's family has come to depend on her income. Although the family has health insurance, Laurie did not arrange for ABC Marketing to offer its employees disability insurance.

After the motor vehicle accident Laurie received rehabilitation services to recover from a left-upper-limb above-elbow amputation, extensive internal injuries, and multiple abrasions to her face and upper body. Occupational therapy intervention was primarily directed toward learning to use a prosthesis in her left dominant extremity. By the time she was discharged Laurie was able to use her prosthesis to independently dress herself and cook a meal. Twelve months following her accident Laurie visited her family physician at the request of her husband. The doctor prescribed antidepressant medication. Two weeks later Laurie had her 40th birthday, attempted suicide by ingesting over-the-counter sleeping pills, and was admitted to the hospital. (See Table 1 for a discussion of major depressive disorders and occupational therapy's role in its treatment.)

During the occupational therapy evaluation Laurie was quiet and slow to respond to questions. She wore a long-sleeve shirt and sweat pants, held her left upper arm with her right hand, and did not have her prosthesis. Laurie indicated that her interest and energy level was very low and that she would prefer to sleep all day rather than go home. Although

prompted to discuss her personal goals, Laurie avoided this request and did not respond. She indicated that she had full intentions of returning to work, but she sustained her business by working out of her home for 2 months after her accident. Laurie has not worked since then. She described her marriage as turbulent and her husband and daughter as the only "constants" in her life. Laurie suggested that her relationship with her husband is "strained" and indicated that "he probably is just not attracted to me." "I don't blame him … look at me I'm useless." "I often wonder why he stays with me." "I always went to parties alone and he would stay at home with our daughter." "He's always hated my friends." "I know they need me to work but I just can't do it. Things won't change." "I just don't feel like seeing anyone." The couple has a 14-year-old daughter who wants to be a photographer.

Table 1: Major Depressive Disorder

Major depressive disorder is characterized by a sustained internal emotional state of depressed mood or loss of interest or pleasure that is a change from previous functioning and that causes distress or disability in social or occupational functioning (American Psychiatric Association, 1994). The first episode occurs before the age of 40 in approximately 50% of patients. Untreated episodes last 6 to 13 months; most treated episodes last approximately 3 months. The lifetime prevalence of major depressive disorder is 15% for the general population and 25% for women. Mood disorders are the psychiatric diagnoses most associated with suicide; and suicide among depressed male patients is more prevalent than among depressed female patients (Kaplan & Sadock, 1996).

Depression changes one's capacity to "engage in goal-directed use of time, energy, interest, and attention" (Devereaux & Carlson, 1992, p. 175). Occupational therapy intervention should be directed at actively engaging clients in structured activities related to goal-setting, future-planning, stress management, and adaptation skills; and defining desired roles (DeCarlo & Mann, 1985; Good-Ellis, Fine, Haas, Spencer, & Glick, 1986; Stein & Smith, 1989).

The information that follows will (a) provide students and instructors with resources to enhance the learning experience and (b) assist the students in completing the assignment.

Learning Resources

Gage, M. (1992). The appraisal model of coping: An assessment and intervention model for occupational therapy. *American Journal of Occupational Therapy, 46,* 353–362.

Gage, M., & Polatajko, H. (1994). Enhancing occupational performance through an understanding of perceived self-efficacy. *American Journal of Occupational Therapy, 48,* 452–461.

Helfrich, C., & Kielhofner, G. (1994). Volitional narratives and the meaning of therapy. *American Journal of Occupational Therapy, 48,* 326.

Helfrich, C., Kielhofner, G., & Mattingly, C. (1994). Volition as narrative: Understanding motivation in chronic illness. *American Journal of Occupational Therapy, 48,* 311–317.

King, L. J. (1978). Toward a science of adaptive responses: 1978 Eleanor Clark Slagle Lecture. *American Journal of Occupational Therapy, 32,* 429–437.

Polkinghorne, D. E. (1996). Transformative narratives: From victim to agentic life plots. *American Journal of Occupational Therapy, 50,* 299–305.

Price-Lackey, P., & Cashman, J. (1996). Jenny's story: Reinventing oneself through occupation and narrative configuration. *American Journal of Occupational Therapy, 50,* 306–314.

Waters, D., (1995). Recovering from a depressive episode using the Canadian Occupational Performance Measure. *Canadian Journal of Occupational Therapy, 62,* 278–282.

Study Questions

1. Define the terms **personal causation**, **self-efficacy**, and **self-concept**.
2. How does self-efficacy affect adaptation?
3. Identify some reasons why there might be disparity between client skills and actual performance.
4. Describe an activity that actively engages a client in identification of therapy goals.
5. Describe an activity that actively engages a client in reconstructing their life history.
6. Describe an activity that actively engages a client in constructing a life plan.

References

American Occupational Therapy Association (AOTA). (1993). Position paper: Purposeful activity. *American Journal of Occupational Therapy, 47,* 1081–1082.

AOTA. (1994). *Uniform terminology for occupational therapy* (3rd ed.). Bethesda, MD: Author.

American Psychiatric Association. (1994). *Diagnostic and statistical manual of mental disorders* (4th ed.). Washington, DC: Author.

Bandura, A. (1986). *Social foundations of thought.* Englewood Cliffs, NJ: Prentice Hall.

DeCarlo, J. J., & Mann, W. C. (1985). The effectiveness of verbal versus activity groups in improving self-perceptions of interpersonal communications skills. *American Journal of Occupational Therapy, 39,* 20–27.

Devereaux, E., & Carlson, M. (1992). Health policy: The role of occupational therapy in the management of depression. *American Journal of Occupational Therapy, 46,* 175–180.

Frank, G. (1996). Life histories in occupational therapy practice. *American Journal of Occupational Therapy, 50,* 251–264.

Gage, M., & Polatajko, H. (1994). Enhancing occupational performance through an understanding of perceived self-efficacy. *American Journal of Occupational Therapy, 48,* 452–461.

Good-Ellis, M., Fine, S. B., Haas, G. L., Spencer, J. H., & Glick, I. D. (1986). Quantitative role and performance assessment: Implications and application to treatment of major depressive disorders. In *Depression assessment and treatment update, proceedings* (pp. 26–48). Bethesda, MD: American Occupational Therapy Association.

Kaplan, H. I., & Sadock, B. J. (1996). *Concise textbook of clinical psychiatry.* Baltimore: Williams & Wilkins.

Kielhofner, G. (1985). *A model of human occupation: Theory and application* (2nd ed.). Baltimore: Williams & Wilkins.

King, L. J. (1978). Toward a science of adaptive responses: 1978 Eleanor Clark Slagle Lecture. *American Journal of Occupational Therapy, 32,* 429–437.

Mosey, A. C. (1986). *Psychosocial components of occupational therapy.* New York: Raven.

Polkinghorne, D. E. (1991). Narrative and self-concept. *Journal of Narrative and Life-History, 1*(2, 3), 135–153.

Polkinghorne, D. E. (1996). Transformative narratives: From victimic to agentic life plots. *American Journal of Occupational Therapy, 50,* 299–305.

Stein, G., & Smith, J. (1989). Short-term stress management programme with acutely depressed in-patients. *Canadian Journal of Occupational Therapy, 56,* 185–191.

Trombly, C. A. (1995). Occupation: Purposefulness and meaningfulness as therapeutic mechanisms. *American Journal of Occupational Therapy, 49,* 960–972.

ACTIVITIES OF DAILY LIVING: THE CASE OF DAWN

"Individuals are independent when they perform tasks themselves, when they perform tasks in an adapted environment, and when they appropriately oversee task completion by others on their own behalf"

(American Occupational Therapy Association, 1995, p. 1014).[1]

Chapter Objectives

1. Evaluate the effect of an orthopedic condition on an individual's occupational performance profile.
2. Evaluate the task demands and contextual variables of dressing and bathing.
3. Use logical thinking and creative analysis to develop an individualized intervention strategy.
4. Use adapted-equipment supplier catalogues and community resources to select assistive devices for a client.
5. Develop skills in teaching by role-modeling the therapist-client interaction.

Assignment

1. Read the case of Dawn.
2. Evaluate the impact of Dawn's current condition on her physical capabilities and her potential to engage in basic activities of daily living.
   Why did Dawn's nurse raise the hospital bed and place a small pillow between her legs?
   Why is Dawn using a walker, a raised toilet seat, and a toilet grab bar?
   What self-care activities do you think Dawn will have difficulty performing?
3. Work in groups of two to design intervention to address Dawn's therapy goals. One individual will complete Project A, on dressing, while the other completes Project B, for bathing skills.
4. The occupational therapy student who completed Project A will role-play the occupational therapy practitioner, and the student who completed Project B will personify Dawn. Teach Dawn how to become independent in dressing and how to use any recommended adapted equipment.

5. The occupational therapy student who completed Project B will role-play the occupational therapy practitioner, and the student who completed Project A will personify Dawn. Teach Dawn how to become independent in bathing and how to use any recommended adapted equipment.

Optional:

6. Identify other activities of daily living or work or productive activities that you would anticipate Dawn having difficulty performing with the current hip range of motion restrictions?

Project A

1. Identify the task and contextual demands required to dress and undress in the "typical fashion." If you would like some assistance with this challenge, complete the Occupational Performance Analysis—Short Form (Appendix B). Participation in this activity will increase the quality and accuracy of analysis.
2. After evaluating the impact of Dawn's current condition on her physical capabilities, and the task demands and contextual variables required to dress and undress, identify which activities would challenge Dawn beyond her current capabilities.
3. Use this information to document specific, measurable, outcome-oriented objectives for Dawn's goal of independence in dressing. If you would like some assistance with this challenge, use the Client Goals Form (Appendix H).
4. What intervention strategies will you use to enable Dawn to be independent in this task? If you would like some assistance with this challenge, (a) examine supplier catalogues of assistive and

---

[1]From "Position Paper: Broadening the Construct of Independence," the American Occupational Therapy Association, 1995, *American Journal of Occupational Therapy, 49*, p. 1014. Copyright 1995 by the American Occupational Therapy Association. Reprinted with permission.

adapted equipment, and (b) review the various intervention strategies identified in the Occupational Performance Practice Model for Service to Individuals outlined in the chapter "Task Analysis: The Contribution of Occupational Therapy to Health."

Project B

1. Identify the task and contextual demands required to bathe in the "typical fashion." If you would like some assistance with this challenge, complete the Occupational Performance Analysis—Short Form (Appendix B).

2. After evaluating the impact of Dawn's current condition on her physical capabilities, and the task demands and contextual variables required to bathe, identify which activities would challenge Dawn beyond her current capabilities.

3. Use this information to document specific, measurable, outcome-oriented objectives for Dawn's goal of independence in bathing. If you would like some assistance with this challenge, use the Client Goals Form (Appendix H).

4. What intervention strategies will you use to enable Dawn to be independent in this task? If you would like some assistance with this challenge, (a) examine supplier catalogues of assistive and adapted equipment, and (b) review the various intervention strategies identified in the Occupational Performance Practice Model for Service to Individuals outlined in the chapter "Task Analysis: The Contribution of Occupational Therapy to Health."

Case Study: Dawn

Dawn is a 52-year-old woman who is recovering from a recent right total hip replacement. She would like to be independent in basic activities of daily living, particularly dressing and bathing, before being discharged from ABC Rehabilitation Center.

Dawn's occupational therapist completed the evaluation yesterday and treatment will commence this morning.

Dawn was diagnosed with rheumatoid arthritis a number of years ago. She has inflammatory joint involvement in her right dominant hand (wrist, metacarpophalangeal [MCP], and proximal inter-phalangeal [PIP] joints), hip, and ankle, and in her left hand (MCP and PIP joints) and hip. She worked full time as an executive assistant in a publishing firm until approximately four months ago. Dawn was experiencing so much pain, stiffness, and discomfort in her right hip that she reduced her hours to part-time and sought medical intervention. Total hip replacement surgery was recommended. Anticipating that the postsurgical restrictions for hip range of motion (no internal rotation, adduction, or flexion beyond 60 degrees for 3 months minimum) would limit Dawn's ability to independently engage in daily living activities, the physician has sent a referral for occupational therapy services. (Table 1 discusses rheumatoid arthritis.)

Dawn, a mother of two children, lives with her husband in their small, single-level, two-bedroom suburban home. She enjoys reading, cooking, playing with her grandchildren, and walking in the park. She loves tennis but has been a spectator rather than a player of this sport for the last 7 years. Her husband drives her to work 3 days per week and the couple leave the home at 7:30 a.m. Dawn expects to return to work as soon as possible, but indicates that she must dress herself in the morning to allow her husband ample time to prepare their breakfast. When asked to describe the layout of her bedroom and bathroom, Dawn indicates that "the bed is on the far wall as you come in. My husband's dresser is beside the bed, and mine is across the room next to the closet. There is a door to the

Table 1: Rheumatoid Arthritis and Total Joint Replacement

Rheumatoid arthritis (RA) is a chronic systemic disease that causes inflammatory changes of joints. Symmetrical involvement of synovial joints is common, but symptoms may appear in any joint. Low-grade fever, loss of appetite, anemia, and fatigue are some of the symptoms of systemic problems. The clinical course is characterized by exacerbations and remissions and prognosis is unpredictable. Severe disability occurs in 10% of those diagnosed. Women are four times more likely to have RA than men (Damjanov, 1996). The onset of RA is usually gradual, with pain, stiffness, and tenderness in many large joints as well as the small joints of the hands and feet. Range of motion may be limited secondary to edema, pain, and changes in joint integrity; and muscles that act on these joints may have reduced strength secondary to disuse (Morawski et al., 1996).

Patients with rheumatoid arthritis receive total hip replacement when it is deemed necessary in order to alleviate pain, regain joint mobility, and avoid fibrotic damage to the joint and tendon structures (Salter, 1970). Physicians will specify postoperative weight-bearing and hip range of motion precautions. These restrictions vary among patients, depending on their hip pathology, the surgical approach used, type of fixative, type of arthroplasty, severity of joint involvement, and so forth. If a posterolateral approach is used, patients are cautioned not to internally rotate, adduct, or flex the hip beyond 60 to 90 degrees (Morawski et al., 1996).

bathroom from the bedroom. When you enter this room, the bathtub is on your right and the sink and toilet on the left next to the far wall." When probed for more details regarding the bathtub, Dawn indicates, "when you face the tub, the shower head is on the left.… There is a storage closet to the right of the tub behind the bathroom door." Dawn's therapist uses this information to visualize the layout of the bedroom and bathroom and to plan intervention.

When the occupational therapist commences the morning treatment session, Dawn is lying on a raised hospital bed with a small pillow between her legs. She has just finished eating her breakfast and would like to go to the toilet before getting dressed. The therapist provides supervision and verbal cues to Dawn as she uses a standard walker to ambulate 10 to 15 feet toward the hospital's bathroom. A raised toilet seat and side grab bar have been put in place and Dawn uses both devices to assist her in sitting on the toilet. Dawn indicates, "I'm glad the bathroom's so close—that was hard work."

The information that follows will (a) provide students and instructors with resources to enhance the learning experience and (b) assist the students in completing the assignment.

Learning Resources

Books

Morawski, D., Pitbladdo, ..., Bianchi, E. M., Lieberman, S. L., Novic, J. P., & Bobrove, H. (1996). Hip fractures and total hip replacement. In L. W. Pedretti (Ed.), *Occupational therapy: Practice skills for physical dysfunction* (4th ed., pp. 735–746). St. Louis, MO: Mosby.

Platt, J. V., Hahn, R., Kessler, S., & McCarthy, D. Q. (1990). *Daily activities after your hip surgery* (rev. ed.). Bethesda, MD: Authors.

Supplier Catalogues

Maddak, Inc. PO Box 922, Randolph, MA 02368-0922. 800-854-4687.

North Coast Medical, Inc. 187 Stauffer Boulevard, San Jose, CA 95125-1042. 800-821-9319.

Sammons, Inc. PO Box 32, Brookfield, IL 60513. 708-325-1700. 800-323-5547.

Smith & Nephew Rolyan Inc. One Quality Drive, Germantown, WI 53022. 800-228-3693.

This list of suppliers is not intended to be exhaustive, nor does it represent endorsements by the author or AOTA.

Study Questions

1. Identify the sensorimotor components required to fasten a button and describe the degree of challenge to each component.

2. Your client is unable to use her right hand and has difficulty fastening buttons. Identify three intervention strategies to address this problem.

3. Your client is unable to carry garments while ambulating with a walker. Identify two intervention strategies to address this problem.

4. Your client sits on a bath seat to bathe. Identify an intervention strategy that would enable this client to clean her feet.

5. Your client has difficulty tying her shoes despite training and practice. Identify an intervention strategy to address this problem.

6. You must teach your client how to don a shirt with one hand. Describe the steps you will take to teach this skill.

References

Damjanov, I. (1996). *Pathology for the health professions.* Philadelphia: W. B. Saunders.

Morawski, D., Pitbladdo, K., Bianchi, E. M., Lieberman, S. L., Novic, J. P., & Bobrove, H. (1996). Hip fractures and total hip replacement. In L. W. Pedretti (Ed.), *Occupational therapy: Practice skills for physical dysfunction* (4th ed., pp. 735–746). St. Louis, MO: Mosby.

Salter, R. B. (1970). *Textbook of disorders and injuries of the musculoskeletal system.* Baltimore: Williams & Wilkins.

WORKER REHABILITATION AND THE BIOMECHANICAL APPROACH: THE CASE OF RICK

"The Nation's proper goals regarding individuals with disabilities are to assure equality of opportunity, full participation, independent living, and economic self-sufficiency for such individuals"

(Americans With Disabilities Act of 1990).

Chapter Objectives

1. Describe the contributions of task analysis and activity analysis to functional capacity evaluations, work-site analysis, and job simulation.
2. Evaluate the occupational performance profile of an injured worker.
3. Interpret clinical observations of performance.
4. Identify the neuromusculoskeletal performance components that underlie performance of a specific work task.
5. Evaluate whether there is a fit among the characteristics of an individual, employment tasks, and workplace contextual demands.
6. Use client goals and evaluation results to identify and document outcome-oriented objectives.
7. Use logical thinking and creative analysis to develop an individualized intervention strategy to return an employee to work.
8. Develop basic skill in designing and fabricating adaptive equipment.

Using Task Analysis to Rehabilitate a Worker

According to the United States Bureau of the Census, individuals with disabilities made up 13.4% of all employed people in 1991 and 1992. The employment rate for individuals with a severe disability was 23.2%, for individuals with a disability that was not severe was 76%, and for individuals with no disability was 80.5%. Approximately 19.5 million of the 16- to 67-year-old population had a work disability (McNeil, 1993). Occupational therapy practitioners are working in collaboration

with other professional groups to improve these statistics. Occupational therapists provide services to (a) individuals with disabilities who are entering the work place, (b) injured workers who are recovering capacities to return to work, (c) workers who need assistance making the transition from work to retirement activities, and (d) nondisabled workers to prevent workplace injury (Jacobs, 1995).

Occupational therapy practitioners who work in vocational rehabilitation use an occupational performance approach to task analysis to evaluate the dynamic relationship between workers and their job tasks and workplace contexts. Discrepancies between worker capacities, job tasks, and work-site demands are identified after a **functional capacity evaluation** (FCE) and ergonomic work-site analysis are completed. FCEs require a determination of the status of a worker's sensorimotor, cognitive, psychological, and psychosocial performance components. An **ergonomic work-site analysis** assesses work methods, work-station design and worker posture, and handle and tool design (Jacobs, 1995). FCEs and ergonomic work-site analysis both require task and activity analyses skills.

Occupational therapy practitioners collaborate with the client and rehabilitation team to plan intervention. Intervention strategies include (a) counseling and improving physical condition to enhance worker capabilities, (b) adapting tasks and altering physical environments to increase function, and (c) promoting enabling workplace environments. **Work hardening** is a work-oriented treatment program that is designed to improve worker performance through the use of graded job simulation (Matheson, Ogden, Violette, & Schultz, 1985). Work hardening and **job simulation** both require the application of task and activity analyses. Accurate analysis and keen observation are key requirements to selecting meaningful and purposeful evaluation and intervention activities that respect personal interests; habits; and educational, cultural, and ethnic differences (Joannidis, 1996).

Impairments of neuromusculoskeletal performance components are exceedingly common in industry, and the biomechanical approach to evaluation and intervention is often used to address these underlying physical skills and abilities (Jacobs, 1995; Trombly, 1995). The **biomechanical approach** uses the principles of ergonomics, kinetics, and kinematics to (a) determine the strength, endurance, and joint ranges required for motion and performance; (b) identify stressful positions, tool design, and forces and repetitions required; and (c) design appropriate intervention activities (Jacobs, 1995; Kielhofner, 1992; Trombly, 1995).

The American Occupational Therapy Association (1994, p. 3) describes the role of occupational therapy practitioners in worker rehabilitation:

> *"An individual who is injured on the job may have the potential to return to work and productive activities, which is a performance area. In order to achieve the outcome of returning to work and productive activities, the individual may need to address specific performance components, such as strength, endurance, soft tissue integrity, time management, and the physical features of performance contexts, like structures and objects in his or her environment. The occupational therapy practitioner, in collaboration with the individual and other members of the vocational team, uses planned interventions to achieve the desired outcome. These interventions may include activities such as an exercise program, body mechanics instruction, and job site modifications, all of which may be provided in a work hardening program."*

Assignment

1. Read the case about Rick.
2. Evaluate Rick's occupational performance profile. If you would like some assistance with this challenge, use the Occupational Performance Profile form in Appendix G to document information on the occupations that are meaningful to Rick; his unique values, interests, goals, and performance component capabilities; and the contexts in which he performs.
3. Therapists are responsible for determining how a diagnosed condition influences present and future function (Mattingly & Fleming, 1994). Hypothesize about Rick's current and potential ability to perform the tasks of a rehabilitation engineer who makes adapted equipment for children with disabilities. In the clinical context, job simulation is used to evaluate this potential.

To answer this challenge, work in groups of four to six to complete Project A or Project B. Engagement in these projects will increase insight into the task and contextual demands of Rick's workplace. Students' participation in woodworking and sewing will also provide the opportunity to practice designing and fabricating adapted therapeutic equipment (see Figure 1).

Project A

Select, design, and fabricate a piece of adapted equipment or pediatric toy (e.g., corner seat, special chair, wheelchair tray, T-stool, equilibrium board). Contact a local early-intervention program if you would like to make and donate a piece of equipment that is needed by this agency.

Divide into two groups of two or three members (Group One and Group Two). Individuals in Group One will personify a rehabilitation engineer who makes adapted equipment for children by developing a blueprint of the project, designing paper templates, transferring the template patterns onto wood, and cutting the wood. The members of Group Two will complete the Occupational Performance/Biomechanical Analysis Form (located at the end of this chapter) while observing Group One's activities. The members of Group Two will represent an occupational therapist who is conducting the work-site analysis.

Students in registered occupational therapist educational programs should also complete the optional Neuromusculoskeletal Analysis Form.

Individuals in Group Two will sand, assemble, paint, and varnish the project. Group One will complete the Occupational Performance/ Biomechanical Analysis Form (located at the end of this chapter) while observing the members of Group Two performing this activity.
Optional: Work together to design and sew a cushion or slipcover for this project. Practice using a sewing machine and sewing by hand.

Figure 1. Occupational Therapy Students with Adapted Equipment Projects.

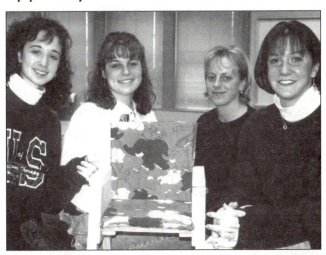

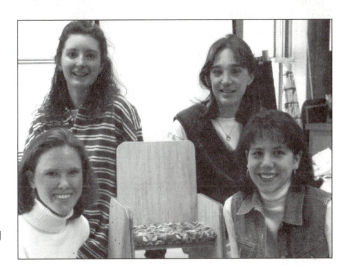

Project B

Design and fabricate a number of beanbags. Try making basic shapes (squares, triangles, circles) or more complex figures (bells, bears, bunnies, hearts, houses, cars, trucks).

Divide into two groups of two or three members (Group One and Group Two). Individuals in Group One will personify a rehabilitation engineer who upholsters adapted equipment for children with disabilities by making one beanbag each. This will require that individuals develop a pattern, transfer the pattern to fabric, cut out fabric pieces, and sew the project together. Practice using a sewing machine and sewing by hand. Individuals in Group Two will complete the Occupational Performance/Biomechanical Analysis Form (located at the end of this chapter) while observing Group One engage in this activity. The members of Group Two will represent an occupational therapist who is conducting the work-site evaluation.

Group Two will then be responsible for making one beanbag each. The individuals in Group One will complete the Occupational Performance/Bio-mechanical Analysis Form (located at the end of this chapter) while observing Group Two members as they engage in this activity.

Students in registered occupational therapist educational programs should also complete the optional Neuromusculoskeletal Analysis Form.

4. After evaluating Rick's occupational performance profile (one of the job tasks performed by the "rehabilitation engineer") and the workplace contextual requirements, identify and list the activities that would challenge Rick beyond his current capabilities.

5. Use the information compiled in Question 4 to prepare a list of specific, measurable, outcome-oriented objectives to help Rick achieve his goal of returning to work. In clinical practice these goals and objectives would be established and priori-tized in collaboration with Rick and the vocational rehabilitation team. The Client Goals Form is located in Appendix H.

6. Use the information collected in Question 5 to identify intervention strategies. If you would like some assistance with this challenge, consider using the various intervention strategies identified in the Occupational Performance Practice Model for Service to Individuals outlined in the chapter "Task Analysis: The Contribution of Occupational Therapy to Health."

Optional:

7. Design a purposeful activity for use with Rick during an individual treatment session.

8. Table 1 provides an alternative method for conducting a biomechanical activity analysis. Compare and contrast this example with the Occupational Performance/Biomechanical Analysis Form.

9. You have been hired by a carpentry firm to assist in designing a workplace that promotes wellness of all workers. What physical environmental design features would you recommend?

10. Donate your project to a local early-intervention program or a pediatric occupational therapy department.

Case Study: Rick

Rick is a 28-year-old rehabilitation engineer who lives on a small ranch with his wife and two young children. In his leisure time Rick enjoys doing mechanical work on his truck and making wood toys for his children. During the week he works at ABC Rehabilitation Center making adapted equipment for children with disabilities. He is involved in the design and fabrication of this equipment and works primarily with thermoplastics and wood. Most of the client positioning devices (e.g., corner seats, adapted chairs, and adapted cushions) made by Rick are covered with upholstery.

Twelve weeks ago Rick fell from his barn roof while replacing shingles, straining the ligaments in his lower back and fracturing his distal right radius and ulna. After weeks of outpatient occupational and physical therapy, Rick is referred to your work hardening clinic. Rick has lower back pain during trunk flexion and rotation. He complains of pain when reaching for objects from the floor and his standing tolerance is 10 minutes. He lifts 3 pounds from the floor, 5 pounds overhead, and carries objects up to 8 pounds. Weeks of immobilization in a cast has caused swelling and weakness throughout his right-dominant hand. Rick has stiffness, pain, and weakness in this hand resulting in limited active and passive flexion range of motion in his wrist and fingers. Rick's active joint range of motion in his right hand is provided in Table 1.

Table 1: Rick's Right Hand Active Range of Motion

Joint	Motion	Active Range	Normal Ranges[a]
Forearm	Pronation	Full	0–80
	Supination	Full	0–80
Wrist	Flexion	0–50	0–80
	Extension	0–30	0–70
	Ulnar Deviation	0–15	0–30
	Radial Deviation	0–10	0–20
Thumb	MP Flexion-Extension	0–20	0–50
	IP Flexion-Extension	0–40	0–80
	Opposition	2 cm	0
Fingers**			
2nd digit	MP/PIP/DIP Flexion	50/80/50	90/100/90
3rd digit	MP/PIP/DIP Flexion	50/80/50	90/100/90
4th digit	MP/PIP/DIP Flexion	40/70/30	90/100/90
5th digit	MP/PIP/DIP Flexion	40/60/20	90/100/90
**Rick has full MP/PIP/DIP extension in the 2nd and 3rd digits. He has lost about 10 degrees of full extension in MP/PIP/DIP extension in his 4th and 5th digits.			

MP–metacarpophalangeal; IP–interphalangeal; PIP–proximal interphalangeal; DIP–distal interphalangeal.

[a]Hislop, H. J., & Montgomery, J. (1995). Daniels and Worthingham's muscle testing: *Techniques of manual examination* (6th ed.). Philadelphia: W. B. Saunders.

Occupational Performance/Biomechanical Analysis Form

Occupational Performance/Biomechanical Analysis

Occupation
Role Performance:
Task: *Work or Job Performance*
Activity: Steps Required to Perform:
1.
2.
3.
4.
5.
6.
7.
8.
9.
10.
Materials, Tools, and Equipment (availability, cost, source...):
Safety Precautions and Contraindications:
Time to Complete:
The Person
Relevance and Meaningfulness: (historical or current personal or social relevance)
Values and Interest:

For each performance component, determine the level of challenge required to perform. (Mod = moderate, Max = maximum).	Level of Challenge		Comments (Indicate N/A if Not Applicable)
	Mod	Max	
A. Sensorimotor Component			
1. Sensory			
Perceptual Skills			
2. Neuromuscular *(OTR students use the last two pages of form)*			
3. Motor			
B. Cognitive Components			
C. Psychosocial & Psychological Components			
1. Psychological			
2. Social			
3. Self-Management			

Performance Context	
	Comments
A. **Temporal Aspects**	
B. **Environmental** 1. Physical	
2. Social	
3. Cultural	

Adaptations, Grading, and Structuring:

Activity	Context	Personal Approach
1.	1.	1.
2.	2.	2.
3.	3.	3.

Assistive and Adaptive Equipment:

1.

2.

3.

How can this activity be graded to increase

Strength?   Range of motion?

1.   1.

2.   2.

3.   3.

Coordination/dexterity?   Endurance?

1.   1.

2.   2.

3.   3.

Optional: Neuromusculoskeletal Analysis[1,2]

Select one of the activity steps from the first page of the Occupational Performance/Biomechanical Analysis form.
Activity step number: _____ performed in _____ (standing, sitting, etc.).

Joint Position or Motion	ROM	Type of Contraction	Primary Muscles	Gravity Assists/ Resists/ No Effect	Minimal Strength Required
Example Dominant Right Side Shoulder Flexion	30°	Isometric	Anterior deltoid Coracobrachialis Pectoralis Major	Resists	4
Dominant Right Side Elbow Flexion	0-90°	Isotonic	Biceps	Resists	4

[1]Note: To be completed with Occupational Performance/Biomechanical Analysis Form
[2]From "Purposeful Activity" (pp. 237-253) by C.A. Trombly, 1995, in *Occupational Therapy for Physical Dysfunction*, edited by C. A. Trombly, Baltimore: Williams & Wilkins. Copyright 1995 by Williams & Wilkins. Reprinted with persmission.

Optional: Neuromusculoskeletal Analysis, continued

Joint Position or Motion	ROM	Type of Contraction	Primary Muscles	Gravity Assists/ Resists/ No Effect	Minimal Strength Required

Table 2: Example of an Alternative Biomechanical Activity Analysis

Example of an Alternative Biomechanical Activity Analysis

1. Name the activity (goal):
   Vacuuming the hallway carpeting using a lightweight vacuum with a 25-foot cord.

2. List the steps.

   a. *Obtain the vacuum cleaner from the closet*

   b. *Unwind the cord*

   c. *Plug cord into wall; turn vacuum on*

   d. *Push the vacuum back and forth*

   e. *Unplug it and wind the cord*

   f. *Return the vacuum to the closet*

3. What capacities and abilities are prerequisite to successful accomplishment of this activity?

   • *Standing balance*

   • *Ability to bend over and straighten up*

   • *Ability to grasp*

   • *Ability to walk forward and backward on carpeting*

   • *Ability to move dominant arm against gravity and moderate resistance*

   • *Vision* [2]

4. Describe the external (contextual) constraints.

   a. Task Constraints: How are the person and the materials positioned, especially in relation to one another?

   • *The vacuum is located in a closet next to the area to be cleaned*

   • *The electrical plug is located halfway between the two ends of the hallway, 5 inches from the floor*

   • *When vacuuming, the person will be directly behind the machine*

   b. Task constraints: What utensils/tools/materials are normally used to do this activity?

   • *A lightweight vacuum*

---

[2]The blind person needs to use adaptive methods for knowing which sections of the carpet have been cleaned and which have not.

Table 2, continued

c. Environmental constraints: Where is the activity usually carried out?

- *The hallway is 20 feet long, 3 feet wide*

- *No furniture is in the way*

- *The carpet is a flat weave*

d. Environmental constraints: Does this activity, or how it is done, hold particular meaning for certain cultures or social roles?

- *The person takes pride in a cleanly vacuumed home*

- *The person is not willing to switch to a nonmotorized carpet sweeper*

5. Describe the internal constraints for step __4__:

Joint Position or Motion	ROM	Primary Muscles	Gravity Assists/ Resists/ No Effect	Minimal Strength Required	Type of Contraction
shoulder flexion	0–75°	anterior deltoid	resists	G– to G	concentric
		coracobrachialis			
		pectoralis major			
elbow extension	90–0°	triceps	assists	G– to G	concentric
scapular protraction	1.5 in.	serratus anterior	no effect	G– to G	concentric
shoulder extension	0–45°	posterior deltoid	assists	G– to G	concentric
		latissimus dorsi	no effect	G– to G	concentric
		teres major	resists	G– to G	concentric
elbow flexion	90–120°	biceps brachialis	resists	G– to G	concentric
scapular retraction	1.5 in.	middle trapezius	no effect	G– to G	concentric
cylindrical grasp		extensors	no effect	G– to G	isometric
		flexors		G– to G	concentric
		interossei			
wrist stabilize		all wrist muscles	no effect	G– to G	isometric
trunk flexion	0–30°	back extensors	assists	F+ to G–	eccentric
trunk extension	30–0°	back extensors	resists	G– to G	concentric

Table 2, continued

6. What must be stabilized to enable certain patients to do this activity and how will the stabilization be provided?
   - *Nothing*

7. For which ages is this activity appropriate?
   - *18+ years primarily*
   - *10–17 years secondarily*

8. What is the estimated metabolic equivalent task (MET) level of this activity?
   - *2–3 METs*

9. What precautions must be considered when using this activity?
   - *Depends on how good the prerequisite abilities (#3) are*

10. For which short-term goal(s) would this activity be appropriate?
    - *Strengthen upper extremity musculature*
    - *Develop functional balance*
    - *Improve grip strength*
    - *Improve central and peripheral endurance*
    - *Learn proper body mechanics*

11. How can this activity be graded to increase
    a. strength?
       - *Heavier vacuum*
       - *Thicker carpet*
    b. active range of motion?
       - *At limit*
    c. passive range of motion?
       - *Not applicable*
    d. coordination/dexterity?
       - *Place furniture in the area*
    e. endurance?
       - *Increase amount of carpeting vacuumed (more rooms)*
    f. reduce edema?
       - *Not applicable*

The information that follows will (a) provide students and instructors with resources to enhance the learning experience and (b) assist the students in completing the assignment.

Learning Resources

Aja, D. (1996). Finding a niche in job-site analysis. *OT Practice, 1*(7), 36–41.

Joannidis, S. (1996). Occupational therapy for skilled workers. *OT Week, 10*(33), 14–15.

Study Questions

1. Identify the sensorimotor performance components required to hammer a nail into a wall.

2. Identify the psychological and self-management performance components that may be affected by chronic pain.

3. What temporal contextual demands could be altered to enhance success of a fatigued worker returning to the workplace?

4. Your client does not have the hand strength or finger flexion range of motion to use a screwdriver. The most appropriate intervention strategy would include which of the following: rest, alternating hot and cold packs, a large-handled screwdriver, a power screwdriver?

5. Your client is unable to carry more than 10 pounds at work. What physical environmental modifications or adaptations would promote continued independence at work?

6. Your 25-year-old client received surgery to repair a tear to the tendon of flexor digitorum profundus. The tear occurred proximal to the wrist. Which of the following activities would be extremely difficult: holding a briefcase with a hook grasp, opening a cupboard door, picking up small objects with a two point pad pinch?

7. Describe how a therapist's skill in task analysis is used to conduct a job simulation.

References

American Occupational Therapy Association. (1994). *Uniform terminology for occupational therapy* (3rd ed.). Bethesda, MD: Author.

Americans With Disabilities Act of 1990, 42 U.S.C. §12101 *et seq.*

Jacobs, K. (1995). Preparing to return to work. In C. A. Trombly (Ed.), *Occupational therapy for physical dysfunction* (4th ed., pp. 329–349). Baltimore: Williams & Wilkins.

Joannidis, S. (1996). Occupational therapy for skilled workers. *OT Week, 10*(33), 14–15.

Kielhofner, G. (1992). *Conceptual foundations of occupational therapy.* Philadelphia: F. A. Davis.

Matheson, L., Ogden, L., Violette, K., & Schultz, K. (1985). Work hardening: Occupational therapy in industrial rehabilitation. *American Journal of Occupational Therapy, 39,* 314–321.

Mattingly, C., & Fleming, M. H. (1994). *Clinical reasoning: Forms of inquiry into a therapeutic practice.* Philadelphia: F. A. Davis.

McNeil, J. M. (1993). *Americans with disabilities: 1991–1992. U.S. Bureau of the Census. Current Population Reports P70-33.* Washington, DC: U.S. Government Printing Office.

Trombly, C. A. (1995). Purposeful activity. In C. A. Trombly (Ed.), *Occupational therapy for physical dysfunction* (4th ed., pp. 237–253). Baltimore: Williams & Wilkins.

DRIVING, SPORTS, AND RECREATION: THE CASE OF JEFF

"Because we freely chose them, our play and leisure activities may be some of the purest expressions of who we are as persons.... If play is the purest expression of who we are as persons, then people who have lost their ability to play in the ways they choose have lost important pieces of themselves" (Bundy, 1993, p. 217, 220).[1]

Chapter Objectives

1. Evaluate the effects of a neurological condition on an individual's occupational performance profile.
2. Compare and contrast a client's premorbid lifestyle and current occupational performance profile and begin to predict a potential future profile.
3. Evaluate the fit between an individual and his or her desired roles, tasks, and activities in the areas of leisure sports or driving a car.
4. Evaluate whether there is a fit between the characteristics of an individual, task demands, and contextual variables.
5. Use logical thinking and creative analysis to develop an individualized intervention strategy.
6. Use community resources to identify assistive technology devices for disabled drivers and paraplegic athletes.
7. Describe the role of occupational therapy practitioners who provide services to individuals with permanent impairments.

Using Task Analysis to Return a Client to a Personally Meaningful Lifestyle

Traumatic injuries such as amputations, spinal cord injuries, and brain injuries may cause permanent, irreversible impairments that alter a person's ability to perform tasks and activities in a manner or within the range considered normal. These disabilities, however, need not negatively affect the person's self-

concept, self-worth, and sense of mastery over life events. The role of occupational therapy practitioners who work with people with permanent disabilities, therefore, is to restructure tasks, alter performance contexts, and teach new methods, thus enabling these clients to envision their potential and reestablish a satisfying lifestyle. By assisting clients in establishing, reconstructing, and controlling their patterns of occupation, therapists facilitate the adaptation process (CAOT, 1994).

Occupational therapy practitioners use their understanding of a client's premorbid lifestyle and knowledge of the effect of the current condition on the client's occupational performance profile to construct an image of future potential. This "possible and desirable future for the patient" gives therapists a starting point and guides intervention (Mattingly & Fleming, 1994, p. 241). The construction, revision, and realization of this future requires active client participation in the therapeutic process (Mattingly & Fleming).

The disability and mobility problems that accompany a permanent spinal cord injury alter many clients' ability to use familiar behaviors to be part of their community, release tension, externalize anger through physical engagement, or gain pleasure from action-oriented activities (Versluys, 1995). Occupational therapy practitioners design intervention to promote engagement and independence in desired roles, tasks, and activities, and to enhance

[1]From "Assessment of Play and Leisure: Delineation of the problem," by A. Bundy, 1993, *American Journal of Occupational Therapy, 47,* pp. 217 and 220. Copyright 1993 by the American Occupational Therapy Association. Reprinted with permission.

clients' participation in activities for which they have high interest but low satisfaction (Yerxa & Baum, 1986).

Successful adaptation requires that the client appraise his or her values and goals and continue to work toward attainment of personal, social, and vocational plans (Versluys, 1995). Therapists who work with clients with traumatic spinal cord injuries or brain injuries define outcome goals and objectives in all occupational performance domains, including activities of daily living, work and productive activities, and play and leisure pursuits. Basic and instrumental activities of daily living are usually addressed initially in therapy. Engagement in productive and leisure pursuits commences when the client has regained enough stamina. Loss of choice in intrinsically motivated play and leisure pursuits affects volition and individuality (Bundy, 1993), whereas participating in sports may increase a disabled person's sense of mastery, self-esteem, adjustment to loss, social interaction, and level of physical fitness (Pasek & Schkade, 1996; Stotts, 1986; Taylor & McGruder, 1996; Valliant, Bezzubyk, Daley, & Asu, 1985). Some clients, however, may benefit from being introduced to novel activities to assist in the construction of a new identity and sense of self (Taylor & McGruder, 1996).

Assignment

1. Read the case about Jeff.
2. Evaluate Jeff's premorbid lifestyle and current occupational performance profile. If you would like assistance with this challenge, use the Occupational Performance Profile form in Appendix G to document information on the occupations that are meaningful to Jeff; his unique values, goals, and performance component capabilities; and the contexts in which he performs.

Why have the initial therapy sessions focused on engagement in activities to enhance skills in the performance components of endurance, postural control, and upper extremity strength? Why might Jeff prefer to put on his undergarments, pants, and shirt while sitting on the bed? Why might Jeff be slow at tying his shoes?

Why were a wheelchair, raised toilet seat, and bath bench seat used to alter the physical environment and promote independence in functional mobility and bathing?

Why did the occupational therapist predict that Jeff would continue to require some type of bath seat?

3. Work in groups of two or three. Use your understanding of Jeff's premorbid lifestyle and knowledge of the effect of his medical diagnoses on his occupational performance profile to construct an image of his future potential. This "possible and desirable future for the patient" gives therapists a starting point and guides intervention (Mattingly & Fleming, 1994, p. 241).

Will Jeff be able to return to living independently? Explain and justify your impressions. Identify potential task demands and contextual variables that might limit independence in this area. Identify and describe possible solutions.

Do you think that Jeff will be able to return to work as a sports commentator? Is there a match among Jeff's performance capabilities, task demands of this job, and contextual variables?

Explain and justify your impressions. Identify potential employment barriers and possible solutions. Is Jeff's employer required to make reasonable accommodations for his new disability? What type of accommodations may be necessary?

4. Complete Project A or B, depending on your interest in Jeff being able to participate in sports or in his ability to drive. Will Jeff be able to actively participate in the sports he is fond of?

Explain and justify your impressions. Identify potential task demands and contextual variables that might limit engagement in these activities. Complete Project A if you would like to explore this domain in more detail.

Will Jeff be able to drive? Explain and justify your impression. Identify potential task demands and contextual variables that might limit Jeff's potential to be independent in this area. Complete Project B if you would like to explore this domain in more detail.

Project A

Assume that you have collaborated with Jeff to define therapy goals and objectives. One of these long-term goals is to independently participate in a recreational sport. Select one leisure sport that Jeff currently enjoys and identify the task and contextual demands required to perform this activity in the "typical fashion." If you would like some assistance with this challenge, complete the Occupational Performance Analysis—Short Form (Appendix B).

After evaluating Jeff's premorbid lifestyle, current occupational performance profile, and the task demands and contextual variables of a selected sport, identify which activities would challenge Jeff beyond his current capabilities.

What intervention strategies will you use to enable Jeff to participate in this sport? If you

would like some assistance with this challenge, (a) use community resources for paraplegic athletes, (b) examine the information provided in the Learning Resources section, and (c) review the various intervention strategies identified in the Occupational Performance Practice Model for Service to Individuals outlined in the chapter "Task Analysis: The Contribution of Occupational Therapy to Health."

Project B

Assume that one of Jeff's goals is to independently drive his car. Identify the task and contextual demands required to perform this activity in the "typical fashion." If you would like some assistance with this challenge, complete the Occupational Performance Analysis—Short Form (Appendix B).

After evaluating Jeff's premorbid lifestyle, current occupational performance profile, and the task demands and contextual variables of driving, identify which activities would challenge Jeff beyond his current capabilities.

What intervention strategies will you use to enable Jeff to drive? If you would like some assistance with this challenge, (a) use community resources for disabled drivers, (b) examine information provided in the Learning Resources section, and (c) review the various intervention strategies identified in the Occupational Performance Practice Model for Service to Individuals outlined in the chapter "Task Analysis: The Contribution of Occupational Therapy to Health."

5. Select and design a purposeful activity for use with Jeff. Treatment sessions in your facility last 30 minutes. Purposeful activities are therapeutic when they (a) are relevant, meaningful, and goal-directed; (b) elicit coordination among sensori-

motor, cognitive, psychological, and psychosocial systems; and (c) promote mastery and feelings of competence (AOTA, 1993; Fidler & Fidler, 1978; Trombly, 1995).

Optional:

6. Read the article by Taylor and McGruder (1996) on *"The Meaning of Sea Kayaking for Persons with Spinal Cord Injuries"* and the activity analysis they provide on page 44 of the article.

7. Read the article by Pierce (1996) titled *"A Road Map for Driver Rehabilitation"* and Lavoot and Gross's (1996) article *"The Role of the COTA in Adaptive Driving Programs."* Describe the role that registered occupational therapists and certified occupational therapy assistants play in driver rehabilitation.

Case Study: Jeff

Jeff is a 32-year-old, single male who sustained a midthoracic, complete spinal cord injury and a mild traumatic brain injury during a recent motor vehicle accident. He plans to return to his job as a sports commentator and has expressed an interest in participating in wheelchair sports. Jeff is fond of baseball, basketball, football, tennis, rugby, fishing, water sports, and camping.

Initial therapy sessions on the rehabilitation unit focus on engagement in activities to build endurance, enhance postural control, increase upper extremity strength, and learn new methods of performing basic activities of daily living. Although Jeff appears to have mild visual-perceptual and short-term-memory problems, his initial lack of independence in basic activities of daily living appears to be primarily secondary to paralysis. After the first few weeks of intervention, Jeff has gained independence in dressing, personal care, and bathing. Jeff puts on his undergarments, pants, and shirt while sitting in bed reclined against the wall.

He puts on his shoes while sitting in his wheelchair and is quite slow tying his shoelaces. Jeff requires supervision to ensure that he safely transfers to a raised toilet seat and a tub bench seat. His occupational therapist predicts that he will eventually transfer independently to a regular-height toilet seat and that he will always require some type of bath seat.

Jeff appears to be very goal-directed and frequently verbalizes his commitment to returning to his previous lifestyle. He has not expressed any other feelings to you about his injury and does not speak much with the other patients in the hospital. Jeff's immediate family does not live nearby. His girlfriend visits regularly and is a physical therapist. Two other people with spinal cord injuries are on the rehabilitation unit at this time. (See Table 1 for a discussion of the prevalence of traumatic spinal cord and brain injury and the role of occupational therapists.)

The information that follows will (a) provide students and instructors with resources to enhance the learning experience and (b) assist the students in completing the assignment.

Learning Resources

Books and Periodicals

Axelson, P. (1988). Hitting the slopes. *Sports 'N Spokes, 14*(4), 22–34.

Axelson, P., & Castellano, J. (1990). Take to the trails. *Sports 'N Spokes, 16*(2), 20–22.

Bernhard, K. F. (1984). Amputee athletes. *Journal of Rehabilitation, 50*(3), 70–71.

Boren, H. A., & Meell, H. (1985). Adolescent amputee ski rehabilitation program. *Journal of the Association of Pediatric Oncology Nurses, 2*(1), 16–23.

Table 1: Spinal Cord and Traumatic Brain Injuries

The incidence of new spinal cord injuries in the United States in 1994 was approximately 200,000. The prevalence during this same year was 38 to 40 per million (Lasfargues, Custis, Morrone, Carswell, & Nguyen, 1995; Price, Makintubee, Herndon, & Istre, 1994). The extent of neurological damage in spinal cord injuries is classified according to the extent and location of injury. A complete spinal cord lesion indicates that there is no motor or sensory function at or below the level of the injury, whereas an incomplete lesion indicates some degree of motor and/or sensory function below the level of the injury (American Spinal Injury Association, 1992). Complete, high, and midthoracic injuries result in paraplegia with motor and sensory loss to the trunk and lower limbs. Occupational therapy practitioners enhance functional performance and psychosocial adjustment by analyzing, retraining, and teaching adapted techniques to provide clients with the tools and resources needed to achieve their potential (Adler, 1996).

Estimates of the incidence of new head-injured people each year approximates 2 million (National Head Injury Foundation, 1993). The major causes of traumatic brain injury (TBI) include motor vehicle accidents, violence, and falls; and surveys suggest that over half of TBI patients were intoxicated at the time of injury (Gordon, Mann, & Willer, 1993). The sequelae of head trauma is broad and ranges from mild (82%), moderate or severe (14%), to fatal (5%) (Kraus, Rock, & Hemyari, 1990). Impairments in sensorimotor, cognitive, psychological, emotional, and psychosocial performance components are common. It is difficult to predict long-term disability as each individual's impairment, character strengths, and social environment are unique (Scott & Dow, 1995).

Colston, L. G. (1991). The expanding role of assistive technology in therapeutic recreation. *Journal of Physical Education, Recreation, and Dance, 62*(4), 39–41.

Hamel, R. (1992). Getting into the game: New opportunities for athletes with disabilities. *Physician and Sports Medicine, 20*(11), 128–129.

Handler, B. S., & Patterson, J. B. (1995). Driving after brain injury. *Journal of Rehabilitation, 61*(2), 43–49.

Kacie, T. (1995). What do you think? Wheelchair sports and the disabled athlete. *SCI Nursing, 12*(2), 66–69.

Kinney, W. B., & Coyle, C. P. (1992). Predicting life satisfaction among adults with physical disabilities. *Archives of Physical Medicine and Rehabilitation, 73,* 863–869.

Krag, M. H., & Messner, D. G. (1982). Skiing for the physically handicapped. *Clinics in Sports Medicine, 1*(2), 319–332.

Lavoot, P., & Gross, M. F. (1996). The role of the COTA in adaptive driving programs. *OT Practice, 1*(10), 32–33.

Lillie, S. M. (1996). Activities of daily living: Driving with a physical dysfunction. In L. W. Pedretti (Ed.), *Occupational therapy: Practice skills for physical dysfunction* (4th ed., pp. 499–506). St. Louis, MO: Mosby.

Longmuir, P. E., & Axelson, P. (1996). Assistive technology for recreation. In J. C. Galvin & M. J. Scherer (Eds.), *Evaluating, selecting, and using appropriate assistive technology* (pp. 162–197). Gaithersburg, MD: Aspen.

Madorsky, J. G. B., & Curtis, K. A. (1984). Wheelchair sports medicine. *American Journal of Sports Medicine, 12*(2), 128–132.

Madorsky, J. G. B., & Kiley, D. P. (1984). Wheelchair mountaineering. *Archives of Physical Medicine and Rehabilitation, 65,* 490–492.

Madorsky, J. G. B., & Madorsky, A. G. (1988). Scuba diving: Taking the wheelchair out of wheelchair sports. *Archives of Physical Medicine and Rehabilitation, 69*(3), 215–219.

Meaden, C. A. (1991). Assessing people with a disability for sport: The profile system. *Physiotherapy, 77,* 360–366.

Pasek, P. B., & Schkade, J. K. (1996). Effects of skiing experiences on adolescents with limb deficiencies: An occupational adaptation perspective. *American Journal of Occupational Therapy, 50,* 24–31.

Pierce, S. (1996). A road map for driver rehabilitation. *OT Practice, 1*(10), 31–38.

Rubin, G., & Fleiss, D. (1983). Devices to enable persons with amputation to participate in sports. *Archives of Physical Medicine and Rehabilitation, 64*(1), 37–40.

Segedy, A. (1996). Unstoppable: 1996 Atlanta Paralympic games. *TeamRehab, 7*(10), 46–55.

Sprigle, S., Morris, B. O., Nowachek, G., & Karg, P. E. (1995). Assessment of the evaluation procedures of drivers with disabilities. *Occupational Therapy Journal of Research, 15*(3), 147–164.

Stevens, C. (1996a, June/July). Fencing hopeful prepares for paralympics. *Rehab Management,* 20.

Stevens, C. (1996b, June/July). Goalball athlete sets sights on Atlanta. *Rehab Management,* 20.

Stotts, K. M. (1986). Health maintenance: Paraplegic athletes and non-athletes. *Archives of Physical Medicine and Rehabilitation, 67,* 109–114.

Taylor, L. P. S., & McGruder, J. E. (1996). The meaning of sea kayaking for persons with spinal cord injuries. *American Journal of Occupational Therapy, 50,* 39–46.

Valliant, P. M., Bezzubyk, I., Daley, L., & Asu, M. E. (1985). Psychological impact of sport on disabled athletes. *Psychological Reports, 56,* 923–929.

Webre, A. W., & Zeller, J. (1990). *Canoeing and kayaking for persons with physical disabilities.* Springfield, VA: American Canoe Association.

Community Resources

Canadian Wheelchair Basketball Association Home Page http://www.cdnsport.ca /~reg/index.html

International Paralympic Committee Home Page http://info.lut.ac.uk/research /paad/ipc/ipc.html

International Wheelchair Aviators Home Page http://www.dsg.cs.tcd.ie /dsg_people/sloubtin/IWA.html

Paralympics HomePage

http://www.uscpaa.org/cppara.htm

Study Questions

1. Identify one local agency that organizes sport activities for individuals with disabilities.

2. Identify assistive technology devices that enable individuals with paraplegia to participate in a sport.

3. Identify two assistive technology devices that enable individuals with disabilities to drive a car.

4. Your client would like to learn to play wheelchair basketball.

   a. How could your client learn about the rules of this sport?

   b. How would you go about linking this individual with a local team?

   c. Design a treatment session to increase your client's endurance for the sport.

5. Your client has a disability and would like to drive. Where does this individual seek a new driver's license?

6. What information do therapists use to construct a vision of a particular client's future potential?

References

Adler, C. (1996). Spinal cord injury. In L. W. Pedretti (Ed.), *Occupational therapy: Practice skills for physical dysfunction* (4th ed., pp. 765–784). St. Louis, MO: Mosby.

American Occupational Therapy Association. (1993). *Position paper: Purposeful activity.* Bethesda, MD: Author.

American Spinal Injury Association. (1992). *Standards for neurological and functional classification of spinal cord injury.* Chicago: Author.

Bundy, A. (1993). Assessment of play and leisure: Delineation of the problem. *American Journal of Occupational Therapy, 47,* 217–222.

Canadian Association of Occupational Therapists. (1994). Everyday occupations and health. *Canadian Journal of Occupational Therapy, 61,* 294–295.

Fidler, G., & Fidler, J. (1978). Doing and becoming: Purposeful action and self-actualization. *American Journal of Occupational Therapy, 32,* 305–310.

Gordon, W. A., Mann, N., & Willer, B. (1993). Demographic and social characteristics of the traumatic brain injury model system database. *Journal of Head Trauma Rehabilitation, 8*(2), 26–33.

Kraus, J. F., Rock, A., & Hemyari, P. (1990). Brain injuries among infants, children, adolescents, and young adults. *American Journal of Diseases of Children, 144,* 684–691.

Lasfargues, J. E., Custis, D., Morrone, F., Carswell, J., & Nguyen, T. (1995). A model for estimating spinal cord injury prevalence in the United States. *Paraplegia, 33*(2), 62–68.

Mattingly, C., & Fleming, M. H. (1994). *Clinical reasoning: Forms of inquiry in a therapeutic practice.* Philadelphia: F. A. Davis.

National Head Injury Foundation. (1993). *Every fifteen seconds.* Washington, DC: Author.

Pasek, P. B. & Schkade, J. K. (1996). Effects of skiing experiences on adolescents with limb deficiencies: An occupational adaptation perspective. *American Journal of Occupational Therapy, 50,* 24–31.

Price, C., Makintubee, S., Herndon, W., & Istre, G. R. (1994). Epidemiology of traumatic spinal cord injury and acute hospitalization and rehabilitation charges for spinal cord injury in Oklahoma, 1988–1990. *American Journal of Epidemiology, 139*(1), 37–47.

Scott, A. D., & Dow, P. W. (1995). Traumatic brain injury. In C. A. Trombly (Ed.), *Occupational therapy for physical dysfunction* (4th ed., pp. 705–733). Baltimore: Williams & Wilkins.

Stotts, K. M. (1986). Health maintenance: Paraplegic athletes and non-athletes. *Archives of Physical Medicine and Rehabilitation, 67,* 109–114.

Taylor, L. P. S., & McGruder, J. E. (1996). The meaning of sea kayaking for persons with spinal cord injuries. *American Journal of Occupational Therapy, 50,* 39–46.

Trombly, C. A. (1995). Occupation: Purposefulness and meaningfulness as therapeutic mechanisms. *American Journal of Occupational Therapy, 49,* 960–972.

Valliant, P. M., Bezzubyk, I., Daley, L., & Asu, M. E. (1985). Psychological impact of sport on disabled athletes. *Psychological Reports, 56,* 923–929.

Versluys, H. P. (1995). Facilitating psychosocial adjustment to disability. In C. A. Trombly (Ed.), *Occupational therapy for physical dysfunction* (4th ed., pp. 377–389). Baltimore: Williams & Wilkins.

Yerxa, E. J., & Baum, S. (1986). Engagement in daily occupations and life satisfaction among people with spinal cord injuries. *Occupational Therapy Journal of Research, 6,* 271–283.

ADULT OCCUPATIONS: THE CASE OF RENA

"Therapists helped people learn or relearn common everyday activities such as bathing, dressing, and working. To do this they had to discover what the functional problem was and how the person could develop strategies for accomplishing desired tasks in the most efficient or effective way, given the limitations of the disability" (Mattingly & Fleming, 1994, p. 337).[1]

Chapter Objectives

1. Evaluate the impact of a neurological condition on an individual's current occupational performance profile.
2. Practice predicting a client's potential future occupational performance profile.
3. Evaluate the fit between an individual and his or her desired roles, tasks, and activities.
5. Use evaluation results and client goals to identify and document outcome-oriented objectives.
6. Use logical thinking and creative analysis to develop an individualized intervention strategy.
7. Identify community resource agencies and social support systems available to individuals with disabilities.
8. Prepare and give a presentation on the intervention strategies used to attain a specific client goal.

Assignment

1. Read the case about Rena.
2. Work in groups of three or four to evaluate Rena's premorbid and current occupational performance profile. If you would like assistance with this challenge, use the Occupational Performance Form in Appendix G to document information on the occupations that are meaningful to Rena; her unique values, goals, and performance component capabilities; and the contexts in which she performs.
3. Therapists are responsible for determining how a diagnosed condition influences present performance and for making accurate predictions about

gains in functional levels (Mattingly & Fleming, 1994). The exercise that follows will help you develop skills in this area.

Estimate how much Rena's cerebral vascular accident (CVA) might influence her current level of independence in occupational performance areas. Complete the column entitled Current Performance in Table 1. This will require you to apply your knowledge of (a) Rena's performance context, and (b) the impact of the CVA on her sensorimotor, cognitive, psychological, and psychosocial performance components. Use Table 1 to assist you in this challenge. In clinical practice Rena's occupational therapist could observe her performance in these domains.

Complete the column titled Long-Term Potential in Table 1 by using your knowledge of (a) Rena's prognosis, (b) her performance context, and (c) the impact of the CVA on Rena's current performance. Some predictions of Rena's long-term potential have been provided. The construction of a "possible and desirable future for the patient" gives therapists a starting point and guides intervention; experienced therapists are able to make quite accurate predictions about potential future functional status (Mattingly & Fleming, 1994, p. 241).

---

[1]From *Clinical Reasoning: Forms of Inquiry in a Therapeutic Practice* (p. 337), by C. Mattingly and M. H. Fleming, 1994, Philadelphia: F. A. Davis. Copyright 1994 by F. A. Davis. Reprinted with permission.

4. During your discussions with Rena, she has identified a number of aspirations, including (a) caring for her children, (b) regaining independence in basic activities of daily living, (c) managing her home, (d) returning to work, and (e) maintaining her relationship with her boyfriend Benjamin.

   Select one of these aspirations and define a specific, measurable, outcome-oriented therapy goal. Compile a list of short-term objectives using the Client Goals Form located in Appendix H. In clinical practice these goals and objectives would be established and prioritized in collaboration with Rena, her family, and members of the rehabilitation team.

   Groups of students within the same occupational therapy class should select different goals.

5. Develop an intervention plan to attain the goal and objectives defined in Question 4. Engagement and independence in these tasks will enable Rena to return to the roles that give meaning and purpose to her life. Prepare to present this intervention plan to your class. If you would like some assistance with this challenge, consider using the intervention strategies identified in the Occupational Performance Practice Model for Service to Individuals outlined in the chapter "Task Analysis: The Contribution of Occupational Therapy to Health."

6. If you have decided to enhance specific performance component skills and abilities (e.g., improve left upper limb strength and fine motor dexterity to be able to prepare a light meal while sitting in the wheelchair), select and design a purposeful activity for use with Rena. Treatment sessions in your facility last 30 minutes.

7. Identify community agencies and social support systems that may provide resources to assist Rena in attaining her therapeutic goals. For example, is there public transportation available to individuals in your city who use a wheelchair for community mobility?

8. Make a presentation to your occupational therapy class: identify the selected goal, delineate objectives, and describe what intervention strategies are used to achieve these therapy outcomes. You may be required to demonstrate adapted techniques or the use of assistive technology devices.

Optional:

9. Almost 5 months have passed and Rena is attending outpatient therapy. She walks short distances with a rolling walker and uses a manual wheelchair for community mobility. She is independent, with equipment and adaptations, in dressing and personal hygiene. Intervention focuses on continuing to improve mobility, vocational preparation, home management, and psychosocial adjustment. Engagement in these tasks requires improvements in the neuromusculoskeletal and motor performance components of postural control, strength, endurance, and left-hand fine motor coordination, and in the cognitive performance components of spatial operations, sequencing, and short-term memory. Rena's left shoulder, elbow, and wrist active range of motion is within 20 to 30 degrees of full range. Her two- and three-point pad grasp strength with this hand is "good."

   Last week Rena announced that her boyfriend Benjamin had proposed marriage. The wedding will take place in 6 months, and Rena is determined to manage all of the arrangements and make her own wedding dress. She wants to have a traditional ceremony with about 20 guests. Select and design a purposeful activity for use with Rena in outpatient therapy.

Case Study: Rena

Rena is a 40-year-old mother who was admitted for rehabilitation following a right ischemic cerebral vascular accident (CVA) from a cardiogenic embolus that lodged in the middle cerebral artery two weeks ago. Rena's medical chart indicates that she has a history of coronary artery disease, arrhythmias, cardiomegaly, and hypercholesteremia. Two years ago Rena was admitted to ABC Medical Center with atrial fibrillation. An echocardiogram showed a dilated aortic root, and a subsequent CT scan of the chest confirmed the diagnosis.

Rena is a divorced parent who has two children, Jacob (11 years old) and Jason (7 years old). She does not have many close friends but has been dating Benjamin for 2 months. The children's grandmother is caring for them until their mother returns home. Prior to her admission to the hospital Rena worked full time as a librarian at the same elementary school that her children attend. The family rode the school bus together each morning. Rena has established a reputation for her literary, art, history, and poetry exhibitions and the school's teachers are very fond of her. Rena enjoys homemaking and occasionally sews clothes for her two children. Prior to admission she attended a continuing education course on advanced computer word processing one night per week. Jacob and Jason play baseball three nights a week and spend very little time at home on the weekends. They spend most of their spare time outdoors watching or participating in neighborhood baseball and basketball games. Rena is known on the boys' baseball team for her great hamburgers and chocolate chip cookies.

Rena, Jacob, and Jason live in a first-floor, two-bedroom apartment, with a 6-inch step at the building entrance. Jacob has provided a graphic illustration of the layout of Rena's bedroom (Figure 1), the family's kitchen (Figure 2), and the bathroom (Figure 3). The laundry room is located on the same floor as the apartment, but it has a 2-inch step at the doorway. The grocery store is 4 blocks away. This family lives in a neighborhood that has a strong social network, but Rena indicates that she prefers not to "get involved" and doesn't like to "depend on anyone."

Figure 1. Rena's Bedroom.

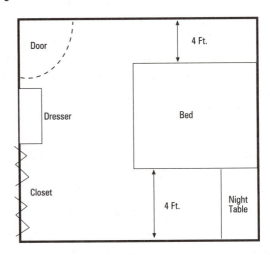

Figure 2. Rena's Kitchen.

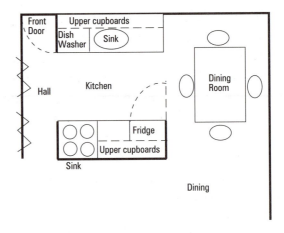

Figure 3. Rena's Bathroom.

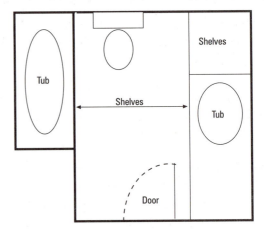

Rena was transferred to rehabilitation from acute care, and the physiatrist expects that she will require 4 more weeks of inpatient services. The physical therapist has indicated that she expects Rena will eventually walk short distances with a rolling walker and use a manual wheelchair for community mobility. The admission note indicates that Rena had a flaccid left trunk, upper and lower extremities; left unilateral sensory loss in her upper limbs more than in her lower limbs; left ptosis; perceptual and cognitive deficits; and impulsivity. The occupational therapy reevaluation is almost complete and you as the occupational therapist must assist the rehabilitation team in preparing Rena for discharge. Rena does not have any cardiac precautions at this time.

During your initial interview, Rena expresses her commitment to care for her two children and indicates, "Although they can help me out around the apartment, I don't want them to have to take care of me." "Sure I love my job, but that will have to come after my children." Rena is fiercely motivated to regain her independence and has full intentions of returning to her previous lifestyle. She is looking forward to preparing her next library exhibition, which will be on Mozart.

Rena has regained some movement in her left shoulder (0 to 90 degrees flexion, no active extension or adduction, 0 to 10 degrees abduction, no internal or external rotation); elbow (0 to 90 degrees flexion, no active extension); and hand (20 degrees wrist flexion; no active wrist extension, ulnar deviation, or radial deviation; approximately 10 to 40 degrees of flexion in all finger joints; no active finger extension). Some resistance to passive range of motion occurs in Rena's left shoulder during external rotation. She is able to grasp large objects with a left cylindrical grasp but does not have the hand strength to carry an object. Her poor distal finger strength does not enable her to use any other

functional prehension pattern. Rena is right dominant and the strength of the right upper and lower extremity is "good."[2]

Rena's left-lower-extremity strength enables her to achieve 90 degrees of hip flexion, 60 degrees of knee flexion, and no active dorsiflexion. Rena's left leg is edematous. Her somatosensory status has improved since initial evaluation, with some gross lower limb tactile and proprioceptive sense. Rena tends to ignore her left side and frequently does not realize when her left arm is hanging over the side of her wheelchair. She is now able to sit unsupported for 10 to 20 seconds; transfers from prone to supine to long sit with minimal assistance; and transfers from sit to stand and bed to wheelchair with moderate assistance.[3]

Rena is alert and oriented. Her long-term memory appears to be at premorbid levels, but her short-term memory is slightly impaired. She does not yet recall the names of her therapists or the last time her children came to visit. She does, however, remember most events that occur within the past 10 minutes. Her visual acuity and field of vision is intact, but testing of visual perception indicates deficits in this area. During morning self-care tasks you have noticed difficulties that likely can be attributed to poor form constancy, figure–ground, spatial relations, and visual closure. She has some difficulty adjusting the position of clothing garments. Rena wears incontinence garments but has not soiled them during the daytime in the last 2 days. She sequences simple or routine activities but has great difficulty with complex unstructured chores or activities. Her topographical orientation around the hospital is also poor. Rena is still able to read and write. The effects of CVA and role of occupational therapists with these clients are described briefly in Table 2.

[2]Muscle strength of "good" means client has full range of motion against gravity but is unable to maintain this position against strong resistance (Hislop & Montgomery, 1995.)
[3]Minimal assistance means that the client performs more than 75% of the task; moderate assistance means that the client performs between 50 and 75% of the task (Hamilton, Granger, Sherwin, Zielezny, & Tashman, 1987).

Table 1: Rena's Current Performance and Long-Term Potential

I: Independent I/E: Independent with Equipment or Adaptations Min A: Minimal Assitance Mod A: Moderate Assistance Max A: Maximum Assitance D: Dependent	Current Performance	Long-Term Potential
Activities of Daily Living		
Grooming, Oral Hygiene, and Medication Routine		
Bathing/Showering		
Toilet Hygiene		
Dressing		
Feeding and Eating		I/E
Functional Mobility		
Community Mobility		
Work and Productive Activities		
Home Management		
Clothing Care		Min A → I/E
Cleaning		Min A
Meal Preparation and Cleanup		
Shopping		Mod A
Money Management		
Household Maintenance		Min A → I/E
Safety Procedures		Mod A
Care of Others		I
Vocational Activities		
Work or Job Performance		
Play or Leisure Performance		
Sewing		
Continuing Education		
Baking		

Table 2: Cerebral Vascular Accidents

Cerebral vascular accident (CVA) is the third-most-common cause of mortality in the United States (Damjanov, 1996). In 1990, 27.1% of registered occupational therapists and 30.3% of certified occupational therapy assistants indicated that the most frequent health problem for which clients were referred to them was CVA (American Occupational Therapy Association, 1991). These statistics indicate that CVA was the most common diagnosis of clients seen by occupational therapy practitioners.

The sequelae following CVA includes hemiplegia or paralysis, sensory disturbances, perceptual deficits, cognitive impairments, and a variety of psychological and psychosocial changes. Damage to the motor cortex results in contralateral impairments: a lesion in the right cerebral hemisphere produces left hemiplegia, and vice versa. Outcome is dependent on the severity of the stroke and the site and extent of damage. Involvement of the middle cerebral artery is most common, and ischemia to the neural tissue supplied by this artery results in contralateral hemiplegia particularly to the arm, face, and tongue; sensory deficits; and cognitive and perceptual deficits such as unilateral neglect, problems with spatial relations and spatial operations, dressing apraxia, and topographical disorientation (Pedretti, Smith, & Pendleton, 1996; Zoltan, Siev, & Freishtat, 1986).

It is difficult to make accurate predictions regarding rate of return, but prognosis for recovery is greater in younger clients and individuals with good sensation, minimal spasticity, and isolated movements on the affected side. The outlook for independence is poor for individuals who have complete sensory loss or fecal or urinary incontinence and do not have any concept of the affected side (Bierman, 1993).

The information that follows will (a) provide students and instructors with resources to enhance the learning experience and (b) assist students in completing the assignment.

Learning Resources

Books

Barnes, K. J. (1991). Modification of the physical environment. In C. Christiansen & C. Baum (Eds.), *Occupational therapy: Overcoming human performance deficits* (pp. 700–745). Thorofare, NJ: Slack.

Foti, D., Pedretti, L. W., & Little, S. (1996). Activities of daily living. In L. W. Pedretti (Ed.), *Occupational therapy: Practice skills for physical dysfunction* (pp. 463–506). St. Louis, MO: Mosby.

Supplier Catalogues

Maddak, Inc. PO Box 922, Randolph, MA 02368-0922. 800-854-4687.

North Coast Medical, Inc. 187 Stauffer Boulevard, San Jose, CA 95125-1042. 800-821-9319.

Sammons, Inc. PO Box 32, Brookfield, IL 60513. 708-325-1700. 800-323-5547.

Smith & Nephew Rolyan Inc. One Quality Drive, Germantown, WI 53022. 800-228-3693.

This list of suppliers is not intended to be exhaustive, nor does it represent endorsements by the author or AOTA.

Study Questions

1. Your client has significant deficits in the area of visual closure and is unable to find certain articles of clothing in a dresser. How would you restructure this task: relocate clothing to another drawer, reorganize clothing by color, or hang garments in the closet?

2. An individual who is unable to see buttons on a printed fabric may have difficulty with: spatial relations, figure–ground, body image, or visual closure?

3. Your client has difficulty monitoring her grilled cheese sandwich as it cooks while simultaneously cutting vegetables for a salad. This skill requires what: attention span, allocation attention, or orientation?

4. Your client would like to bake something for a family member's birthday and you would like to work on controlled grasp and release. Which activity would be most appropriate: mixing muffins with a hand-powered mixer, rolling cookie dough into balls and placing the balls on a tray, mixing cookie dough with a built-up handle spatula?

5. Which meal preparation activity is the simplest: preparing a can of soup, preparing a casserole, or baking brownies?

6. An occupational therapy practitioner would recommend which of the following items for a person with fine motor incoordination who frequently drops objects: shirt with contrasting colors, spray deodorant, toothpaste with flip-top lid, or pants with a drawstring waist?

7. Writing a check to pay for groceries requires which of the following cognitive skills: praxis, figure–ground, orientation, or categorization?

References

American Occupational Therapy Association. (1991). *1990 Membership data survey.* Bethesda, MD: Author.

Bierman, S. N. (1993). Cerebrovascular accident. In R. A. Hansen & B. Atchison (Eds.), *Conditions in occupational therapy: Effect on occupational performance* (pp. 16–49). Baltimore: Williams & Wilkins.

Damjanov, I. (1996). *Pathology for the health-related professions.* Philadelphia: W. B. Saunders.

Hislop, H. J., & Montgomery, J. (1995). *Daniels and Worthingham's muscle testing: Techniques of manual examination* (6th ed.). Philadelphia: W. B. Saunders.

Mattingly, C., & Fleming, M. H. (1994). *Clinical reasoning: Forms of inquiry in therapeutic practice.* Philadelphia: F. A. Davis.

Pedretti, L. W., Smith, J. A., & Pendleton, H. M. (1996). Cerebral vascular accident. In L. W. Pedretti (Ed.), *Occupational therapy: Practice skills for physical dysfunction* (pp. 785–805). St. Louis, MO: Mosby.

Zoltan, B., Siev, E., & Freishtat, B. (1986). *The adult stroke patient: A manual for evaluation and treatment of perceptual and cognitive dysfunction* (2nd ed.). Thorofare, NJ: Slack.

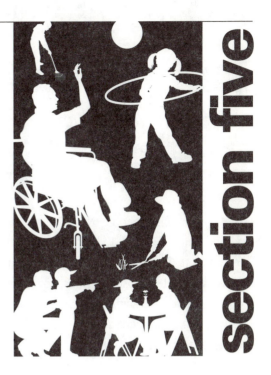

section five

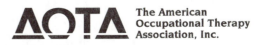

SECTION FIVE: SENIORS

"The occupational therapy practitioner's commitment to those whom he or she serves is to guide them in the use of purposeful activities so as to empower them to enhance the quality of their being in the daily reality where they live as parents, children, students, homemakers, workers, or retirees" (American Occupational Therapy Association, 1993, p. 1082).[1]

The number of people over the age of 65 years will increase from 13% of the population in 2000 to 22% in 2030; and the most rapid increase will be for those individuals over 85 years of age (Institute of Medicine, 1990). As the size of the elderly[2] population increases so does the number of occupational therapy practitioners working in the area of geriatrics. In 1990 approximately 11,000 registered occupational therapists (OTRs), or 28%, and 3,500 certified occupational therapy assistants (COTAs), or 37%, indicated that they worked primarily with geriatric clients (AOTA, 1991). According to the AOTA 1995–1996 Member Update, approximately 19,000, or 43%, of practicing OTRs and 7,700, or 66%, of COTAs indicate that they work primarily in geriatrics (P. F. Burchman, personal communication, January 23, 1997). Occupational therapy practitioners now work more often with people over age 65 than with any other age group (AOTA, 1996).

The likelihood of becoming disabled to some degree increases with age. A survey conducted in 1991 and 1992 by the United States Bureau of the Census found a disability prevalence rate of "29.2% among persons 45 to 64 years old, 44.6% among persons 65 to 74 years old, 63.7% among persons 75 to 84 years old, and 84.2% among persons 85 years old and over." Among persons with a disability, the likelihood that the disability was severe increased from 56.8% among persons 65 to 74 years old to 81.2% among persons 85 and over (McNeil, 1993, p. 8). Maintaining healthy seniors and enhancing the func-

tional performance of disabled seniors has economic, social, and personal benefits to the individuals, their families, and their communities (Bonder & Goodman, 1995; U.S. Department of Health and Human Services, 1992).

Section Five provides occupational therapy students with the opportunity to refine their task analysis skills. By applying this assessment and intervention tool, students will learn to resolve the occupational performance problems demonstrated by seniors in several hypothetical client cases. These cases provide realistic contexts for using task analysis skill to (a) evaluate clients, their desired tasks, and performance contexts; and (b) target intervention at variables that affect occupational performance, health, and well-being. Students will be required to employ preventative, functional, and remedial approaches to intervention and to select and design purposeful activities.

Nelson is a 65-year-old widower who retired at the age of 60. He lives alone in his small farmhouse, but he sold most of his land when he retired. Nelson is receiving rehabilitation services in a skilled nursing facility to recover from a left below-knee amputation and he has significant difficulty maintaining postural control in standing due to peripheral neuropathy in his right leg. Nelson has a number of home maintenance and improvement tasks that he enjoys doing, and his leisure interests are in woodworking and

---

[2]Within this text the terms **elderly**, **seniors**, and **geriatric** refer to those individuals over the age of 65.

horseback riding. Task analysis is required to (a) identify the variables that limit Nelson's ability to perform these meaningful occupations, (b) target intervention strategies toward maximizing Nelson's participation in selected tasks, and (c) design purposeful activities to facilitate adaptation. Students will discuss the role of occupational therapy and the use of purposeful activity in facilitating adaptation and preventing, detecting, and treating depression in the elder population.

Wayne and Minnie have been married for 48 years. While Minnie describes herself as the "planner, organizer, and motivator" of their busy lifestyle, Wayne relies heavily on his wife's assistance for functional and community mobility. Minnie has broken her arm and cannot assist her husband for 6 to 8 weeks. Task analysis is required to identify the variables that limit the occupational performance profiles of these seniors and to target intervention strategies at these barriers. Students will compare Wayne's occupational performance profile with the task and contextual demands of certain functional and community mobility activities. This client case introduces the concepts of work simplification and energy conservation and examines the availability of services to homebound seniors.

Rhonda just celebrated her 89th birthday in a nursing home and her daughter is concerned about Rhonda's level of independence in feeding and eating. Task analysis is required to evaluate (a) the impact of this client's chronic condition on her ability to eat, and (b) the task and environmental

demands of eating and drinking. By participating in eating and drinking during a meal, students can increase the accuracy of their analysis. Students will use logical thinking and creative analysis to target intervention to improve client performance, adapt task demands, and alter contextual variables. The goal is to maximize Rhonda's performance in this self-care task. Students will be required to plan a series of treatment sessions and will role-model intervention strategies.

Maureen and Bert both have cognitive impairments and live in a skilled nursing facility. The staff members who structure evening recreational activities have not been successful in their attempts to work with either client and have asked for assistance. Students will use task analysis to evaluate the sensorimotor, cognitive, psychological, and psychosocial profiles of these seniors; to select an activity, craft, or game for evaluating the client's cognitive capabilities; and to analyze the cognitive requirements required to participate in a task. After completing the analysis, students will offer activity suggestions to the nursing home staff. The Cognitive Disabilities Model is introduced, and the use of crafts in evaluation and intervention is reviewed.

Gladys is a 78-year-old mother of four who has been married for over 50 years. Gladys has led a very active life and shared a social lifestyle with her husband but retired 20 years ago when she was unable to work because of the pain associated with her rheumatoid arthritis. Over the years, as her disease progressed, Gladys became more and more dependent on her husband. Three weeks ago she fell while dancing and fractured her hip and elbow. Gladys is now dependent on her husband for most activities, but she has a number of intervention needs and priorities. Students will be required to evaluate the occupational performance profile of Gladys and analyze the role and contribution of her primary caregiver. Task analysis will be used to understand current and potential functional performance, task demands, and contextual variables, and to design intervention strategies that would enable Gladys to engage in desired roles and activities.

ABC township is planning to develop an **Accessible Seniors Center.** Three occupational therapy practitioners in private practice are providing consultation services for design of the facility and for program planning. The seniors center will be built adjacent to the local library and will offer day programs and respite services to seniors with disabilities. The community response has been positive. A number of well elderly would like to volunteer once the center is open. Occupational therapy students will work in small groups to consult on environmental design and activities programming to facilitate the successful implementation of this community-based project. Students will use task analysis to (a) assess the occupational performance profiles, needs, and occupations of local seniors; and (b) structure the center's activity program and environment in order to maintain or promote the health of the elder community.

By completing the assignments in Section Five, students will learn to apply the Occupational Performance Practice Model to address the health needs of individuals and elder communities. The model was introduced in the chapter "Task Analysis: The Contribution of Occupational Therapy to Health." The clinical cases provided in this section introduce the role of caregivers in supporting the health of seniors, the application of task analysis to the promotion of health, and the contribution made by occupational therapy to the geriatric population.

References

American Occupational Therapy Association (AOTA). (1991). *1990 membership data survey.* Bethesda, MD: Author.

AOTA. (1996). OT practitioners work with more elderly patients. *OT Practice 1*(3), 17.

Bonder, B. R., & Goodman, G. (1995). Preventing occupational dysfunction secondary to aging. In C. A. Trombly (Ed.), *Occupational therapy for physical dysfunction* (4th ed., pp. 391–404). Baltimore: Williams & Wilkins.

Institute of Medicine. (1990). *The second fifty years: Promoting health and preventing disability.* Washington, DC: National Academy Press.

McNeil, J. M. (1993). *Americans with disabilities: 1991–1992 U.S. Bureau of the Census. Current population reports, P70-33.* Washington, DC: U.S. Government Printing Office.

U.S. Department of Health and Human Services. Public Health Service. (1992). *Healthy people 2000: National health promotion and disease prevention objectives.* Boston: Jones and Bartlett.

HOME IMPROVEMENT: THE CASE OF NELSON

"The role of the occupational therapist is to facilitate individuals' engagement with their environment. An essential component of the therapeutic relationship is the therapist/client interaction and the exchange which occurs throughout the learning situation created by the occupational therapist. Purposeful activity is used to develop and refine task skills, to explore alternative roles, and to promote positive change in areas of occupational performance" (*Health Canada, 1983*).[1]

Chapter Objectives

1. Describe the relevance of role adaptation to geriatric occupational therapy practice.
2. Evaluate the impact of a client's health status on his or her occupational performance profile.
3. Identify and document outcome-oriented objectives.
4. Use logical thinking and creative analysis to target intervention to enhance client skills, adapt a task, or alter performance context.
5. Select and design a purposeful activity to address client needs.
6. Discuss the role of occupational therapy and the use of purposeful activity in prevention, detection, and treatment of depression in the elderly.

Using Purposeful Activity to Facilitate Adaptation

The roles that people assume provide a sense of identity, guide behavior, communicate performance expectations, add pleasure or enjoyment to life, contribute to achievement, and help maintain the self and family life (Christiansen, 1991; Kielhofner, 1992; Trombly, 1995). As individuals age, the roles they assume change. Children become students when they enter school, adolescents become employees when they enter the workforce, adults become parents when they have children, and seniors become retirees when they leave the workplace.

Seniors may relinquish or experience a progressive loss of roles as they age because of decreased personal capacities (Blau, 1973). Disengagement theory proposes that the elderly withdraw physically and psychologically from activities in preparation for death (Cummings & Henry, 1961). Other theorists, however, suggest that the activity repertoire of the elderly reflects the activity history of the individual (Atchley, 1989) or the developmental stages of this life stage (Erikson, 1963; Levinson, 1978). Ratings of life satisfaction by elderly people appear to (a) relate to the number and meaningfulness of their occupational roles (Elliott & Barris, 1987); and (b) positively correlate with interests, values, personal causation, recreation, and work (Smith, Kielhofner, & Watts, 1986). Maintaining occupational behavior can prevent the loss of roles, habits, and skills and create a positive self-image among retirees (Gregory, 1983).

Bonder (1994a) integrates the theories of activity engagement in the elderly by proposing that the meaning an individual ascribes to engagement in his or her roles and activity choices is a function of the social and cultural contexts and of the individual's needs and perceptions. Bonder's model is a preliminary attempt to construct a "comprehensive description of individual creation of meaning," because finding meaning in life is a "central human motive" (Bonder, 1994a, pp. 28 & 38; Frankel, 1962).

[1] From *Guidelines for the Client-Centred Practice of Occupational Therapy*, by Health Canada, 1983. Reproduced with permission of the Minister of Public Works and Government Services Canada, 1997.

The elderly experience many life changes that place them at risk of increased social isolation (U.S. Department of Health and Human Services, 1992). Retirement, changes in social roles, and the loss of spouses and friends can affect the breadth and depth of social support mechanisms. Individuals differ, however, in the ways in which they respond to growing old. This variability may be due to personal experiences, societal expectations of appropriate roles, cohort effects, or personality factors that influence attitudes toward aging (Bonder, 1994b).

Assignment

1. Identify some of the new roles that seniors engage in after they retire.

   Elliott and Barris (1987) surveyed 158 members of senior-citizen organizations. The individuals surveyed indicated that differences exist between their past and present roles. While the most common roles performed in the past included religious participant, worker, student, and hobbyist or amateur, the most common occupational roles performed in the present included home maintainer, friend, family member, religious participant, and hobbyist or amateur.

2. Read the case about Nelson.

3. Work with a partner to evaluate Nelson's occupational performance profile. If you would like assistance with this challenge, use the Occupational Performance Profile Form (Appendix G) to document information on the roles and occupations that are meaningful to Nelson; his values, interests, goals, and performance components; and the contexts in which he performs.

   Occupational therapy practitioners are responsible for determining how a diagnosed condition influences performance. These determinations or judgments, however, frequently are based on limited information. To develop skill in this area, use the information provided in the case to predict the effect of Nelson's condition on his ability to be independent in various instrumental activities of daily living, in the productive activities that he enjoys, and in play and leisure pursuits. For example, given his current capabilities, will Nelson be able to do the projects he would like to do after he leaves ABC Skilled Nursing Facility (ABC SNF)?

4. Use the information compiled in Question 3 to identify, prioritize, and document outcome-oriented goals and objectives for Nelson that are more current than his goals in the domain of basic activities of daily living. If you would like some assistance with this challenge, use the Client Goals Form (Appendix H). In clinical practice Nelson's occupational therapy practitioner would be able to facilitate the development of these goals and objectives collaboratively with Nelson.

5. Develop an intervention plan to attain the goals and objectives defined in Question 4. Independent engagement in these tasks will enable Nelson to return to the roles that give meaning and purpose to his life. If you would like some assistance with this challenge, consider using the intervention strategies identified in the Occupational Performance Practice Model for Service to Individuals outlined in the chapter "Task Analysis: The Contribution of Occupational Therapy to Health."

6. Select one of the projects that Nelson would like to do after leaving ABC SNF. Contrast Nelson's occupational performance profile with the task and contextual demands of this project to identify the activities within this task that would challenge Nelson beyond his current capabilities. Use task analysis skills to design an intervention strategy to enable Nelson to participate in this project. Intervention could be directed at improving Nelson's skills and abilities, adapting task demands, or altering performance contexts. If you

would like assistance with the task analysis, use the Occupational Performance Analysis—Short Form (Appendix B).

OR

Select and design a purposeful activity to facilitate Nelson's adaptation. Treatment sessions in your facility last 30 minutes. Purposeful activities are therapeutic when they (a) are relevant, meaningful, and goal directed; (b) elicit coordination among sensorimotor, cognitive, psychological, and psychosocial systems; and (c) promote mastery and feelings of competence (AOTA, 1993; Fidler & Fidler, 1978; Trombly, 1995).

OR

Describe how an occupational therapy practitioner could work with Nelson to resolve his limitations regarding use of the lawn mower. Direct your attention toward improving Nelson's skills and abilities, adapting the task demands, or altering performance contexts. If you would like assistance with the task analysis, use the Occupational Performance Analysis—Short Form (Appendix B).

7. A relationship appears to exist between medical illness, functional disabilities, decreased levels of daily activity, and symptoms of depressed mood in seniors (Berkman et al., 1986; Riley, 1994; Shoskes & Glenwick, 1987). Discuss the role of occupational therapy and the use of purposeful activity in preventing, detecting, and treating depression in the elderly. Table 1 provides an overview of depression in the elderly.

Case Study: Nelson

Nelson is a 65-year-old widower whose wife died 3 years ago from a cardiac arrest. The couple did not have children, but Nelson is very fond of his nieces, nephews, and their children. Nelson was a wheat farmer until he retired at the age of 60. He lives alone in his small farmhouse, which is approximately 10 miles from the closest township. He sold most of his land 5 years ago. During his leisure time Nelson enjoys woodworking and riding his horse.

Nelson has been receiving occupational and physical therapy rehabilitation services at ABC Skilled Nursing Facility (ABC SNF) to recover from a left below-knee amputation. His medical history includes diabetes mellitus, peripheral vascular

Table 1: Depression and the Elderly

> Depression is the most common psychiatric syndrome of seniors in institutions and the community. Estimates of prevalence of clinical depression, dysthymic disorders, and depressed mood range from 15 to 25% (Berkman et al., 1986). Undetected or untreated depression in seniors can lead to impairments in social functioning, interpersonal relationships, and occupational performance; the most serious consequence is attempted or completed suicide (Riley, 1994). While the national rate of suicide is 12.5 deaths per 100,000, the rate for men age 65 and older is 40 deaths per 100,000 (Kaplan, Sadock, & Grebb, 1994).

disease, hypertension, cataracts, atherosclerosis, and peripheral neuropathy. Table 2 provides an overview of diabetes. Nelson's physician has suggested that Nelson be discharged home within the next 2 weeks.

Although Nelson is walking with his temporary prosthesis in physical therapy, he mobilizes around the facility in a wheelchair that belongs to ABC SNF. Yesterday he walked 5 to 10 feet but relied very heavily on a standard walker because of poor standing balance. Both the physical and the occupational therapist feel that this problem with postural control is secondary to peripheral neuropathy in Nelson's right leg. When Nelson is not in therapy, he spends most of his time sleeping or sitting alone in his room. He rarely converses with the other residents and has had few visitors. His affect during therapy sessions is flat.

Occupational therapy has been involved with this client since his admission, and services have been directed primarily toward achieving functional goals in basic activities of daily living (ADL). Nelson is now independent in these areas using some adapted equipment (e.g., bath chair). He performs these ADL, however, from a wheelchair. The entrance to Nelson's home is not wheelchair-accessible, nor is he interested in purchasing or renting "one of those clunkers."

Over the past week Nelson has commented that he has achieved all of his occupational therapy goals. When instrumental ADL, productive work, and leisure interests are discussed, Nelson indicates that he plans to get to and from town by driving his truck. This vehicle has an automatic transmission. "Once I am able to push the clutch down on my lawn mower I can do the chores at home." Nelson indicates that he has a number of projects that he would like to do after leaving ABC SNF, including

painting the garage, tuning up the lawn mower, replacing the rain gutters, fixing the snow blower, and chopping wood for the winter.

The information that follows will (a) provide students and instructors with resources to enhance the learning experience and (b) assist the students in completing the assignment.

Learning Resources

American Occupational Therapy Association. (1996). *Role of occupational therapy with the elderly* (2nd ed.). Bethesda, MD: Author.

Bonder, B. R. (1994). The psychosocial meaning of activity. In B. R. Bonder and M. B. Wagner (Eds.), *Functional performance in older adults* (pp. 28–40). Philadelphia: F. A. Davis.

Cummings, E. M., & Henry, W. E. (1961). *Growing old: The process of disengagement.* New York: Basic Books.

Eilenberg, A. O. (1986). An expanding community role for occupational therapy: Preventing depression. *Physical and Occupational Therapy in Geriatrics, 5*(1), 47–58.

Riley, K. P. (1994). Depression. In B. R. Bonder & M. B. Wagner (Eds.), *Functional performance in older adults* (pp. 256–268). Philadelphia: F. A. Davis.

Table 2: Diabetes

Diabetes mellitus (DM) is one of the most prevalent chronic conditions among Americans. Although non-insulin dependent DM (NIDDM or Type II) is most common, the more severe diabetes, insulin dependent DM (IDDM or Type I), occurs in 10% of all cases. The most prominent complications of inadequately controlled or uncontrolled DM include coronary atherosclerosis, glomerulosclerosis, cataracts, retinal microaneurysms, atherosclerosis in the lower extremities, neuropathy, and gangrene (Damjanov, 1996). Diabetes accounts for approximately 30% of kidney failure cases and 50% of all nontraumatic amputations (U.S. Department of Health and Human Services, 1992).

Study Questions

1. Describe the potential relationship between activity adaptation and role adaptation.
2. Describe the potential relationship between role adaptation and health.
3. Identify and describe five characteristics of roles.
4. What is the role of occupational therapy in the prevention of depression in the elderly?
5. Your client must hold onto his walker with two hands to ambulate.

   a. Identify five instrumental activities of daily living that would be difficult to perform.

   b. Select one of these activities and describe an intervention strategy to promote participation or independence.

   c. Describe two methods that this client could use to carry objects.

References

American Occupational Therapy Association. (1993). *Position paper: Purposeful activity.* Bethesda, MD: Author.

Atchley, R. C. (1989). *Continuity theory of normal aging. Gerontologist, 29,* 183.

Berkman, L. F., Berkman, C. S., Kasl, S., Freeman, D. H., Leo, L., Ostfield, A. M., Cornono-Huntingley, J., & Brody, J. A. (1986). Depressive symptoms in relation to physical health and functioning in the elderly. *American Journal of Epidemiology, 124,* 372–388.

Blau, Z. (1973). *Old age in a changing society.* New York: New Viewpoints.

Bonder, B. R. (1994a). The psychosocial meaning of activity. In B. R. Bonder & M. B. Wagner (Eds.), *Functional performance in older adults* (pp. 28–40). Philadelphia: F.A. Davis.

Bonder, B. R. (1994b). Growing old in the United States. In B. R. Bonder & M. B. Wagner (Eds.), *Functional performance in older adults* (pp. 4–14). Philadelphia: F.A. Davis.

Christiansen, C. (1991). Occupational therapy: Intervention for life performance. In C. Christiansen & C. Baum (Eds.), Occupational therapy: *Overcoming human performance deficits* (pp. 2–43). Thorofare, NJ: Slack.

Cummings, E. M., & Henry, W. E. (1961). *Growing old: The process of disengagement.* New York: Basic Books.

Damjanov, I. (1996). *Pathology for the health professions.* Philadelphia: W. B. Saunders.

Elliott, M. S., & Barris, R. (1987). Occupational role performance and life satisfaction in elderly persons. *Occupational Therapy Journal of Research, 7,* 215–224.

Erikson, E. H. (1963). *Childhood and society.* New York: W. W. Norton.

Fidler, G., & Fidler, J. (1978). Doing and becoming: Purposeful action and self-actualization. *American Journal of Occupational Therapy, 32,* 305–310.

Frankel, V. E. (1962). *Man's search for meaning.* New York: Touchstone.

Gregory, M. D. (1983). Occupational behavior and life satisfaction among retirees. *American Journal of Occupational Therapy, 37,* 548–553.

Kaplan, H. I., Sadock, B. J., & Grebb, J. A. (1994). *Synopsis of psychiatry: Behavioral sciences clinical psychiatry* (7th ed.). Baltimore: Williams & Wilkins.

Kielhofner, G. (1992). *Conceptual foundations of occupational therapy.* Philadelphia: F. A. Davis.

Levinson, D. L. (1978). *The seasons of a man's life.* New York: A. A. Knopf.

Riley, K. P. (1994). Depression. In B. R. Bonder & M. B. Wagner (Eds.), *Functional performance in older adults* (pp. 256–268). Philadelphia: F. A. Davis.

Shoskes, J., & Glenwick, D. S. (1987). The relationship of the Depression Adjective Check List to positive affect and activity level in older adults. *Journal of Personality Assessment, 51,* 565–571.

Smith, N. R., Kielhofner, G., & Watts, J. H. (1986). The relationships between volition, activity pattern, and life satisfaction in the elderly. *American Journal of Occupational Therapy, 40,* 278–283.

Trombly, C. A. (1995). Occupation: Purposefulness and meaningfulness as therapeutic mechanisms. *American Journal of Occupational Therapy, 49,* 960–972.

U.S. Department of Health and Human Services. Public Health Service. (1992). *Healthy people 2000: National health promotion and disease prevention objectives.* Boston: Jones and Bartlett.

DINING OUT:
THE CASE OF WAYNE AND MINNIE

"A vision of health as the possession of a repertoire of skills to achieve one's own purposes fits with occupational therapy's traditional emphasis on skill, mastery, and competence that can be attained regardless of pathology or impairment. It also suggests that occupation that develops skills can prevent illness and influence health by developing competency and making life worth living" (Yerxa, 1994, p. 587).[1]

Chapter Objectives

1. Evaluate the effect of two clients' health status on their functional and community mobility.
2. List the activities involved in functional and community mobility.
3. Use logical thinking and creative analysis to develop intervention strategies to enable two seniors to safely mobilize around their home and community.
4. Identify community resource agencies and social support systems available to enable seniors to maintain their independence.

Using Task Analysis to Ensure Community Access

Occupational therapy practitioners, in collaboration with other professionals and service agencies, address the health needs of the growing number of elderly people in our communities. According to the United States Bureau of the Census, 15.2 million noninstitutional elderly in the United States in 1991 and 1992, or close to 50%, had difficulty with or were unable to perform one or more functional activities. These individuals reported having the most difficulty with tasks that require community and functional mobility including getting outside of the home, doing light housework, taking a bath or shower, or getting in or out of bed or a chair. Table 1 provides information on the prevalence of

disability in persons 65 or older who do not live in nursing homes or other institutions (McNeil, 1993).

Functional and community mobility contributes to an individual's ability to participate in other activities of daily living, work and productive activities, play, and leisure pursuits. Functional mobility refers to ambulation, transporting objects, and "moving from one position or place to another, such as in-bed mobility, wheelchair mobility, [and] transfers (wheelchair, bed, car, tub, toilet, tub/shower, chair, floor)" (AOTA, 1994, p. 1051). Community mobility refers to moving in "the community and using public or private transportation, such as driving, or accessing buses, taxi cabs, or other public transportation systems" (AOTA, 1994, p. 1052). Unfortunately over 40% of seniors are not able to or do not engage in leisure-time physical activity, and less than 35% participate in regular moderate exercise such as walking or gardening (Caspersen, 1989; U.S. Department of Health and Human Services, 1992). Physical activity is one of the key ingredients to healthy aging (U.S. Department of Health and Human Services, 1992).

Occupational therapy practitioners provide services to individuals who have difficulty with functional and community mobility. Task analysis is used to (a) identify clients' performance problems, task demands, and contextual variables that limit engage-

---

[1]From "Dreams, Dilemmas, and Decisions for Occupational Therapy Practice in a New Millennium: An American Perspective," by E. J. Yerxa, 1994, *American Journal of Occupational Therapy, 48,* p. 587. Copyright 1994 by the American Occupational Therapy Association. Reprinted with permission.

Table 1: Prevalence of Disability in Persons 65 Years of Age or Older

	Percentage of Seniors	Number of People (millions)
Has difficulty with or is unable to perform one or more functional activities	49.6	15.215
Activities of Daily Living (ADL)		
Has difficulty with or needs personal assistance with one or more ADL	14.6	4.478
Taking a bath or shower	9.5	2.909
Getting in or out of bed or a chair	9.5	2.905
Getting around inside the home	7.7	2.357
Dressing	6.2	1.907
Toileting	4.4	1.358
Eating	2.1	646
Instrumental Activities of Daily Living (IADL)		
Has difficulty with or needs personal assistance with one or more IADL	21.6	6.614
Getting around outside the home	16.0	4.924
Doing light housework	12.2	3.747
Preparing meals	9.3	2.850
Keeping track of money and bills	7.5	2.303
Using the telephone	6.5	1.990

Note: Figures do not include those individuals who live in nursing homes or other institutions.

From *Americans with Disabilities: 1991–1992 U.S. Bureau of the Census. Current population reports, P70-33,* (pp. 6–8), by J. M. McNeil, 1993, Washington, DC: U.S. Government Printing Office.

ment; and (b) target intervention strategies at these barriers. Intervention may be directed at improving an individual's skills and abilities, adapting task demands, or altering performance contexts. The occupational therapy profession supports the attitude that all individuals should be able to take part in the "naturally occurring activities of society" (AOTA, 1996, p. 855). Providing services directed at enhancing seniors' access to daily activities within their community parallels this tradition.

Assignment

1. Read the case about Wayne and Minnie.
2. Work with a partner to evaluate Wayne's and Minnie's occupational performance profiles. If you would like assistance with this challenge, use two copies of the Occupational Performance Profile Form (Appendix G) to document information on the occupations that are meaningful and relevant to each senior; their respective values, interests, goals, and performance components; and the contexts in which they perform.

Occupational therapy practitioners are responsible for determining how a diagnosed condition influences present performance. These determinations or judgments, however, are frequently made with limited information. To develop skill in this area, use the information provided in the case to predict the impact of Wayne and Minnie's conditions on their ability to be independent in various activities of daily living, work and productive activities, play, and leisure pursuits. For example, will the couple be able to go on their community outings with the car? In clinical practice Wayne's occupational therapy practitioner could either observe or ask about their performance in these domains.

3. Use the information compiled in Question 2 to identify, prioritize, and document some specific, measurable, outcome-oriented goals and objectives for Wayne and Minnie. Minnie has provided some information about her needs and priorities. If you would like some assistance with this challenge, use the Client Goals Form (Appendix H).

4. One of the services requested by Minnie relates to assisting Wayne in bathing. Contrast Wayne's occupational performance profile with the task and contextual demands of bathing to identify the activities within this task that challenge Wayne beyond his capabilities. Imagine that the layout and design of Wayne and Winnie's bathroom is the same as your own.

ABC Home Health offers personal care attendants to assist clients in bathing. What occupational therapy intervention might be appropriate to try before recommending that Wayne and Minnie be provided with this service? Be specific in your description of intervention strategies.

5. One of the services requested by Minnie relates to assisting Wayne in toileting. Contrast Wayne's occupational performance profile with the task and contextual demands of toileting to identify the activities within this task that challenge Wayne beyond his capabilities. What occupational therapy intervention might be appropriate to reduce Wayne's reliance on his wife to safely perform this activity? Be specific in your description of intervention strategies.

If you would like some assistance with the challenges presented in Questions 4 and 5, consider using the intervention strategies identified in the Occupational Performance Practice Model for Service to Individuals outlined in the chapter "Task Analysis: The Contribution of Occupational Therapy to Health."

6. Minnie has expressed her need for assistance with light housework but ABC Home Health does not offer this service. Identify and describe intervention strategies in this area.

From discussions with Minnie it is apparent that she would like assistance with housework to enable her to devote time to more meaningful tasks. How might this home management task, or other tasks that Wayne and Minnie perform in a day, be simplified to reduce their work load? Identify and describe work simplification or energy conservation techniques that would assist Wayne and Minnie in this area.

What environmental supports or community services might assist Wayne and Minnie in this area? Would this couple benefit from any services that are available to homebound seniors?

7. What other services might occupational therapy offer this couple to address their health needs and support their continued success in the community? Consider preventive, functional, and remedial approaches to health.

Case Study: Wayne and Minnie

Wayne and Minnie have been married for 48 years and have four children and eight grandchildren. The couple are both in their mid-70s. Four days ago Minnie fell while gardening and fractured her humerus; her right arm is in a cast and will be in a sling for approximately 6 to 8 weeks. Minnie has great difficulty caring for her husband in this condition, and her family and physician arranged for home-health services. Wayne was diagnosed with Parkinson's disease (PD) almost 20 years ago.

Minnie answers the door and introduces herself and her husband; Wayne lifts his tremulous hand as if to wave hello from his seat at the dining room table. He is sitting in front of playing cards that are arranged in a row, face up, on the tabletop. The couple appear to have been playing a game. As the interview proceeds, Minnie contributes to most of the conversation while her husband watches. Minnie

has a list of services that she wants, including an assistant to come and bathe Wayne twice a week, someone to assist with housework, and a grab bar next to the toilet. Once provided with this assistance, Minnie expects that she will once again be able to take care of her husband.

When asked about her concerns regarding bathing and access to the toilet, Minnie indicates that she is unable to get her husband into the bathtub with her broken arm. Although she assists him on and off the toilet, this task is very difficult for both Minnie and Wayne. Since Minnie injured herself, the task has become close to impossible. Wayne has begun to wear incontinence pads. The couple do not use any assistive devices in the bathroom. Minnie indicates that Wayne was given a walker 5 years ago, but it is her opinion that he walks better with her than with the walker.

Wayne relies very heavily on his wife's assistance and support to get up and down from furniture and to walk. When the couple walk together from the dining room to the living room, the most difficult activity is getting up from the dining room chair. Minnie indicates that "getting up is always the hardest.... After he gets going we are pretty good together." Wayne walks into the living room with a stooped posture and slow, shuffling gait; and his wife holds him close to her using her left arm. Once in the living room the couple slow their pace before turning toward the piano. Wayne sits on the piano bench and says in a quiet monotone, "It's easier to get up from here." Table 2 provides an overview of falls and fractures in the elderly while Table 3 provides an overview of clinical features of PD.

Minnie indicates that she is the "planner, organizer, and motivator of the family." "My husband and I spend every second Monday afternoon at the library.

Wayne doesn't read very much because he has trouble with the pages, but I love to read. On the way home we stop for dinner at a restaurant. On Tuesday or Wednesday we go out to the bank and the grocery store. My husband stays in the car while I do the running around…. Friday is our day for swimming [and] my husband takes me out for an afternoon dinner date every Saturday. We often go to our favorite garden terrace restaurant. Sunday is our day of rest, although I am usually busy in the yard. By the end of the day we are usually ready to go out for a light dinner."

The couple live in a small, two-bedroom home in the suburbs. The property has a very large lawn and a small garage. Prior to her fall Minnie drove the couple around in their small, two-door car. Wayne watches his wife as she describes their week together. Although he does not smile, he seems to be very interested in the conversation.

Table 2: Falls and Fractures in the Elderly

Falls are common in the elderly and are the leading cause of unintentional injuries in this population. Approximately one third of seniors who live in the community fall each year. Women fall three times more often than men, and the likelihood of falling increases with age. Of those persons hospitalized for a fall, only 50% are alive 1 year later (Tideiksaar, 1994). The alterations in posture and gait and absence of righting reactions and protective responses in individuals with Parkinson's disease place them at high risk for falling (Alta, 1982).

The treatment of fractures in the elderly costs Medicare upward of $4 billion annually, and as the size of the elderly population increases, safety and injury prevention programs will become more important (Steib, 1996b). Approximately 15% of registered occupational therapy practitioners and 10% of certified occupational therapy assistants provide services to clients with fractures (Steib, 1996a; Steib, 1996b).

Table 3: Parkinson's Disease

Parkinson's disease (PD) is a degenerative disorder of posture and movement characterized by pathological changes in the motor system nuclei of the midbrain (Damjanov, 1996). Approximately one in every 100 men and women over the age of 50 in the United States have PD (Washington, 1993). The clinical features of PD include resting tremor, rigidity, bradykinesia, postural instability, and loss of righting reactions and protective responses. Initiating and executing movement, turning, and backing up are particularly difficult. Facial and speech involvement occurs in more advanced stages, and thought processing may be slow (Hooks, 1996). Approximately 40% of people with PD are depressed, and it is estimated that 10 to 30% exhibit dementia (Cummings, 1992; Damjanov, 1996).

Hooks (1996) suggests that occupational therapy practitioners who work with clients with PD should direct services at (a) educating families and caregivers, (b) teaching clients to compensate, (c) providing guidelines to prevent musculoskeletal impairments, (d) offering graded activity to facilitate function, (e) adapting environments to maximize sensory input and accommodate for immobility, and (f) linking families with support groups.

The information that follows will (a) provide students and instructors with resources to enhance the learning experience and (b) assist the students in completing the assignment.

Learning Resources

Hasselkus, B. R. (1993). Functional disability and older adults. In H. L. Hopkins & H. D. Smith (Eds.), *Willard and Spackman's occupational therapy* (8th ed., pp. 742–752). Philadelphia: J. B. Lippincott.

Hooks, M. L. (1996). Parkinson's disease. In L. W. Pedretti (Ed.), *Occupational therapy: Practice skills for physical dysfunction* (4th ed., pp. 845–851). St. Louis, MO: Mosby.

Tideiksaar, R. (1989). *Falling in old age: Its prevention and treatment.* New York: Springer.

Tideiksaar, R. (1994). Falls. In B. R. Bonder & M. B. Wagner (Eds.), *Functional performance in older adults* (pp. 224–239). Philadelphia: F. A. Davis.

Study Questions

1. List four functional mobility activities.
2. List four community mobility activities.
3. Describe why functional mobility may affect a person's level of independence in other activities of daily living, work and productive activities, play, and leisure pursuits.
4. Describe three community services that are available to homebound seniors.
5. How might a senior go about finding someone to assist with light housework?

References

Alta, J. E. (1982). Why patients with Parkinson's disease fall. *Journal of the American Medical Association, 247,* 515.

American Occupational Therapy Association (AOTA). (1994). Uniform terminology for occupational therapy (3rd ed.). *American Journal of Occupational Therapy, 48,* 1047–1054.

AOTA. (1996). Occupational therapy: A profession in support of full inclusion. *American Journal of Occupational Therapy, 50,* 855.

Caspersen, C. J. (1989). Physical activity epidemiology: Concepts, methods, and applications to exercise science. *Exercise and Sports Sciences Reviews, 17,* 423–473.

Cummings, J. L. (1992). Depression and Parkinson's disease: A review. *American Journal of Psychiatry, 149,* 443–448.

Damjanov, I. (1996). *Pathology for the health-related professions.* Philadelphia: W. B. Saunders.

Hooks, M. L. (1996). Parkinson's disease. In L. W. Pedretti (Ed.), *Occupational therapy: Practice skills for physical dysfunction* (4th ed., pp. 845–851). St. Louis, MO: Mosby.

McNeil, J. M. (1993). *Americans with disabilities: 1991–1992 U.S. Bureau of the Census. Current population reports, P70-33.* Washington, DC: U.S. Government Printing Office.

Steib, P. A. (1996a). Growth in geriatric care reflected in OTR survey. *OT Week 10*(46), 16–17.

Steib, P. A. (1996b). Skilled nursing facilities: Top employment setting for COTAs. *OT Week, 10*(47), 16–17.

Tideiksaar, R. (1994). Falls. In B. R. Bonder & M. B. Wagner (Eds.), *Functional performance in older adults* (pp. 224–239). Philadelphia: F. A. Davis.

U.S. Department of Health and Human Services. Public Health Service. (1992). *Healthy people 2000: National health promotion and disease-prevention objectives.* Boston: Jones and Bartlett.

Washington, H. (1993, July). Parkinson's disease. *Harvard Health Letter,* 1.

DINING IN: THE CASE OF RHONDA

"Occupational therapy is founded on the premise that man has a need to be purposefully engaged in meaningful activity in order to successfully fulfill the mental, physical, sociocultural, and spiritual roles appropriate to his chosen lifestyle" (Canadian Association of Occupational Therapists, 1990, p. 1).[1]

Chapter Objectives

1. Evaluate the effect of an individual's health status on his or her ability to participate in eating.
2. List the tasks and activities involved in feeding and eating.
3. Alter task and environmental demands to enable a client to participate in eating.
4. Design practice opportunities to enhance a client's performance in eating.
5. Use logical thinking and creative analysis to develop an intervention strategy to maximize a client's participation in eating.

Using Task Analysis to Enhance Participation in Self-Care

Seniors have diverse wishes and perceptions about independence in self-care, but most accommodate their limitations by locating and accepting assistance (Bonder & Goodman, 1995). While 95% of the elderly live in the community, approximately 10% of these individuals have difficulty with or require personal assistance for preparing a meal and 2% have difficulty with or require personal assistance with eating (McNeil, 1993; U.S. Congress, 1991). Approximately 3% of the noninstitutional elderly over the age of 85 require personal assistance for eating (McNeil, Lamas, & Harpine, 1986). The prevalence of disabilities in the institutional elderly is higher than in the community, which may be suggestive of higher rates of eating problems in this population.

Self-maintenance tasks involving feeding and eating can be separated into four phases. First, food must be introduced into the mouth, which requires setting up food; selecting and using appropriate utensils and tableware; cleaning one's face, hands, and clothing; bringing food or drink to the mouth; or managing alternative methods of nourishment. Second, oral manipulation of food in preparation for swallowing involves sucking, masticating, coughing, and forming a bolus. These first two phases are called the **oral preparatory** phase and the **oral** phase (O'Sullivan, 1990). The third phase, or **pharyngeal,** requires triggering of the swallowing response, and the final phase, **esophageal,** involves the bolus traveling through the esophagus into the stomach (AOTA, 1994; AOTA, 1996).

Occupational therapy practitioners are involved in the evaluation of and intervention with clients who have feeding and eating problems because these tasks are essential to health and well-being (AOTA, 1996). Dysphagia, or having difficulty swallowing, may lead to dehydration and malnutrition. Pulmonary complications may occur secondary to aspiration (Konosky, 1995). Registered occupational therapists (OTR) are trained in many approaches to evaluating and planning intervention for eating dysfunction. Certified occupational therapy assistants may contribute observations and implement treatment programs under the supervision of an OTR, but dysphagia intervention requires advanced learning opportunities (AOTA, 1996).

Task analysis is used by therapists as an assessment and intervention tool to promote independence in feeding and eating. Assessment of the client involves consideration of his or her past experiences, values,

---

interests, and goals, as well as of sensorimotor, cognitive, psychosocial, and psychological performance components. Assessment of the task requires determination of the specific activities that require intervention. Assessment of the environment encompasses temporal variables (e.g., disability status) and environmental factors that influence engagement. Intervention is directed at developing client skills and abilities or modifying the task and environmental demands to promote higher levels of safe, functional independence in eating. Evaluation and intervention services may be provided in conjunction with a rehabilitation team.

An example of intervention directed at developing client skills is the occupational therapy practitioner using techniques to normalize the client's oral sensitivity or facilitate the swallow response. Practitioners select and design purposeful activities to enable clients to strengthen weak oral musculature, practice compensatory strategies, learn self-monitoring skills, or develop more advanced oral-motor movements (AOTA, 1996). Examples of intervention directed at modifying task and physical environmental demands include (a) the use of positioning devices to provide head and trunk alignment and stability to those clients who lack the required degree of postural control, (b) the selection and adaptation of food consistencies to maximize functional independence in eating for those individuals who lack the required degree of oral-motor control, and (c) the selection and use of adapted devices and orthoses to promote independence in eating (AOTA, 1996). The social and cultural environment can also be structured to be relevant and meaningful, and caregivers may be trained to perform specific feeding activities or use certain feeding techniques with the client (AOTA, 1996).

Assignment

1. Read the case about Rhonda.
2. Work with a partner to evaluate Rhonda's occupational performance profile. If you would like some assistance with this challenge, use the Occupational Performance Profile Form (Appendix G) to document information on the occupations that are important to Rhonda; her past experiences, values, interests, goals, and performance component capabilities; and the contexts within which she performs.
3. Obtain three bowls, one plate, utensils, and three cups. Fill the first bowl with liquid (e.g., broth), the second bowl with food with varied textures (e.g., vegetable soup or fruit cocktail), and the third bowl with pureed food (e.g., apple sauce or pudding). Place solid food on the plate (e.g., cheese, vegetable, meat). Fill the first cup with regular liquid (e.g., water), the second cup with a thicker liquid (e.g., apricot nectar, tomato juice, prune juice), and the third cup with a thick liquid drink (e.g., gravy or a milk shake).

   Eat food from the bowls and plate, drink each of the liquids, and analyze the task of eating. Identify and describe the task and contextual demands placed on an individual who is independent in eating by completing the Occupational Performance Analysis—Short Form (Appendix B).

   Rank the foods according to the degree of sensorimotor skill required to eat. Rank the liquids according to the degree of sensorimotor skill required to drink. Why has Rhonda been placed on a pureed food diet with thickened liquids?
4. Feeding and eating tasks can be separated into four phases. Each phase includes a number of activities. After comparing Rhonda's occupational performance profile with the task and contextual demands of eating and drinking, identify the activi-

ties Rhonda has difficulty performing and explain why these activities are difficult. It is these activities that will be targeted for intervention.

Does Rhonda's posture during feeding affect her ability to bring food to her mouth or orally manipulate her food and drink in preparation for swallowing? Would Rhonda have difficulty holding and manipulating regular utensils?

If Rhonda were able to sit upright at the table and hold a utensil would she be able to (a) locate and obtain the food on her plate, or (b) bring food or drink to her mouth? Does Rhonda have difficulty orally manipulating food? If so, specify what is difficult.

Given the information presented in the case, does Rhonda appear to have difficulty during the pharyngeal and esophageal phase of swallowing? In clinical practice, registered occupational therapists and other members of the dysphagia team use advanced assessment techniques to validate this determination.

5. After targeting which eating activities require intervention, reflect on the skills and abilities, task demands, and environmental variables that limit Rhonda's ability to perform these specific activities. Review the treatment plan described in the occupational therapy notation on Rhonda's chart. The analysis conducted in response to Questions 2, 3, and 4 should explain the rationale for the occupational therapy plan.

6. Plan a 30-minute midmorning treatment session to practice increasing Rhonda's independence in bringing food and drink to her mouth. One student partner will role-play the occupational therapy practitioner and the other will personify Rhonda.

Obtain a small bowl of pureed food and a glass of thickened liquid. What intervention strategies will be used to enhance Rhonda's independence in

eating these foods? Refer to the occupational therapy plan (i.e., 1A, 1B, 1C, 1D, 2A, and 2B) on Rhonda's chart.

7. How could the complexity of this treatment session be gradually increased over the next week to promote more and more independence? Plan the next three or four treatment sessions.

8. After 1 week Rhonda is able to feed herself approximately 25% of her meal with the appropriate positioning, adapted equipment, and setup. Plan a lunch-hour treatment session to assist Rhonda in generalizing this new level of independence.

Describe how the dining room environment will be structured to (a) promote generalization of learning and performance, and (b) attain other therapy goals.

Case Study: Rhonda

Rhonda had a right cerebral vascular accident (CVA) 5 years ago and has been living in a nursing home ever since. She is a mother of three children and has six grandchildren. Rhonda's husband was admitted to the same nursing home two years after she was, but he passed away within 6 months.

Rhonda just celebrated her 89th birthday. One of Rhonda's daughters expressed concern to the attending physician regarding her mother's inability to eat birthday cake. Although Rhonda fed herself on admission, she has progressively become more and more dependent on staff in this domain. The occupational therapy department received a referral and initiated evaluation and intervention in this area. Rhonda's chart notation reads:

Yesterday's Date

   Subjective:

   This client's daughter expressed concern regarding her mother's inability to eat birthday cake. The nursing staff indicated that this 89-year-old woman has been fed by the staff for the past 6 months. Physician was not concerned about nutrition or body weight but reported that the client has a recent history of dehydration. Rhonda expressed an interest in eating more independently. Rhonda reported that she misses eating "candy, potato chips, pretzels, cookies, cake, fresh fruit, and meat." She indicated that she enjoys meals at the nursing home and is particularly fond of their desserts. When asked about her reliance on staff to eat, Rhonda replied "It's all right ... the ladies enjoy helping me at dinnertime. They are very nice."

Objective:
This client was fed pureed foods and thickened liquids while sitting in her wheelchair in approximately 40 degrees of recline. Rhonda cleaned her spoon primarily with the right side of her mouth. She was slow to create a bolus and swallowed within 1 minute of receiving food. Rhonda coughed occasionally (four times during one lunch meal) on both food and liquid. Cough was productive and quickly cleared the airway. Took 25 minutes to eat an entire lunch meal. After lunch was served Rhonda had some food pocketed under the left lower lip. This therapist taught the client how to clear this pocketed food. Rhonda was given a small piece of cracker which she grasped from the therapist and ate with a rotary chewing pattern. Sensorimotor status: Wears glasses but visual acuity remains poor. Has hearing aids but does not always wear them. Left homonymous hemianopsia.

Unilateral neglect of left side. Right-hand dominant with some metacarpal and interphalangeal bony changes in this hand secondary to arthritis. Weak right cylindrical grasp with mild right tremor. Spastic left hemiplegia with little voluntary movement. Left arm primarily held in a flexor synergy pattern when sitting upright. Does not appear to have tactile or proprioceptive awareness of this extremity. Rhonda sat in a wheelchair that has recline and tilt-in-space position options. When positioned in upright sitting, Rhonda indicated that she prefers to be reclined. When reclined in her wheelchair, this client's neck and upper and lower extremities extended.

Cognitive status: Oriented to person and place but not date, month, or year. Oriented to time of day. Remembered that her family came to celebrate her recent birthday, but Rhonda was unable to remember who came, when the party was, or which birthday she celebrated. Recognized and labeled all food items on tray. Attended to meal during the entire meal and engaged in casual conversation with staff. Did not converse with other residents at the dinner table.

Psychological and psychosocial status: During this evaluation Rhonda did not converse with the resident in her room or any of the residents in the hallway on the way to the dining room. Although she verbally indicated an interest in eating more independently, she appeared to be very fond of the staff that assist her.

Contextual variables: Current health condition is chronic. Dined at a table with five other residents who were fed by two staff members. Three of these residents were located to Rhonda's left side. All five residents were also fed pureed food. Socialization did not occur between residents before or after the meal and conversations primarily occurred between staff and residents.

Assessment:
This client's participation in eating has declined over the past 6 months and she is currently dependent in this occupational performance area. She has a number of sensorimotor deficits that alter her ability to eat in the typical fashion. These

include left spastic hemiplegia with sensory loss, left homonymous hemianopsia and unilateral neglect, arthritic and tremulous right hand, and left oral-motor paralysis. Primitive postural reflexes appear to be elicited in recline, which is the position this client is fed in. She tolerates pureed foods and appears to have a productive, protective cough. During meals this client socializes primarily with staff.

Plan:

1. Increase independence in bringing food to mouth by
    A. Recommending alternative sitting position during meals.
    B. Providing adapted equipment to reduce sensorimotor requirements to feed self with right hand.
    C. Providing practice opportunities to increase independence in bringing food and drink to mouth.
    D. Providing appropriate setup and teaching compensatory techniques for homonymous hemianopsia and unilateral neglect.

2. Enhance efficiency of performance and safety regarding oral manipulation by
    A. Teaching techniques to avoid food pocketing.
    B. Providing practice opportunities to avoid food pocketing and ensure mouth is clear when leaving the table.

3. Reduce reliance and attention to staff during meals by
    A. Enhancing independence.
    B. Facilitating conversations with other residents before and after meals.

4. Communicate with nursing home staff regarding
    A. Changing levels of independence.
    B. Training in patient setup.
    C. Facilitating conversations between this patient and other residents before and after meal.

5. Use videofluoroscopy for confirmation of swallow status and evaluation of swallow status with semisolids, solids, and regular liquids when client is in a comfortable, upright sitting position.

6. Provide intervention five times per week for 30 minutes for 3 weeks and reevaluate.
    ABC Practitioner, OTR/L

As an occupational therapy practitioner working in this nursing home, you have read this notation and must plan and initiate treatment. Rhonda's medical chart indicates that she has a history of depression, transient ischemic attacks, two right cerebral vascular accidents, arthritis, hypertension, cardio-megaly, atherosclerosis, dentures, and bilateral cataracts. She has glasses, bilateral hearing aids, and dentures. Table 1 discusses cerebral vascular accidents.

Table 1: Cerebral Vascular Accidents

Cerebral vascular accident (CVA) is the third-most-common cause of mortality in the United States (Damjanov, 1996) and the number one health problem treated by occupational therapy practitioners (Steib, 1996a; Steib, 1996b). Transient ischemic attack (TIA) refers to focal neurological ischemic events of sudden onset and brief duration; and most are due to cerebral emboli arising from plaque or atherosclerotic ulcers involving the carotid or vertebral arteries (Berkow, 1987). In 1995 approximately 30% of registered occupational therapists and 45% of certified occupational therapy assistants provided services to clients with CVA (Steib, 1996a; Steib, 1996b).

The sequelae following CVA include hemiplegia or paralysis, sensory disturbances, perceptual deficits, cognitive impairments, and a variety of psychological and psychosocial changes. Outcome is dependent on the severity of the stroke and the site and extent of damage. It is difficult to make accurate predictions regarding prognosis, but recovery is greater in younger clients and individuals with good sensation, minimal spasticity, and isolated movements on the affected side. The outlook for independence is poor for individuals who have complete sensory loss or fecal or urinary incontinence and do not have any concept of the affected side (Bierman, 1993).

Damage to the motor cortex results in contralateral impairments; a lesion in the right cerebral hemisphere produces left hemiplegia and vice versa. Homonymous hemianopsia refers to a loss of one side of the visual field. Left homonymous hemianopsia occurs when the right optic tract is damaged. This type of damage causes individuals to lose the ability to see objects placed on the left side of their body midline because this position is outside of the remaining visual field. Intervention involves teaching patients head-turning or postural adjustment compensatory strategies and providing practice opportunities to enable clients to incorporate these techniques into their daily routine (Dunn, 1991). Unilateral neglect occurs when there is either sensory or attention deficits that cause individuals to fail to report, respond, or orient to stimuli presented to the side of the body contralateral to a cerebral lesion (Bierman, 1993).

The information that follows will (a) provide students and instructors with resources to enhance the learning experience and (b) assist the students in completing the assignment.

Learning Resources

Books and Periodicals

American Occupational Therapy Association. (1996). Position paper: Eating dysfunction. *American Journal of Occupational Therapy, 50,* 846–847.

Supplier Catalogues

Maddak, Inc. PO Box 922. Randolph, MA 02368-0922. 800-854-4687.

North Coast Medical, Inc. 187 Stauffer Boulevard, San Jose, CA 95125-1042. 800-821-9319.

Sammons, Inc. PO Box 32, Brookfield, IL 60513. 708-325-1700. 800-323-5547.

Smith & Nephew Rolyan Inc. One Quality Drive, Germantown, WI 53022. 800-228-3693.

This list of suppliers is not intended to be exhaustive, nor does it represent endorsements by the author or AOTA.

Study Questions

1. Define the term **dysphagia.**
2. What is the optimal sitting position for feeding and eating?
3. Your client can use only one hand during meals.
   a. Identify an activity(s) that may be difficult for this client.
   b. Identify an assistive technology device(s) that could be used to cut meat.
   c. Identify an assistive technology device(s) that could be used to scoop food from a plate onto a fork.
4. How can food consistencies be altered to accommodate for varying levels of sensorimotor skills and oral-motor coordination?
5. Your client is on a puree diet. Which of the following foods would this person be able to eat: cookies, apple sauce, or juice?

References

American Occupational Therapy Association (AOTA). (1994). *Uniform terminology for occupational therapy* (3rd ed.). Bethesda, MD: Author.

AOTA. (1996). Position paper: Eating dysfunction. *American Journal of Occupational Therapy, 50,* 846–847.

Berkow, R. (Ed.). (1987). *The Merck manual of diagnosis and therapy* (15th ed.). Rahway, NJ: Merck Sharp & Dohme Research Laboratories.

Bierman, S. N. (1993). Cerebrovascular accident. In R. A. Hansen & B. Atchison (Eds.), *Conditions in occupational therapy: Effect on occupational performance* (pp. 16–49). Baltimore: Williams & Wilkins.

Bonder, B. R., & Goodman, G. (1995). Preventing occupational dysfunction secondary to aging. In C. A. Trombly (Ed.), *Occupational therapy for physical dysfunction* (4th ed., pp. 391–404). Baltimore: Williams & Wilkins.

Damjanov, I. (1996). *Pathology for the health professions.* Philadelphia: W. B. Saunders.

Dunn, W. (1991). Sensory dimensions of performance. In C. Christiansen & C. Baum (Eds.), *Occupational therapy: Overcoming human performance deficits* (pp. 228–257). Thorofare, NJ: Slack.

Konosky, K. A. (1995). Dysphagia. In C. A. Trombly (Ed.), *Occupational therapy for physical dysfunction* (4th ed., pp. 893–904). Baltimore: Williams & Wilkins.

McNeil, J. M. (1993).*Americans with disabilities: 1991–1992 U.S. Bureau of the Census. Current population reports, P70-33.* Washington, DC: U.S. Government Printing Office.

McNeil, J. M., Lamas, E. J., & Harpine, C. J. (1986). *Disability, functional limitation, and health insurance coverage.* Washington, DC: U.S. Government Printing Office.

O'Sullivan, N. (Ed.). (1990). *Dysphagia care: Team approach with acute and long-term patients.* Los Angeles: Collage Square.

Steib, P. A. (1996a). Growth in geriatric care reflected in OTR survey. *OT Week 10*(46), 16–17.

Steib, P. A. (1996b). Skilled nursing facilities: Top employment setting for COTAs. *OT Week, 10*(47), 16–17.

U.S. Congress. House of Representatives, Committee on Ways and Means, Subcommittee on Health. (1991). *Long-term care: Proposals to improve Medicare's skilled nursing facility and health care benefits.* Washington, DC: U.S. Government Printing Office.

CRAFTS FOR ASSESSMENT AND INTERVENTION: THE CASE OF BERT AND MAUREEN

"As the dementia progresses and performance becomes more difficult, the occupational therapy practitioner simplifies the demands of everyday tasks. Each task is analyzed in terms of its component parts, and each part is then evaluated in terms of the person's ability to continue to perform it"

*(American Occupational Therapy Association, 1994, p. 1030).*1

Chapter Objectives

1. Evaluate the effects of a chronic condition on an individual's occupational performance profile.
2. Describe the role of occupational therapy practitioners who provide services to individuals with cognitive disabilities or dementia.
3. Identify the cognitive performance components that underlie task engagement.
4. Use creative analysis to target intervention at adapting task demands and altering performance contexts to facilitate an individual's engagement in productive and leisure activities.
5. Apply concepts from the Cognitive Disabilities Model of practice to evaluate and provide intervention services to individuals with cognitive impairments.

Using Task Analysis to Enhance Participation in Productive Activities and Leisure Pursuits

Age-related changes in cognition occur normally in the elderly, but when impairments in this area cause disability, the services of occupational therapy practitioners become necessary. An estimated 15% of the elderly have mild dementia. Approximately 5% of all elderly and 20% of those over the age of 80 have severe dementia (Kaplan, Sadock, & Grebb, 1994). Dementia is a progressive and irreversible impairment of intellect that increases in prevalence with the age of a population. Dementia involves changes in cognition, memory, language, visuospatial functions, behavior, and functional performance (Kaplan, Sadock, & Grebb, 1994).

The type of occupational therapy service provided to individuals with irreversible dementia is dependent on the stage of cognitive decline and the resultant disability. Initially, evaluation and intervention is directed toward maintaining client participation in the activities in which a decline is first noticed. As impairments progress and occupational performance becomes more impaired, attention shifts to maintaining functional mobility, communication, self-care, and leisure pursuits and eventually to basic life functions such as feeding, dysphagia, and positioning. Although the cognitive impairment cannot be reversed, performance can be improved by modifying task requirements, adapting the environment, and supporting and educating caregivers (AOTA, 1994a).

As the dementia progresses and performance becomes more difficult, the occupational therapy practitioner simplifies the demands of everyday tasks. Each task is analyzed in terms of its component parts, and each part is then evaluated in terms of the person's ability to continue to perform it.... Even though the person may not complete all steps of the task, the person is not deprived of using the abilities that remain. In treating cognitively impaired individuals in groups, task analysis may be combined with an assembly-line approach. Each group member may complete only one step of the task, while the group as a whole accomplishes the total task. In making holiday decorations, for example, one member may trace the decorations, another cut them, and a third glue the parts together" (AOTA, 1994a, p. 1030).

The Cognitive Disabilities Model is one of the approaches used by occupational therapy practitioners to provide evaluation and intervention services to individuals with cognitive disabilities. The approach proposes that a continuum of cognitive levels exists, ranging from level 1 to level 6, and that an individual's cognitive level can be identified by examining functional performance, assessing the type of assistance required, and observing social dysfunction (Allen & Allen, 1987). Crafts are used for screening and diagnostic purposes, and both task and activity analysis are employed during evaluation and intervention (Allen, Earhart, & Blue, 1992; Allen, Kehrberg, & Burns, 1992). Services are directed toward maximizing the client's use of residual capabilities, adapting task demands, or altering the environment to facilitate best performance and enable successful participation in routine tasks (Levy, 1993).

Assignment

1. Read the case about Maureen and Bert.
2. Work individually or with a partner to evaluate Maureen's and Bert's occupational performance profiles. If you would like assistance with this challenge, use two copies of the Occupational Performance Profile Form (Appendix G) to document information on the occupations that are meaningful and relevant to each senior; their respective values, interests, goals, and performance components; and the contexts in which they perform.

Use the information provided in the case to begin to make a determination about the cognitive capabilities and sensorimotor, psychosocial, and psychological profiles of both clients. Consider the cognitive performance components defined in *Uniform Terminology for Occupational Therapy* (AOTA, 1994b) (Appendix E) and the cognitive levels proposed by the Cognitive Disabilities Model (Allen, Earhart, & Blue, 1992).

If you would like some assistance understanding the effects of different cognitive levels on the daily living skills of individuals with Alzheimer's disease, review the article by Levy (1986) listed in the Learning Resources section.

3. After evaluating the occupational performance profiles of these two seniors, select an activity, craft, or game that could be used to evaluate the cognitive capabilities of these clients in more detail. If you would like some assistance with this challenge, refer to the Allen, Kehrberg, and Burns (1992) chapter or the Earhart, Allen, and Blue (1995) manual listed in the Learning Resources section.

Identify and describe the task and contextual demands required to engage in this activity and discuss how the activity will be used to assess cognition. If you would like assistance with this challenge use the Occupational Performance Analysis—Short Form (Appendix B); consult the book by Allen, Earhart, and Blue (1992); or refer to the Earhart, Allen, and Blue (1995) manual listed in the Learning Resources section.

4. After making a determination about the cognitive levels of Maureen and Bert, identify five to 10 recreational activities that could be used by the nursing-home staff in the evening.
5. Describe the specific features of the activities you selected that make them appropriate for use with Maureen and Bert. For example, does the activity

require Maureen or Bert to learn new skills or can they rely on previous experience?

If you would like some assistance with this challenge, review the article by Levy (1990) listed in the Learning Resources section. This article provides an overview of how the analysis process is used to adapt activities to address therapeutic goals for clients with cognitive disabilities.

6. The department of occupational therapy has decided to offer therapy group sessions for the residents with dementia. The group will be designed to meet the sensorimotor, cognitive, psychosocial, and psychological needs of these individuals. Work with a partner to write a proposal for this occupational therapy group. Discuss, identify, and document the goals and objectives for the group. If you would like assistance with this challenge, use the Client Goals Form (Appendix H).

Develop a weekly treatment plan by listing the activities that will be provided in each therapy group session. Determine the time of day and length of time that the session will be scheduled.

Case study: Maureen and Bert

Maureen and Bert have lived in the same nursing home for almost a decade. Both residents have cognitive impairments; Maureen's impairments are secondary to Alzheimer's disease, and Bert has a history of multiple cerebral vascular infarcts. Table 1 provides an overview of dementia, Alzheimer's disease, and cognitive impairments in the elderly.

Table 1: Dementia, Alzheimer's Disease, and Cognitive Impairments

Dementia is a progressive and irreversible impairment of intellect that increases in prevalence relative to the age of the population. Dementia involves changes in cognition, memory, language, visuospatial functions, and behavior. Cognitive impairments in the elderly may be caused by primary degenerative central nervous system disease, brain injuries, cerebral vascular accidents, cerebral tumors, acquired immune deficiency syndrome, alcohol consumption, medications, infections, chronic pulmonary diseases, inflammatory diseases, vascular diseases, and Alzheimer's disease. Between 10 and 15% of individuals with dementia have reversible conditions (Kaplan, Sadock, & Grebb, 1994).

Between 50 and 60% of individuals with dementia have Alzheimer's disease (AD). AD is characterized by gradual onset and progressive decline of cognition and by personality changes; learning difficulty; and memory loss. The disease affects 5% of all seniors and 15 to 25% of those over the age of 85 years (Kaplan, Sadock, & Grebb, 1994). Longitudinal research suggests that a relationship exists between cognition, social functioning, and activities of daily living in seniors with AD who live in the community. The research also suggests these individuals lose the ability to perform instrumental activities of daily living before basic activities of daily living and that social function is determined less by cognition than by declining functional status (Carswell & Eastwood, 1993). Individuals with AD who remain active in their instrumental, leisure, and social activities of daily living require less help with their basic activities of daily living, demonstrate fewer disturbing behaviors, and cause less stress in their caregivers (Baum, 1995).

The occupational therapy department received referrals to see both clients. The nursing-home staff members that structure evening recreation activities have not been able to work with either client and they have asked for assistance in this area. Many of the craft, game, or group interaction activities provided appear to be beyond the sensorimotor, cognitive, and social capabilities of these two residents.

Maureen is a 77-year-old mother and grandmother. Her husband visits once or twice a week. Maureen does not recognize her husband, although the couple will celebrate their 57th wedding anniversary next month. Maureen is ambulatory and well known by staff and residents for her tendency to wander. She spends most of her day exploring the rooms and drawers of other residents, which adds to her unpopularity with her peers. Maureen enjoys talking with the other nursing-home residents but she tends not to stay on topic during these conversations. Most of the residents appear to deliberately ignore or avoid Maureen.

In preparation for her daily activities, Maureen will get out of bed between 4 and 7 o'clock in the morning. Maureen selects the garments she would like to wear but does not consider weather or seasonal conditions. She tends to choose her favorite sweater and pants every day. Maureen requires assistance in dressing. If she is left alone for this task, Maureen often puts her clothes on backwards, inside out, or over her pajamas. She is able to fasten large buttons but has difficulty with small fasteners and zippers.

Maureen is not able to find her way around the nursing home when she is asked to go to a specific location, but she follows people to the dining room at mealtime. Once her meal is served, Maureen eats on her own but is unable to open the sugar packages or small coffee creamers. Maureen is the last to arrive for meals and the first person to leave the dining room.

When Maureen feels the need to use the toilet during her daily adventures around the facility, she is able to find her way into someone's bathroom. Unfortunately, when Maureen is not supervised she often forgets to clean her perineal area or wash her hands. Once a week, on average, the staff find her sitting on the toilet with 10 to 20 feet of toilet paper on the floor. She has difficulty pulling sheets of paper off the toilet paper roll.

Maureen's husband indicates that she attended church on a regular basis, taught Sunday school, and sang in the church choir. She has experience as a volunteer with a women's auxiliary at a local hospital. On Saturday afternoons she often went out for tea with her girlfriends. Over the course of her life, Maureen has had a range of leisure interests including baking, knitting, gardening, and woodworking.

Bert is a 75-year-old widower who has two children and one grandchild. He spends most of his day at the nursing home sitting in a large, comfortable, reclining chair in the corridor. Bert has a long history of transient ischemic attacks and has had two strokes. He has right hemiplegia and expressive aphasia. Bert is dependent on the nursing staff for most of his morning care, but he helps the staff position his body during dressing and hygiene activities. He combs his own hair, uses his electric razor, and feeds himself in the dining room. Although Bert has a wheelchair, he gets very frustrated when trying to maneuver himself. He pushes the left wheel forward or propels the wheelchair with his left foot but is unable to determine how to steer around obstacles. He inevitably ends up stuck against the wall in the corridor.

Many of the residents and most of the staff talk to Bert as he sits in his large reclining chair in the corridor. Although he understands their comments, Bert has difficulty replying. Bert's friends enjoy his warm smile, inquisitive glares, and occasional speech. He speaks in very short, dysarthric phrases and has word-finding difficulties. Bert's most frequent visitor is "Socks," the nursing home's pet cat. Although Socks does not stay very long, she jumps onto Bert's lap for a visit once or twice a day. Bert appears to be very fond of petting this animal.

Bert remembers the names of his children but has difficulty recalling when they last visited. His children indicate that their father was a construction worker and project site supervisor. Over the course of his life Bert also had a range of leisure interests. "His first love was our mother ... but after that it's fly fishing." Bert apparently spent most of his spare time fishing. When he wasn't fishing, Bert was tying flies or talking about his next vacation. He has taken many classes in zoology and has spent time exploring photography. Bert's children wonder whether he can recognize his old photographs.

The information that follows will (a) provide students and instructors with resources to enhance the learning experience and (b) assist the students in completing the assignment.

Learning Resources

Allen, C. K., Earhart, C. A., & Blue, T. (Eds.). (1992). *Occupational therapy treatment goals for the physically and cognitively disabled.* Bethesda, MD: American Occupational Therapy Association.

Allen, C. K., Kehrberg, K., & Burns, T. (1992). Evaluation instruments. In C. K. Allen, C. A. Earhart, & T. Blue (Eds.), *Occupational therapy treatment goals for the physically and cognitively disabled.* Bethesda, MD: American Occupational Therapy Association

American Occupational Therapy Association (AOTA). (1994a). Statement: Occupational therapy services for persons with Alzheimer's disease and other dementias. *American Journal of Occupational Therapy, 48,* 1029–1031.

AOTA. (1994b). *Uniform terminology for occupational therapy* (3rd ed.). Bethesda, MD: Author.

Bowlby, C. (1993). *Therapeutic activities with persons disabled by Alzheimer's disease and related disorders.* Gaithersburg, MD: Aspen.

Earhart, C. A., Allen, C. K., & Blue, T. (1995). *Allen diagnostic module: Instruction manual.* Colchester, CT: S & S Worldwide.

Hatter, J. K., & Nelson, D. L. (1987). Altruism and task participation in the elderly. *American Journal of Occupational Therapy, 41,* 379–381.

Hellen, C. R. (1992). *Alzheimer's disease: Activity-focused care.* Boston: Andover Medical Publishers.

Kiernat, J. M., (1982). Environment: The hidden modality. *Physical and Occupational Therapy in Geriatrics, 2,* 3–12.

Levy, L. L. (1986). A practical guide to the care of the Alzheimer's disease victim: The cognitive disability perspective. *Topics in Geriatric Rehabilitation, 1*(2), 16–26.

Levy, L. L. (1987). Psychosocial intervention and dementia. Part 2. *Occupational Therapy in Mental Health, 7,* 13–36.

Levy, L. L. (1989). Activity adaption in rehabilitation of the physically and cognitively disabled aged. *Topics in Geriatric Rehabilitation, 4*(4), 53–66.

Levy, L. L. (1990). Activity, social role retention, and the multiply disabled aged: Strategies for intervention. *Occupational Therapy in Mental Health, 10*(3), 1–30.

Schemm, R. L., & Gitlin, L. N. (1993). A model to promote activity competency in elders. *American Journal of Occupational Therapy, 47,* 147–153.

Study Questions

1. Describe the approach to cognitive evaluation proposed by the Cognitive Disabilities Model.
2. Describe the approach to intervention proposed by the Cognitive Disabilities Model.
3. Identify a purposeful group activity designed to engage the long-term-memory capabilities of elder clients.
4. Identify a purposeful activity that is designed to engage a client who has a cognitive level of 3.
5. Rank the following activities in terms of the degree to which they challenge an individual's cognitive capabilities: assembling a bird feeder, placing stickers on a card, making a tile trivet, sewing a doll.
6. Describe the role of occupational therapy with clients with mild dementia and with severe dementia.

References

Allen, C. K., & Allen, R. E. (1987). Cognitive disabilities: Measuring the social consequences of mental disorders. *Journal of Clinical Psychiatry, 48*(5), 185–190.

Allen, C. K., Earhart, C. A., & Blue, T. (Eds.). (1992). *Occupational therapy treatment goals for the physically and cognitively disabled.* Bethesda, MD: American Occupational Therapy Association.

Allen, C. K., Kehrberg, K., & Burns, T. (1992). Evaluation instruments. In C. K. Allen, C. A. Earhart, & T. Blue (Eds.), *Occupational therapy treatment goals for the physically and cognitively disabled.* Bethesda, MD: American Occupational Therapy Association.

American Occupational Therapy Association (AOTA). (1994a). Statement: Occupational therapy services for persons with Alzheimer's disease and other dementias. *American Journal of Occupational Therapy, 48,* 1029–1031.

AOTA. (1994b). *Uniform terminology for occupational therapy* (3rd ed.). Bethesda, MD: Author.

Baum, C. M. (1995). The contribution of occupation to function in persons with Alzheimer's disease. *Journal of Occupational Science, 2*(2), 59–67.

Carswell, A., & Eastwood, R. (1993). Activities of daily living, cognitive impairment, and social function in community residents with Alzheimer's disease. *Canadian Journal of Occupational Therapy, 60,* 130–136.

Kaplan, H. I., Sadock, B. J., & Grebb, J. A. (1994). *Synopsis of psychiatry: Behavioral sciences clinical psychiatry* (7th ed.). Baltimore: Williams & Wilkins.

Levy, L. L. (1993). Section 3C: Cognitive disability frame of reference. In H. L. Hopkins & H. D. Smith (Eds.), *Willard and Spackman's occupational therapy* (8th ed., pp. 67–71). Philadelphia: J. B. Lippincott.

SENIOR OCCUPATIONS: THE CASE OF GLADYS

"This [professional care giving] relationship can be viewed as a partnership involving the exchange of expertise, values, and interests. Sensitivity to the spatial, temporal, and evaluative components of meaning in care giving will enable professionals to work more comfortably with family care givers and thereby be more supportive of the family unit's role as a health provider for frail elderly people in the community"

(Hasselkus, 1989, pp. 654-655).[1]

Chapter Objectives

1. Evaluate the effects of a chronic condition on a client's occupational performance profile.
2. Analyze the role and contribution of a caregiver to the health status of a client.
3. Evaluate task demands and contextual variables.
4. Use logical thinking and creative analysis to target intervention at enhancing client skills, adapting tasks, and altering performance context.
5. Select and design a purposeful activity to address client needs.

Assignment

1. Read the case about Gladys and her husband.
2. Work individually or with a partner to evaluate Gladys's occupational performance profile. If you would like assistance with this challenge, use the Occupational Performance Profile Form (Appendix G) to document information on the roles and occupations that are meaningful to Gladys; her values, interests, goals, and performance components; and the contexts in which she performs.

Occupational therapy practitioners are responsible for determining how a diagnosed condition influences performance. These determinations or judgments, however, frequently are made with limited information. To develop skills in making such determinations, use the information provided in the case to predict the effect of Gladys's condition on her ability to participate in various activities of daily living, productive activities, play, and leisure pursuits. For example, what effect do Gladys's current limitations in functional mobility have? What dressing activities was Gladys probably able to perform prior to fracturing her arm?

3. Sexual expression or engagement in desired sexual and intimate activities is included as an activity of daily living in *Uniform Terminology for Occupational Therapy* (AOTA, 1994) (Appendix E). What is the role of the occupational therapy practitioner regarding the sexual concerns of his or her disabled clients?

Evans (1987) illustrates how occupational therapy practitioners can use their skills in activity analysis to assist clients with physical disabilities in maintaining intimacy with their sexual partners.

A case example of a client with rheumatoid arthritis is provided in Evans's article. This article is listed in the Learning Resources section.

4. Use the information provided in the case to make a judgment about Gladys's husband Gene's occupational performance profile. Hypothesize about the occupations that are meaningful to Gene. How could these judgments be validated? How does Gene's occupational performance profile influence the health and well-being of this couple?

---

[1]From "The Meaning of Daily Activity in Family Caregiving for the Elderly," by B. R. Hasselkus, 1989, *American Journal of Occupational Therapy, 43*, pp. 654–655. Copyright 1989 by the American Occupational Therapy Association. Reprinted with permission.

5. How could Gladys's husband be more involved in the evaluation and intervention process to ensure that occupational therapy services support his role as a caregiver while promoting the heath and well-being of the couple?

6. Gladys has agreed to the following occupational therapy objectives:

   a. Increase functional mobility, including ascending and descending six stairs, in order to get to and from the bedroom (3 weeks).

   b. Select, obtain, and practice using an assistive technology device(s) to increase participation in dressing and eating (2 weeks).

   c. Increase bilateral hand strength and endurance to increase participation in more activities of daily living (3 weeks).

   d. Select, obtain, and practice using an assistive technology device(s) to independently participate in a card game (2 weeks).

   e. Identify and alter any environmental hazards within the home to prevent falls (1 week).

   Develop an intervention plan to attain these objectives. Enhancing Gladys's participation in these activities will enable this couple to return to their previous lifestyle. If you would like some assistance with this challenge, consider using the intervention strategies identified in the Occupational Performance Practice Model for Service to Individuals outlined in the chapter "Task Analysis: The Contribution of Occupational Therapy to Health."

   OR

   Select and design a purposeful activity to facilitate Gladys's achievement of one or more of these objectives. Purposeful activities are therapeutic when they (a) are relevant, meaningful, and goal directed; (b) elicit coordination among sensorimotor, cognitive, psychological, and psychosocial systems; and (c) promote mastery and feelings of competence (AOTA, 1993; Fidler & Fidler, 1978; Trombly, 1995).

7. What other services might occupational therapy offer this couple to address their health needs and support their continued success in the community? Consider preventative, functional, and remedial approaches to health. Identify other community support services that might assist Gladys and her husband.

Case Study: Gladys

Gladys was celebrating her 78th birthday 3 weeks ago when she fell and fractured her right elbow and hip while dancing with her husband. She was admitted to the hospital, received rehabilitation services for 3 weeks, and has just started to receive occupational and physical therapy services from ABC Home Health. Gladys has had rheumatoid arthritis (RA) for many years and her medical history includes gastritis, peptic ulcer, and anemia. She is not currently in an acute episode of arthritis. Her right arm is casted with the elbow at 90 degrees of flexion and the forearm in a neutral position. This cast will not be removed for at least 4 more weeks. Gladys is able to tolerate full weight through her legs when standing and walking but can only ambulate 10 to 15 feet and ascend and descend three stairs with minimal assistance from her husband.[2] Table 1 provides an overview of the clinical features of RA. Table 2 summarizes the prevalence of falls in the elderly and treatment of fractures by occupational therapy practitioners.

As soon as the registered occupational therapist arrived at Gladys and her husband Gene's home to begin the initial evaluation session, Gene asked his wife what he should make for lunch. Gladys sat in an overstuffed antique chair that was positioned next to a window. From this position she could see the front entrance to the house and the garden. The chair was surrounded by magazines, two candy dishes, a radio, and a television. Gladys gave her husband specific directions about lunch. Gene

---

[2]Minimal assistance means that the client performs over 75% of the task; moderate assistance means that the client performs between 50 and 75% of the task; and total assistance means that the client performs between 0 to 25% of the task (Hamilton, Granger, Sherwin, Zielezny, & Tashman, 1987).

Table 1: Rheumatoid Arthritis

Rheumatoid arthritis (RA) is a chronic, systemic disease that causes inflammatory changes of joints. Symmetrical involvement of synovial joints is common, but symptoms may appear in any joint. Low-grade fever, loss of appetite, anemia, and fatigue are some of the symptoms of systemic problems. The clinical course is characterized by exacerbations and remissions, and prognosis is unpredictable. Severe disability occurs in 10% of those diagnosed. Women are 4 times more likely than men to have RA. The onset of RA is usually gradual with pain, stiffness, and tenderness in many large joints as well as in the small joints of the hands and feet (Damjanov, 1996).

Approximately 55% of the elderly have arthritis (Yelin, 1992); and 30% of the elderly cite arthritis as the most frequent cause of physical limitations and difficulties with activities of daily living (ADL) and instrumental ADL (IADL) (McNeil, 1993). Of those seniors who have arthritis and no other chronic conditions, 66% experience physical limitations and 25% encounter limitations in ADL and IADL. Of those seniors with arthritis and at least one other chronic condition, 82% experience physical limitations and 41% encounter limitations in ADL (Yelin & Katz, 1990).

Elderly persons with arthritis have the greatest difficulty in the areas of functional and community mobility, reaching, stooping, endurance, and strength (Verbrugge, Lepkowski, & Konkol, 1991). A survey of home-based elderly indicates that they experience a decline in health status, pain, depression, and reduced independence (Mann, Hurren, & Tomita, 1995). These seniors have high rates of use of assistive technology devices (about 10 per person) and indicate a need for additional devices. The most frequently cited activities that these individuals miss include doing crafts, walking, shopping, socializing, doing housework, gardening, and playing sports.

walked over to the candy dish, put two small peppermints in his wife's mouth, and left the room.

During the evaluation interview Gladys identified the self-care, productive work, and leisure tasks that she wants to be able to do during her day: feed herself, dress, socialize with friends, watch Gene and her daughter in the garden, and read home and garden magazines. She expressed dissatisfaction with her current dependency on her husband for meals and dressing and dislikes having to sleep in the den. When asked about the new sleeping arrangements, Gladys indicated that the bedroom is upstairs. Gene and Gladys's home is a split-level design with the

Table 2: Falls and Fractures

> Falls are common in the elderly and are the leading cause of unintentional injuries in this population. Approximately one third of seniors who live in the community fall each year. Women fall three times more often than men, and the likelihood of falling increases with age. Of those persons hospitalized for a fall, only 50% are alive 1 year later (Tideiksaar, 1994).
>
> The treatment of fractures in the elderly costs Medicare upward of $4 billion annually, and as the size of the elderly population increases, safety and injury prevention programs will become more important (Steib, 1996b). Approximately 15% of registered occupational therapy practitioners and 10% of certified occupational therapy assistants provide services to clients with fractures (Steib, 1996a; Steib, 1996b). His range of motion may be limited after a fracture secondary to edema and pain, and muscles that act on these joints may have reduced strength secondary to disuse. (Morawski, Pitbladdo, Bianchi, Lieberman, Novic, & Bobrove, 1996).

kitchen, dining room, living room, den, and bathroom on the main level and the bedrooms and a full bath on the upper level.

When asked about the garden Gladys commented, "My oldest daughter comes over to help her father in the garden throughout the summer. I can't help with the gardening anymore…. It takes my husband over 20 minutes to get me up and down those steps." Gladys's driveway and sidewalk are surrounded by wildflowers, large rosebushes, and a rock garden. As the conversation progressed, Gladys was asked about her hospitalization. She indicated that Gene visited every day. "He came to visit early in the morning because he wanted to dress me. When I had my afternoon nap he would sneak in beside me." Gladys explained that she spent most of her time at the hospital sitting in "one of those old wheelchairs." "When I was able to walk short distances they let me go!… The ambulance drivers carried me up the front steps and into the house."

Gladys retired at the age of 58 because of arthritic hand pain that significantly affected her ability to perform her work duties as an accountant. Her husband Gene retired 5 years later. Prior to the progression of her RA the couple enjoyed a very active life of gardening, hiking, traveling, and socializing with friends. Today Gene and Gladys socialize on a regular basis and host a bridge tournament at their home once a month. Gladys watches while Gene and their guests play the game.

Prior to her fall Gladys required total assistance from Gene for other basic activities of daily living including grooming, oral hygiene, sponge bathing, toilet hygiene and transfers, dressing, and feeding. Gladys used her right hand, however, to serve herself large finger foods (e.g., grapes), eat small portions of food at the dinner table, and contribute to dressing activities. She primarily used lateral prehension or a weak cylindrical grasp with her right hand and held her left hand in a fisted position. She used her left arm to stabilize or carry objects (e.g., magazines). Holding onto a fork with her right hand was not easy, and Gladys's hands fatigued after she ate large meals. Gene often fed her the majority of their lunch and dinner meal. Table 3 provides a summary of the growing demand for caregiving services in the United States.

Prior to her fall Gladys walked very slowly around her home. She ascended and descended the six steps inside and eight steps outside her home with moderate assistance from Gene. Fortunately, Gladys has a very small build and weighs just over 100 pounds. The arthritic changes in Gladys's hands, however, limit her ability to hold onto a cane or walker. Gladys did not use any assistive devices with the exception of a raised toilet seat. She has a pair of hand splints but does not wear them any more and owns a reacher but has been unable to use it because of the amount of finger extension required to grasp the trigger.

Gladys indicated that she feels very weak and stiff in the mornings. "My hip bothers me and it is painful when I move it out"; Gladys put her hand on her femur and demonstrated abduction. She explained, "The doctor said my hip is healing just fine.... My elbow doesn't hurt but I can't use my right hand in this cast." Gladys has limited extension in all metacarpophalangeal (MP) joints and an ulnar drift bilaterally. Although she holds her left MP and proximal interphalangeal (IP) joints in flexion, she

Table 3: Caregiving in the United States

As the size of the elder population and the level of dependency of this cohort increase, so does the demand for caregiver assistance in the community. Culver (1994) estimates that the size of this demand will increase 175% between 1984 and 2010. Caregivers of the elderly are typically women from 55 to 64 years of age who are primarily adult daughters or daughters-in-law who find themselves simultaneously caring for their children and parents. If we assume that all women between the ages of 55 and 64 are available to care for their parents, the supply of caregivers will increase by only 60% between 1984 and 2010 (Cutler, 1994). This growing discrepancy between demand and supply of caregiving services has tremendous implications regarding (a) access to care; (b) the cost, quality, and use of caregiving services; and (c) public policy.

has enough active extension in these fingers to hold an object 1 inch in diameter with a cylindrical grip. Her left elbow extension is limited and elbow flexion is weak. Gladys continued, "I hope you can help us.... I spend most of my day sitting in this chair."

The information that follows will (a) provide students and instructors with resources to enhance the learning experience and (b) assist the students in completing the assignment.

Learning Resources

Books and Periodicals

Evans, J. (1987). Sexual consequences of disability: Activity analysis and performance adaptation. *Occupational Therapy in Health Care, 4*(1), 149–155.

Hasselkus, B. R. (1989). The meaning of daily activity in family caregiving for the elderly. *American Journal of Occupational Therapy, 43,* 649–656.

Mann, W. C., Hurren, D., & Tomita, M. (1995). Assistive devices used by home-based elderly persons with arthritis. *American Journal of Occupational Therapy, 49,* 810–820.

Tideiksaar, R. (1989). *Falling in old age: Its prevention and treatment.* New York: Springer.

Tideiksaar, R. (1994). Falls. In B. R. Bonder & M. B. Wagner (Eds.), *Functional performance in older adults* (pp. 224–239). Philadelphia: F. A. Davis.

Supplier Catalogues

Maddak, Inc. PO Box 922. Randolph, MA 02368-0922. 800-854-4687.

North Coast Medical, Inc. 187 Stauffer Boulevard, San Jose, CA 95125-1042. 800-821-9319.

Sammons, Inc. PO Box 32, Brookfield, IL 60513. 708-325-1700. 800-323-5547.

Smith & Nephew Rolyan Inc. One Quality Drive, Germantown, WI 53022. 800-228-3693.

This list of suppliers is not intended to be exhaustive, nor does it represent endorsements by the author or AOTA.

Study Questions

1. Your client's elbow (dominant extremity) is casted at 90 degrees of flexion. Identify three basic activities of daily living that would be difficult to perform independently.

2. Your client has very limited hand strength and range of joint motion.
   a. Describe an assistive technology device that could be used to play cards.
   b. Describe an assistive technology device(s) that would enable this client to use a walker.

3. How could gardening be adapted to enable a nonambulatory client to participate in this activity?

4. Describe how the physical environment can be adapted to prevent an elderly client from falling.

References

American Occupational Therapy Association (AOTA). (1993). *Position paper: Purposeful activity.* Bethesda, MD: Author.

AOTA. (1994). *Uniform terminology for occupational therapy* (3rd ed.). Bethesda, MD: Author.

Culver, N. E. (1994). Functional limitation and the need for personal care. In B. R. Bonder & M. B. Wagner (Eds.), *Functional performance in older adults* (pp. 210–222). Philadelphia: F. A. Davis.

Damjanov, I. (1996). *Pathology for the health professions.* Philadelphia: W. B. Saunders.

Fidler, G., & Fidler, J. (1978). Doing and becoming: Purposeful action and self-actualization. *American Journal of Occupational Therapy, 32,* 305–310.

Hamilton, B. B., Granger, C. V., Sherwin, F. S., Zielezny, M., & Tashman, J. S. (1987). A uniform national data system for medical rehabilitation. In M. J. Fuhrer (Ed.), *Rehabilitation outcomes: Analysis and measurement* (pp. 135–147). Baltimore: Paul H. Brookes.

Mann, W. C., Hurren, D., & Tomita, M. (1995). Assistive devices used by home-based elderly persons with arthritis. *American Journal of Occupational Therapy, 49,* 810–820.

McNeil, J. M. (1993). *Americans with disabilities: 1991–1992 U.S. Bureau of the Census. Current population reports, P70-33.* Washington, DC: U.S. Government Printing Office.

Morawski, D., Pitbladdo, K., Bianchi, E. M., Lieberman, S. L., Novic, J. P., & Bobrove, H. (1996). Hip fractures and total hip replacement. In L. W. Pedretti (Ed.), *Occupational therapy: Practice skills for physical dysfunction* (4th ed., pp. 735–746). St. Louis, MO: Mosby.

Steib, P. A. (1996a). Growth in geriatric care reflected in OTR survey. *OT Week 10* (46), 16–17.

Steib, P. A. (1996b). Skilled nursing facilities: Top employment setting for COTAs. *OT Week, 10*(47), 16–17.

Tideiksaar, R. (1994). Falls. In B. R. Bonder & M. B. Wagner (Eds.), *Functional performance in older adults* (pp. 224–239). Philadelphia: F. A. Davis.

Trombly, C. A. (1995). Occupation: Purposefulness and meaningfulness as therapeutic mechanisms. *American Journal of Occupational Therapy, 49,* 960–972.

Verbrugge, L. M., Lepkowski, J. M., & Konkol, L. L. (1991). Levels of disability among U.S. adults with arthritis. *Journal of Gerontology, 46*(2), 67–83.

Yelin, E. (1992). Arthritis: The cumulative impact of a common chronic condition. *Arthritis and Rheumatism, 35,* 489–497.

Yelin, E. & Katz, P. P. (1990). Transitions in health status among community dwelling elderly people with arthritis: A national, longitudinal study. *Arthritis and Rheumatism, 33,* 1205–1215.

ACCESSIBLE SENIORS CENTER: THE VOLUNTEER AGENCY

" ... Adult day-care programs exist to provide respite for families of disabled elderly people, to restore or rehabilitate the person to his or her highest level of function, to maintain the person's present level of function as long as possible, to provide socialization and meaningful activity, and to serve as an integral part of the community social service network"

(Hasselkus, 1992, p. 199).[1]

Chapter Objectives

1. Apply skills in task analysis to promote the health of an elder community.
2. Evaluate the needs of seniors living in a local community.
3. Delineate the expected outcomes of a proposed day program for seniors.
4. Identify and describe appropriate educational sessions and activity programs to achieve proposed program objectives.
5. Design an enabling environment for a social and physical day program for seniors with disabilities.
6. Write a proposal for a seniors day program to document initiatives in facility design and program activities.

Assignment

1. Read the case about the Accessible Seniors Center: The Volunteer Agency. Work in groups of three to develop and write a proposal for a seniors day program. The proposal will contain Tables 2, 3, and 4 and a facility layout plan.
2. Use your own community as a surrogate location for the center's day program. Evaluate the needs of local seniors by hypothesizing about their occupational performance profiles. Consider the values, interests, desires, performance capabilities, and needs of seniors in your community; their occupations and meaningful tasks; and temporal and environmental variables. Use this information to complete Table 1, Profile of the Elder Community. Table 1 has been started. In practice, these variables could be assessed by conducting research, interviews, and focus group discussions with seniors, their families, and professionals in various agencies that serve this clientele. If you would like some assistance with this assessment and the day program proposal, review the Occupational Performance Model for Service to People in Communities introduced in the chapter "Task Analysis: Occupational Therapy's Contribution to Health."

3. Delineate and document the expected outcomes of the day program by defining the center's vision, values, mission, goals, and objectives. Use this information to complete Table 2, Seniors Day Program.

The center's vision should be the image it holds for the future of the community; the values should describe the ideals and beliefs that will form the foundation for the center's programs. For example, the document *Core Values and Attitudes of Occupational Therapy Practice* describes the ideals and beliefs that are shared by practitioners of the profession (American Occupational Therapy Association, 1993). The mission statement should provide the center with a clear, focused strategy as it summarizes and communicates what the center will contribute to the community. Program goals and objectives should be achievable, verifi-

---

[1]From "The Meaning of Activity: Day Care for Persons with Alzheimer Disease," by B. R. Hasselkus, 1992, *American Journal of Occupational Therapy, 46,* p. 199. Copyright 1992 by the American Occupational Therapy Association. Reprinted with permission.

able, specific, and explicit (Whyte & Blair, 1995). The center's vision, values, mission, goals, and objectives should be congruent and complement each other.

4. Design a weekly schedule of group sessions for the center's day program. One example has been provided. If you would like assistance with this challenge, use Table 3, Schedule of Weekly Program Sessions. The days and times listed in the table can be changed. One example activity group is provided.

   The tasks and activities of the center's day program sessions should be designed to meet the goals, priorities, and needs of the elder community and should parallel the objectives delineated in Question 3. For example, the center could offer educational sessions in promoting health and preventing disease. The center could also provide caregiver support or offer activity groups targeted toward promoting increased levels of engagement in self-care, productive work, play, and leisure pursuits. In addition, these activity groups could be structured to maintain or enhance sensori-motor, cognitive, psychosocial, and psychological performance components. If you would like some suggestions about potential educational and remedial activities for seniors, review the Learning Resources section.

5. Make extra copies of Table 4, Program Sessions: Purpose, Rationale, and Potential Activities. Complete this table by documenting the purpose and rationale for every session and give examples of potential activities. One example has been provided.

6. After designing tasks to meet the characteristics of the program's target client population, determine how the center will create an enabling context for occupational performance. Consider temporal variables and features of the social, cultural, political, economic, and physical environ-

ment. Include a facility layout plan with your proposal.

For example, if one of the program's objectives is to provide respite services to caregivers who work, the center's schedule must meet the temporal needs of these individuals. If one of the program's objectives is to provide services to seniors with disabilities, the physical environment of the facility must accommodate the mobility needs of these individuals. If one of the program's objectives is sustainability, economic variables must be considered.

7. Complete and submit your proposal. Be prepared to give a 5-minute presentation to the proposal review committee.

Case Study: Accessible Seniors Center: The Volunteer Agency

Three occupational therapy practitioners who work together in private practice read a "Request for Proposals" notice for a new Accessible Seniors Center. ABC Township is planning to build a 1,000-square-foot center for seniors adjacent to the local library. The center will offer day programs and respite care to promote the health of seniors. Meals will not be provided, but those clients who stay over the lunch hour may bring a meal. The center will be staffed with one full-time director, one program assistant, and an itinerant nurse. ABC Township anticipates that the project will receive a rather large initial endowment for capital expenditures and a modest yearly operating budget. It is expected that there will be a number of well elderly who will volunteer once the center is open. Proposal submissions must not exceed 10 pages, including accompanying illustrations and appendices. The organization, agency, or business with the most appropriate proposal will be offered a contract to oversee the development, implementation, and management of the center's program. The terms of the contract (e.g., referrals, eligibility, staffing, program evaluation, budgets) will be discussed by both parties at a later date.

One of the practitioners attends a roundtable discussion with other proposal writers and the head librarian. The group discusses the project and its potential effect on the library. ABC Library provides services 6 days a week (9:00 a.m. to 8:00 p.m.) to a small community of 30,000 residents; and employs full-time librarians, part-time staff members, and a number of volunteers. Although the library serves a number of seniors, the primary customers are young families and mothers with small children. In addition to the book collection, the library staff are very proud of their new multimedia center and assortment of educational videos. As the interview progresses the head librarian indicates, "We are supportive of the idea, although my staff do not have the expertise to work with people who are sick. I'm concerned about patients wandering outside or into the library," but adds, "The seniors at the center could have access to any large-print or auditory books available in the library."

The three practitioners study the profiles of the local elder community and the services offered by other community agencies. Seniors account for close to 18% of the community, which is slightly higher than the national average. The prevalence of disabilities in the noninstitutional elderly parallels national averages: (a) the prevalence of disability increases with increased age as does the severity of the disability; (b) 50% of seniors have difficulty with or are unable to perform one or more functional activities; (c) 17.5% of seniors need personal assistance with activities of daily living (ADL) and instrumental ADL (IADL), (d) 3% use a wheelchair; (e) 9% have used a cane, crutch, or walker for at least 6 months; and (f) 4% have a mental or emotional disability (U.S. Congress, 1991). The

tasks that seniors report having the most difficulty performing include climbing stairs, mobilizing in the community, doing light housework, mobilizing in the bathroom, and dressing; conditions cited as causing these limitations include arthritis, heart trouble, back or spine problems, lung or respiratory problems, and hypertension (McNeil, 1993). Although 95% of older people do not live in nursing homes (U.S. Congress, 1991), most of the people over the age of 85 in this community live in a nursing home.

The medical facilities in the area offer some preventative clinical services, including immunization against influenza and screenings for high blood pressure and cancers. ABC Rehabilitation Center provides inpatient and outpatient services, and ABC Home Health provides nursing, therapy, and hospice services to clients with medical needs. The local skilled nursing facilities offer residential care and inpatient rehabilitation services. The community apparently does not have an agency that provides respite or caregiver support.

Table 1: Profile of the Elder Community

Occupational Performance Profile		
Occupations	**Person**	**Contexts**
Roles	Health Status	Temporal
Friends	*Conditions that seniors cite as the primary cause of their disabilities include arthritis, heart trouble, back/spine problems, hearing and vision problems, and stroke (McNeil, 1993); 55% have arthritis (Yelin, 1992)*	
Parents		
Grandparents		
Community elders		
Tasks and Activities	Values, Interests, and Goals	Social
Activities of Daily Living	*Loves animals, the circus, gymnastics, and parties.*	
Greatest difficulty with community and functional mobility, doing light housework	Performance Components	Cultural
	Sensorimotor Components	
	3% use a wheelchair *9% use a cane, crutch, or walker*	
Work and Productive Activities	Cognitive Integration and Cognitive Components	Physical
	5% have severe dementia, 15% have mild dementia (Kaplan, Sadock, & Grebb, 1994)	
Play or Leisure Activities	Psychological and Psychosocial Components	
	15 to 25% are depressed (Riley, 1994).	

Table 2: Seniors Day Program

Vision

Values and Principles

Mission

Goals and Objectives

Table 3: Schedule of Weekly Program Sessions

Morning	Monday	Tuesday	Wednesday	Thursday	Friday
8:30 - 9:00	New Arrivals and Welcome Group	New Arrivals and Welcome Group	New Arrivals and Welcome Group	New Arrivals and Welcome Group	New Arrivals and Welcome Group
9:00 - 9:30					
9:30 - 10:00					
10:00 - 10:30					
10:30 - 11:00					
11:00 - 11:30					
11:30 - 12:00					

Afternoon	Monday	Tuesday	Wednesday	Thursday	Friday
12:00 - 12:30					
12:30 - 1:00					
1:00 - 1:30					
1:30 - 2:00					
2:00 - 2:30					
2:30 - 3:00					
3:00 - 3:30					
3:30 - 4:00					
4:00 - 4:30					

Table 4: Program Sessions: Rationale and Potential Activities

Program Session and Purpose	Rationale	Potential Activities
New Arrivals and Welcome Group *Provide socialization opportunities with peers and daily orientation.*	*Seniors with disabilities have great difficulty accessing their community. Many have lost peers as a result of mobility limitations or death. These individuals would benefit from socialization with other seniors. Those with dementia will benefit from daily activities to orient them to person, place, and time.*	*Introduce new and continuing group members using name games, etc. Make name tags. Review or make a calendar of the day's schedule. Do individual or small group journal writing. Have a morning fitness session.*

The information that follows will (a) provide students and instructors with resources to enhance the learning expericompleting the assignment.

Learning Resources

American Occupational Therapy Association (AOTA). (1986). *Role of occupational therapy with the elderly* (2nd ed.). Bethesda, MD: Author.

American Occupational Therapy Association (AOTA). (1986). Occupational therapy in adult day care. *American Journal of Occupational Therapy, 40,* 814–816.

AOTA. (1986). Roles and functions of occupational therapy in adult day care. *American Journal of Occupational Therapy, 40,* 817–821.

Eilenberg, A. O. (1986). An expanding community role for occupational therapy: Preventing depression. *Physical and Occupational Therapy in Geriatrics, 5*(1), 47–58.

Hoff, S. (1987). The occupational therapist as case manager in an adult day health care setting. *Physical and Occupational Therapy in Geriatrics, 6*(1), 21–32.

Kaufmann, M. M. (1994). Activity-based intervention in nursing home settings. In B. R. Bonder & M. B. Wagner (Eds.), *Functional performance in older adults* (pp. 306–321). Philadelphia: F. A. Davis.

Kirchman, M. M., Reichenbach, V., & Giambalvo, B. (1982). Preventive activities and services for the well elderly. *American Journal of Occupational Therapy, 36,* 236–242.

Levine Schemm, R., & Gitlin, L. N. (1993). A model to promote activity competence in elders. *American Journal of Occupational Therapy, 47,* 147–153.

Levy, L. L. (1990). Activity, social role retention, and the multiply disabled aged: Strategies for intervention. *Occupational Therapy in Mental Health, 10*(3), 1–30.

Mann, M., Edwards, D., & Baum, C. M. (1986). OASIS: A new concept for promoting the quality of life for older adults. *American Journal of Occupational Therapy, 40,* 784–786.

Mazor, R. (1982). Drama therapy for the elderly in a day care center. *Hospital and Community Psychiatry, 33,* 577–579.

Neustadt, L. E. (1985). Adult day care: A model for changing times. *Physical and Occupational Therapy in Geriatrics, 4*(1), 53–66.

Norman, A. N., & Crosby, P. M. (1990). Meeting the challenge: Role of occupational therapy in geriatric day hospital. *Occupational Therapy in Mental Health, 10*(3), 65–78.

Osorio, L. P. (1993). Adult day care. In H. L. Hopkins & H. D. Smith (Eds.), *Willard and Spackman's occupational therapy* (8th ed., pp. 812–815). Philadelphia: J. B. Lippincott.

Schemm, R. L., & Gitlin, L. N. (1993). A model to promote activity competence in elders. *American Journal of Occupational Therapy, 47,* 147–153.

Speake, D. L. (1987). Health promotion activity in the well elderly. *Health Values: Achieving High-Level Wellness, 11*(6), 25–30.

Valentine-Garzon, M. A., Maynard, M., & Selznick, S. Z. (1992). ROM dance program effects on frail-elderly women in an adult day care center. *Physical and Occupational Therapy in Geriatrics, 11*(1), 63–83.

Study Questions

1. Seniors with severe arthritis use many different assistive technology devices to perform their basic activities of daily living (Mann, Hurren, & Tomita, 1995). How might a seniors center educate this population about the availability and use of adapted equipment?

2. Between 12 and 16% of seniors with disabilities indicate that they have difficulty getting around outside the home and doing light housework (McNeil, 1993). How might a volunteer service program be structured to address this need?

3. Identify a purposeful activity to increase the physical activity level of seniors with disabilities.

4. Describe a purposeful group activity to increase the cognitive level of seniors with severe dementia.

5. Describe an educational program that might be valued by caregivers of severely physically disabled seniors.

6. How might the time of day affect the interest and energy levels of different seniors with disabilities?

References

American Occupational Therapy Association. (1993). Core values and attitudes of occupational therapy practice. *American Journal of Occupational Therapy, 47,* 1085–1086.

Kaplan, H. I., Sadock, B. J., & Grebb, J. A. (1994). *Synopsis of psychiatry: Behavioral sciences clinical psychiatry* (7th ed.). Baltimore: Williams & Wilkins.

Mann, W. C., Hurren, D., & Tomita, M. (1995). Assistive devices used by home-based elderly persons with arthritis. *American Journal of Occupational Therapy, 49,* 810–820.

McNeil, J. M. (1993). *Americans with disabilities: 1991–1992 U.S. Bureau of the Census. Current population reports, P70-33.* Washington, DC: U.S. Government Printing Office.

Riley, K. P. (1994). Depression. In B. R. Bonder & M. B. Wagner (Eds.), *Functional performance in older adults* (pp. 210–222). Philadelphia: F. A. Davis.

U.S. Congress. House of Representatives, Committee on Ways and Means, Subcommittee on Health. (1991). *Long-term care: Proposals to improve Medicare's skilled nursing facility and health-care benefits.* Washington, DC: U.S. Government Printing Office.

Whyte, E. G., & Blair, J. D. (1995). Strategic planning for health care provider organizations. In L. F. Wolper (Ed.), *Health care administration: Principles, practices, structure, and delivery* (2nd ed., pp. 289–301). Gaithersburg, MD: Aspen Publishers.

Yelin, E. (1992). Arthritis: The cumulative impact of a common chronic condition. *Arthritis and Rheumatism, 35,* 489–497.

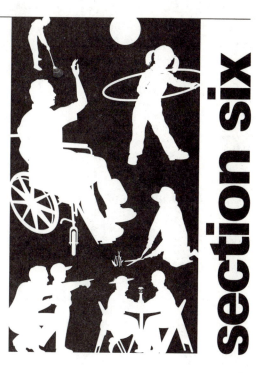

section six

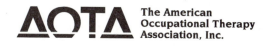

SECTION SIX: STUDENT OCCUPATIONAL PERFORMANCE ANALYSES

Section Six contains a collection of Occupational Performance Analysis - Short Forms that have been completed by sophomore occupational therapy students. These samples demonstrate how the Short Form can be used to conduct a generic analysis before an activity or task is graded, adapted, and applied to a particular client. The activities analyzed include:

- *Downhill skiing*

- *Beginning swimming*

- *Oil and watercolor painting*

- *Parachute games*

- *Puppetry*

- *Tea party*

Occupational Performance Analysis Form–Short Form
Erin Panciera, Occupational Therapy Student, Class of 1998

Occupation
Role Performance: *Friend, Mother, Father, Sister, Brother*
Task: *Outdoor leisure/play activity during the winter months (weather permitting)*

Activity: *Downhill skiing*

Steps Required to Perform:

1. *Obtain a map of the mountain and become oriented to the layout of the slopes and lifts.*
2. *Get dressed.*
3. *Put ski boots on and tighten if necessary.*
4. *Step into skis (audible snap when skis are on correctly).*
5. *Ski to the desired chair lift.*
6. *Load onto the chair lift and pull safety bar down.*
7. *Once the unloading area is in sight, raise safety bar and prepare to unload.*
8. *Unload the chair (be cautious of other skiers that may be congregated around the unloading area).*
9. *Choose the desired trail, paying close attention to the level-of-challenge markings denoted on each trail.*
10. *Ski down the trail.*

Materials, Tools, and Equipment (availability, cost, source . . .):

Warm clothing (e.g., ski pants, jacket, hat, gloves, and goggles), ski boots, ski poles, and skis. Ski equipment can be purchased new or used, or can be rented.

Safety Precautions and Contraindications:

Skiing is a dangerous sport and the skier must be in control at all times to ensure the safety of self and others. Skiers must be alert and aware of their surroundings while skiing down the mountain and getting on and off the chairlift. It is extremely important that the safety bar be lowered into position when riding the chairlift. Ski equipment must be fitted to the individual. It is important to wear warm clothing and leave as little skin exposed as possible to prevent frostbite.

Time to Complete: *Depending on the individual.*

The Person

Relevance and Meaningfulness: (historical or current personal and social relevance)

Thousands of years ago humans skied across the frozen, snow-covered ground to find food during the cold winter months. Today, skiing is no longer used for survival and is a pleasurable and competitive sport for people of all ages. Norwegians are credited with introducing skiing as a sport to the world in the late 18th century (Brasch, 1970). Since then its popularity has grown tremendously.

Skiing can be an individual or group activity. Although skiing is not specific to one culture, there are geographic limitations for some populations. It is necessary to be in or around a mountainous area where the climate is snowy and cold for part of the year. Skiing may hold personal meaning if it is a family or holiday tradition, favorite leisure sport, or peer group activity. Skiers must enjoy cold temperatures and the outdoors.

Values and Interests:

The skiing population is growing rapidly because skiing is a sport that can be enjoyed by all individuals. Skiing is a great way to exercise, enjoy the outdoors, and achieve personal gratification. Interest levels may vary among individuals.

For each performance component, determine the level of challenge required to perform. (Mod = moderate, Max = maximum).	Level of Challenge		Comments (Indicate N/A if Not Applicable)
	Mod	**Max**	
A. Sensorimotor Component			
1. Sensory			
a. Awareness and Processing	X		*Requires awareness and integration of proprioceptive, vestibular, visual, and tactile information.*
Proprioception		X	*Awareness of arm and leg position while on slope.*
Vestibular		X	*Very high in linear and angular movement.*
Visual	X		*To identify location of obstacles. Required for depth perception.*
b. Perceptual Skills *Kinesthesia*		X	*Force is required when using poles and to begin momentum.*
Body Scheme		X	*Constant internal awareness of body positions.*
Depth Perception	X		*Determine distance between self and other individuals and objects.*
2. Neuromuscular *Strength*		X	*Requires strength in arms, legs, and trunk.*
Endurance	X		*Depends upon the length of the trail and the number of rest periods.*
Postural Control		X	*Requires ability to maintain the trunk in upright position for an extended period.*
3. Motor *Gross Coordination*		X	*Necessary to get on and off a chairlift and to ski down slope.*
Bilateral Integration		X	*Contralateral use of arms and legs.*

For each performance component, determine the level of challenge required to perform. (Mod = moderate, Max = maximum).	Level of Challenge		Comments (Indicate N/A if Not Applicable)
	Mod	Max	
Praxis		X	To get on and off chairlift and to plan movements on skis.
Visual-Motor Integration	X		To maneuver self down the mountain.
B. Cognitive Integration and Cognitive Components Sequencing		X	Preparation steps, getting on and off the chairlift, and planning route down the slope.
Level of Arousal	X		Must respond to changing environmental obstacles.
Spatial Operations		X	Getting equipment on, loading and unloading chairlift, and maneuvering around objects.
Recognition	X		Recognize objects, familiar trails, and level-of-challenge markings.
C. Psychosocial Skills & Psychological Components 1. Psychological Self-Concept	X		Successful participation will improve the self-concept of the individual.
2. Social Social Conduct	X		Must respect others on the mountain.
Self-Expression	X		Allows individual to be creative in an open environment.
3. Self-Management Self-Control	X		Individual must be able to manage his or her behavior in the environment. Dependent on novelty of activity.
Coping Skills	X		Depends upon the individual demands of the environment.

Performance Context

	Comments
A. **Temporal Aspects** Chronological Age	*Begin in middle childhood at the earliest. May start at any age thereafter.*
B. **Environmental**	
1. Physical	*Many stationary and moving objects. Chairlift must be used as transportation up the mountain.*
2. Social	*Can be an individual or group activity.*
3. Cultural	*Certain populations may experience geographic limitations.*

Adaptations, Grading, and Structuring:

Activity	Environment	Personal Approach
1. *Poma lift to get up mountain*	1. *Slalom or mogul skiing*	1. *Shorter duration*
2. *Cross-country skiing*	2. *Difficulty of slope*	2. *Ski without poles*
3. *Snow boarding*	3. *Length of slope*	
	4. *Presence of friends*	

Assistive and Adaptive Equipment:

1. *Canadian hand-held outriggers*
2. *Sit-ski*
3. *Ski bra or bungee cord*

References and Learning Resources

Brasch, R. (1970). *How did sports begin?: A look at the origins of man at play.* New York: David McKay.

McCree, S. (1993). *Leisure and play in therapy: Theory, goals, and activities.* Tucson, AZ: Therapy Skill Builders.

O'Leary, H. (1987). *Bold tracks: Skiing for the disabled.* Evergreen, CO: Cordillera Press.

Raible, R. (1995). Skiing: A therapeutic lift. *OT Week, 9*(14), 16–19.

Occupational Performance Analysis Form–Short Form
Karin Sandstrom, Occupational Therapy Student, Class of 1998

Occupation
Role Performance: *Friend, Sister, Brother, Daughter, Son*
Task: *(a) leisure/play or competitive activities for indoor or outdoor (b) functional mobility in the pool (c) dressing, if including change of garments*
Activity: *Beginner swimming*   Steps Required to Perform: 1. *Get into 3-foot-deep water by using the stairs at the end of the pool.*   2. *Walk around the shallow end and swing your arms.*   3. *Walk over to the wall and hold onto it with two hands.*   4. *While holding the wall, flutter kick for 20 seconds. Repeat six times with a 30-second rest.*   5. *Repeat step 4 putting your head in the water and holding your breath for as long as possible. Repeat six times with as long a rest as needed.*   6. *Swim from one side of the shallow end to the other while holding onto the kick board and flutter kicking with your head out of the water. Repeat five times.*   7. *Repeat step 6. Put your head in the water for as long as possible, lift your head up when you need a breath, and continue to flutter kick. Repeat five times.*
Materials, Tools, and Equipment (availability, cost, source . . .):   *A pool, kick board, bathing suit, towel, open space, water (water temperature has to be considered when dealing with physically disabled children), and toys (optional).*
Safety Precautions and Contraindications: *A lifeguard, life jackets, life rings, safety poles, and a first-aid kit must be present at all times. Horseplaying, running, or diving is not allowed in the pool area. Children should not swim alone.*
Time to Complete: *Approximately 45 minutes to 1 hour*

The Person

Relevance and Meaningfulness: (historical or current personal and social relevance)

The origin of swimming is somewhat of a mystery, but it is believed that man learned to swim from animals. The English in 1837 were the first to compete in swimming rather than use it as a survival skill. The two strokes the English used were the sidestroke and the breaststroke (Vickers & Vincent, 1984).

As time went on, swimming became a key component in the Olympics and also a part of the Ironman race and triathlons. Swimming is now a major event in the Special Olympics, in which children and adults with disabilities can compete in diving, breaststroke, backstroke, butterfly, and freestyle swimming. Events have also been adapted so severely disabled individuals can participate in such events as a walk race, a flotation race, and an assisted and unassisted swim.

Swimming is necessary for survival, but it is also a recreational and leisure activity. It is an activity that can be done throughout the life span, beginning around the age of 3 or 4. Swimming may hold personal meaning if it is a favorite leisure activity, a family sport tradition, or part of a holiday ritual to visit the beach. A number of swimming-related games may hold significant meaning and an individual may have fond memories of group swimming events.

Values and Interests:

Swimming is a very self-gratifying activity and a great way to build confidence. It is an activity that can be fun or be taken seriously. For example, many children and adolescents enjoy swimming competitively whether at school or on a club swim team. It is also a great cardiovascular activity and a good way to socialize and interact with others. Finally, swimming is a form of independence that many people cherish.

For each performance component, determine the level of challenge required to perform. (Mod = moderate, Max = maximum).	Level of Challenge		Comments (Indicate N/A if Not Applicable)
	Mod	Max	
A. Sensorimotor Component			
1. Sensory			
a. Awareness and Processing *Tactile*		X	*Water movement across the skin. Light touch, temperature, and pressure of the water.*
Proprioception		X	*Kicking, moving the arms, and walking down the stairs.*
Vestibular		X	*Moving the head in the water when breathing or propelling forward.*
b. Perceptual Skills *Kinesthesia*		X	*Determine how hard to kick your legs.*
Body Scheme	X		*Knowing which foot or arm to move next. Internal awareness of body position without looking.*
2. Neuromuscular *Endurance*	X		*Kicking and holding your breath for a long period of time.*
Range of Motion		X	*Midrange in the hips, knees, and elbows. Full shoulder flexion.*
Postural Control		X	*Holding the flutter board in the water and staying balanced. Getting into and out of the water.*
3. Motor *Bilateral Integration*		X	*Using both hands to hold onto the board and both feet to kick.*
Praxis		X	*Planning how to use your body to swim to the other side.*

For each performance component, determine the level of challenge required to perform. (Mod = moderate, Max = maximum).	Level of Challenge		Comments (Indicate N/A if Not Applicable)
	Mod	Max	
B. Cognitive Integration and Cognitive Components *Spatial Operations*	X		*Correctly orient flutter board.*
C. Psychosocial Skills & Psychological Components 1. Psychological *Self-Concept*		X	*Feeling good about what you have accomplished.*
Interest		X	*Enjoyable and fun. Learning a new leisure activity.*
2. Social *Interpersonal Skills*	X		*Talking and communicating with the teacher and other classmates.*
3. Self-Management *Coping Skills*	X		*Realizing that you may not be able to swim. Letting others help.*

Performance Context

A. **Temporal Aspects**	Comments
Chronological Age	*Typically between 5 and 7 years of age, but may start at any age.*

B. **Environmental**	
1. Physical	*Accessibility to a pool. Temperature of the water. Allow only a few distractions. Use a flotation device.*
2. Social	*An opportunity to socialize but also to learn to swim. Learn in groups or with peers.*
3. Cultural	*Swimming is a universal activity that every child can learn.*

Adaptations, Grading, and Structuring:

Activity	Environment	Personal Approach
1. *Number of repetitions*	1. *Depth of water*	1. *Amount of time*
2. *Thickness of the kick board*	2. *Number of people*	2. *Include dressing*
3. *Type of swim stroke*	3. *Temperature of water*	3. *Freestyle stroke*
4. *Dressing requirement*		

Assistive and Adaptive Equipment:

1. *Kick board*
2. *Floating bathing suits*
3. *Goggles*
4. *Lumbar-sacral flotation device*
5. *Inner tubes*
6. *Transfer boards*
7. *Special seats and belts*
8. *Pull buoy*
9. *Flippers*
10. *Full body board*
11. *Flotation ring*
12. *Life jacket*
13. *Hydrostatic lift*

References and Learning Resources

Compton, D., Goode, P., Town, B., & Motheral, L. (1988, Jan–Feb). Project PAIRS: A peer-assisted swimming program for the severely handicapped. *Children Today*, 28–30.

Jamison, L., & Ogden, D. (1996). Aquatic therapy: Enhancing rehabilitation through teamwork. *OT Practice, 1*(5), 26–31.

Vickers, B., & Vincent, W. (1984). *Swimming.* Dubuque, Iowa: William Brown.

Occupational Performance Analysis Form—Short Form
Megan Early, Occupational Therapy Student, Class of 1998

Occupation
Role Performance: *Artist*
Task: *Work, play, or leisure activity*
Activity: *Work, play, or leisure activity*   Steps Required to Perform: 1. *Decide if you want to reproduce a subject or create your own from your imagination.*   2. *Secure all necessary supplies.*   3. *Choose the setting in which you want to work, preferably free from distraction.*   4. *Plan design on paper.*   5. *Choose colors, texture, etc.*   6. *If needed, blend and mix colors on palette.*   7. *Reproduce plan onto canvas using actual paints.*   8. *Modify activity according to errors, change of mind, or time constraints.*   9. *If layering colors to create texture, you may have to allow drying time. Thus, you will have to wait for another session to complete the activity.*   10. *Place artwork in a safe place to dry, wash brushes, allow to dry, clean self and area.*
Materials, Tools, and Equipment (availability, cost, source . . .):   *Canvas, paper, easel, paintbrushes, cup of water, paints, smock, chair, cloth, and palette.*
Safety Precautions and Contraindications: *Nontoxic paints as necessary; smocks to prevent unwanted stains; goggles if the client has decreased visual-motor control or a spastic condition that could cause poking in the eye; a cloth to dry any spilled water or paint to decrease the hazard of slipping.*
Time to Complete: *45 minutes*

The Person

Relevance and Meaningfulness: (historical or current personal and social relevance)

The earliest known paintings date back to 10,000–30,000 b.c. and are on the walls in the caves of Lascoux, France (Encyclopedia Americana, 1995). Artisans used raw materials such as manganese dioxide and ferrous oxide mixed with grease to create their colors, and applied them with either their fingers, sticks, or leaves (The New Encyclopaedia Britannica, 1993). Figures in the paintings are believed to represent various aspects of cultural ceremonies, rituals, and magic spells (Mazet, 1993; Encyclopedia Americana, 1995).

Paintings are also used to convey an artist's feelings and emotions, to arouse the audience's attention, or to accompany a text, as in an illustration (Encyclopedia Americana, 1995). More recently painters used their crafts to commemorate an event or a person. In the Middle Ages it was not uncommon for the wealthy to have portraits made, thus ensuring their status in society would be recognized by future generations (Encyclopedia Americana, 1995).

Painting may hold personal meaning due to the pleasure derived from the process or outcome of this leisure or productive activity. Many artists enjoy the creative process of painting or the evolving content of their work. A completed picture may hold quite significant meaning to the painter, family members, or significant others. The content of the work, the method of assembly, and the tools and techniques used may hold significant meaning to the artist or viewer. The location, objects, people painted, or the intended owner of the finished work may also hold significance to the painter.

Values and Interests:

Painting is available as an outlet of creative expression for all ages across the life span and for those of varying degrees of ability. Paint-by-numbers, finger painting, and body painting (using colored soap that is dispensed from a container resembling a tube of acrylic paint) are available for children. They may also choose to "paint" using a wet brush and pictures that are speckled with water-soluble, colored dots. Older children and adults may experiment with watercolors, oil paints, and acrylics. Tempera paints are used for painting posters, puffy paints are used for decorating clothing and shoes, and specialized paints are available for use on ceramic and wood craft projects. People choose to participate in this art form for various reasons: to accomplish the task of painting a bedroom wall, to create a gift, for self-expression, and for relaxation.

Those who need assistance in painting can find a number of adaptive devices: built-up brushes, lift-up lids as opposed to screw-top jars, washable paints, and brushes that can be manipulated orally or with the digits of the feet. One can paint on a variety of surfaces as well, such as easels, paper, framed canvases, and scrolls (Encyclopedia Americana, 1995).

For each performance component, determine the level of challenge required to perform. (Mod = moderate, Max = maximum).	Level of Challenge		Comments (Indicate N/A if Not Applicable)
	Mod	**Max**	
A. Sensorimotor Component			
1. Sensory a. Awareness and Processing		X	Requires sensory awareness and integration of visual, tactile, and proprioceptive systems.
Tactile	X		Gripping pencil, paintbrush; if finger painting, actually touching the paint, feeling the canvas.
Proprioception		X	Throughout the activity: sitting, reaching, and blending paints.
Visual		X	Looking at subject, selecting colors, and seeing colors on the artwork.
b. Perceptual Skills Kinesthesia	X		Squeezing paint from the tube. How hard to apply brush strokes.
Right/Left Discrimination	X		With regard to replicating a subject.
Form Constancy	X		Paint in a tube is still paint when it is applied to a canvas. Objects illustrated.
2. Neuromuscular Range of Motion	X		0–110 degrees shoulder and elbow flexion. Finger flexion to hold brush.
Endurance		X	This activity lasts approximately 45 minutes.
3. Motor Gross Coordination	X		Setting up the easel, situating oneself in a chair, and painting the piece of art.
Laterality		X	Drawing the design on paper, transferring it to the canvas, unscrewing the lid to the paint, gripping and moving the paintbrush.

For each performance component, determine the level of challenge required to perform. (Mod = moderate, Max = maximum).	Level of Challenge		Comments (Indicate N/A if Not Applicable)
	Mod	**Max**	
Praxis		X	Constructive praxis as demonstrated by reconstructing an idea onto paper with paint, securing and organizing all supplies, and carrying out the objective.
Fine Coordination		X	Grasping the pencil to draw the initial design, unscrewing the tube of paint, blending colors, and grasping paintbrush.
Visual-Motor Integration		X	Throughout the entire activity.
Motor Control		X	When mixing the paints, going from palette to canvas, and moving along the surface of the canvas.
B. Cognitive Integration and Cognitive Components Attention Span		X	Client must stay focused on the subject or concept he or she is trying to produce in the painting, and how to go about doing so.
Sequencing	X		Order is important to ensure success in this activity. Client must know to let base color dry before applying any additional coats.
Spatial Operations	X		When planning, recognizing the adjustments of figures to adequate proportions and dimensions.
Concept Formation	X		Deciding to paint, with what medium, and of what subject. Envisioning the finished product.
C. Psychosocial Skills & Psychological Components 1. Psychological Values		X	Is this painting a gift for someone else? Is it a painting of something that is significant to the client?

For each performance component, determine the level of challenge required to perform. (Mod = moderate, Max = maximum).	Level of Challenge		Comments (Indicate N/A if Not Applicable)
	Mod	Max	
Self-Concept	X		*The artist could potentially learn something new about himself or herself through attempting the task of painting.*
2. Social Self-Expression		X	*Artists often paint a subject about which they have strong feelings.*
3. Self-Management Coping Skills	X		*Adjusting actions according to errors in planning and judgment.*

Performance Context

A. **Temporal Aspects**	Comments
Chronological Age	*Can be performed throughout the entire life span.*
B. **Environmental**	
1. Physical	*One can engage in this activity indoors, outdoors, and in a variety of settings.*
2. Social	*Painting can be done by oneself or in a group context.*
3. Cultural	*Styles of painting are very often representative of the artist's cultural background and influences.*

Adaptations, Grading, and Structuring:

Activity	Environment	Personal Approach
1. *Time constraint*	1. *Presence of others*	1. *Artists' position altered*
2. *Paint made from raw materials*	2. *Indoors or outdoors*	2. *Brush in mouth*
3. *Types of brushes or surface*	3. *Reproduce scene or object*	3. *Painting of idea vs. object*
4. *Paint-by-numbers kit*	4. *Location of supplies*	4. *Painting of something from childhood*
5. *Predrawn picture*		5. *Finger paint*
6. *Sponge painting*		

Assistive and Adaptive Equipment:

1. *Built-up brushes*

2. *Pudding or shaving cream used as a finger paint*

3. *Vegetables dipped in nontoxic paint to use as stamps*

4. *Pop-up lids on containers*

5. *Brushes placed in mouth, feet or orthoses, or prosthetics*

References and Learning Resources

Cope, M. (Ed.). (1995). *Encyclopedia Americana: 100th anniversary library edition* (100th ed., Vol. 21). Danbury, CT: Grolier.

Davis, C. B. (1989). The use of therapeutic and group processes with grieving children. *Issues in Comprehensive Pediatric Nursing, 4,* 269.

Encyclopaedia Britannica. (1993). *The New Encyclopaedia Britannica* (15th ed., Vol. 9). Chicago: Author.

LaMore, K. L., & Nelson, D. L. (1993). The effects of options on performance of an art project in adults with mental disabilities. *American Journal of Occupational Therapy, 47,* 397–401.

Mazet, J. (1993). *Cougnac.* Gourdon: Imp. Pierre Domene Sarl.

Occupational Performance Analysis Form—Short Form
Alison Devers, Occupational Therapy Student, Class of 1998

Occupation
Role Performance: *Friend*
Task: *Leisure and play activity indoors and outdoors; socialization*
Activity: *Parachute games; umbrella exchange* Steps Required to Perform: 1. *Take parachute out of bag, unfold, and place group members equally spaced around the parachute.* 2. *Instruct group as to how to inflate the parachute and practice doing so.* 3. *Start the game. Participants count aloud numbers one to three, going around circle.* 4. *The therapist calls out a number from one to three. All people with that assigned number run underneath the parachute and exchange places with another person with that number.* 5. *Repeat step 4, calling out other numbers. Put the parachute away when finished with the game.*
Materials, Tools, and Equipment (availability, cost, source . . .): *Parachute (around $20, depending on size) or large blanket; large room with high ceiling and floor space, or outdoors; balls or comparable objects (can be used with other parachute games).*
Safety Precautions and Contraindications: *Colliding with others while under the parachute can be dangerous.*
Time to Complete: *15 minutes*

The Person

Relevance and Meaningfulness: (historical or current personal and social relevance)

Parachute games are noncompetitive, collaborative, social activities that provide fun while being therapeutic. Socialization results when the common purpose is inflating the parachute. Parachutes or the people engaged in this activity may be particularly meaningful to group members.

Values and Interests:

Parachute games can be made gender- or ethnically relevant. Many games have been created using the parachute, or you can just use your imagination to create a new game.

For each performance component, determine the level of challenge required to perform. (Mod = moderate, Max = maximum).	Level of Challenge		Comments (Indicate N/A if Not Applicable)
	Mod	**Max**	
A. Sensorimotor Component			
1. Sensory			
a. Awareness and Processing			
Proprioception		X	*Moving parachute up and down. Changing places under parachute.*
Visual		X	*Seeing a place to move to, and moving around the parachute. Synchronization of movement of parachute, and seeing different colors of the chute.*
Auditory		X	*Listening to directions. Hearing the numbers of people who should switch position.*
b. Perceptual Skills			
Kinesthesia		X	*How hard to move the parachute up and down. How fast to run.*
Position in Space		X	*Interpret instructions: go under the parachute and raise it above your head.*
Depth Perception	X		*Getting to your destination around the parachute. Reaching for handles of chute when you get there.*
Body Scheme	X		*Awareness of body when raising parachute up and down and going under the chute.*
2. Neuromuscular *Range of Motion*		X	*Walking under parachute. Raising and opening parachute requires shoulder and finger range.*
Endurance		X	*Continuous movement with arms and legs. Depends on activity duration.*
Postural Control	X		*Standing while raising chute. Walking or running under parachute.*

For each performance component, determine the level of challenge required to perform. (Mod = moderate, Max = maximum).	Level of Challenge		Comments (Indicate N/A if Not Applicable)
	Mod	**Max**	
3. Motor			
Gross Coordination		X	*Opening parachute. Raising parachute. Walking or running.*
Visual-Motor Integration		X	*Moving parachute in synchronized fashion. Walking or running to designated position around the parachute. Reaching to grasp the chute handles.*
Motor Control	X		*Entire activity.*
Praxis		X	*Unfolding and folding parachute. What to do and where to go when your number is called.*
B. Cognitive Integration and Cognitive Components			
Level of Arousal		X	*Fast-paced activity.*
Recognition	X		*Realizing that the number called may pertain to you.*
Attention Span	X		*Dependent on activity duration.*
Spatial Operations	X		*Unfolding the parachute. Figuring out the place to move to when your number is called.*
C. Psychosocial Skills & Psychological Components			
1. Psychological *Interest*	X		*Play.*
2. Social *Social Conduct*	X		*Social Behavior.*
Interpersonal Skills	X		*Group and teamwork lead to socialization.*
3. Self-Management *Self-Control*	X		*Responding to activity demands and feedback from others to be successful in a group.*

Performance Context	
	Comments
A. **Temporal Aspects**	
Chronological Age	*This activity is typically used between ages of 4 and 10 years, but can be used throughout the life span.*
Life Cycle	*Early to middle childhood play and possibly early learning process. Socialization for young and older adults.*
B. **Environmental**	
1. Physical	*Large room with high ceilings without obstacles. Outdoors.*
2. Social	*Teamwork leads to an activity that can be used in a therapy setting.*
3. Cultural	*Popular in a preschool setting.*

Adaptations, Grading, and Structuring:

Activity	Environment	Personal Approach
1. *Chute size and shape*	1. *More or less people*	1. *Duration of activity*
2. *One person runs*	2. *Indoors or outdoors*	2. *One-handed grasp*
3. *Different "calls"*	3. *Retrieving objects under chute*	3. *Person unable to move can call out*
4. *Calls by name or attribute*		

Assistive and Adaptive Equipment:

1. *Use a blanket instead of a parachute. It is harder to hold on to because blankets have no handles.*

2. *Velcro-type mitt to keep hand in position around parachute with handles. It is ideal for the person who stands around the parachute but is not able to switch places.*

References and Learning Resources

New Games Foundation. (1976). *The new games book.* New York: Doubleday.

Orlick, T. (1982). *Cooperative sports and games book.* New York: Pantheon Books.

Witoski, M. L. (1992). *It's not just a parachute.* Tucson, AZ: Therapy Skill Builders.

Occupational Performance Analysis Form—Short Form
Carolyn Silva, Occupational Therapy Student, Class of 1998

Occupation
Role Performance: *Friend, Student*
Task: *Leisure and play activity, socialization*

Activity: *Puppetry*

Steps Required to Perform:

1. *Decide what you would like the puppet to look like (color, length of hair, etc.) and collect all necessary materials.*

2. *Put sock on one hand and with the other mark with a pencil where you would like to put the nose and mouth.*

3. *Draw nose and mouth on felt and cut them out.*

4. *Use yarn for hair. Measure and cut 12 pieces of yarn whatever length you prefer.*

5. *Glue eyes, nose, mouth, and hair (6 pieces on each side) on puppet.*
   Allow glue to dry.

Materials, Tools, and Equipment (availability, cost, source . . .):

Yarn, a sock (any color), fabric glue, two plastic eyeballs, scissors, felt, ruler, and pencil.

Safety Precautions and Contraindications:

Use caution when using scissors. Keep glue away from mouth and eyes.

Time to Complete: *30 to 45 minutes*

The Person

Relevance and Meaningfulness: (historical or current personal and social relevance)

Expressive arts can assist a child in working through conflicts that are not expressed verbally. Puppets are used to help children express an emotion or feeling or to teach children important concepts. For example, the Kids on the Block puppet show is used throughout 29 countries worldwide to teach tolerance and sensitivity toward people with disabilities (Hettinger, 1996). Puppets serve as a communication vehicle that children may be able to identify with. Puppets can be adapted to fit the culture or the specific needs of the child.

On a personal level, puppetry or storytelling may have unique meaning to different people. The types of puppets used or the characters and stories portrayed may reflect memories, motivations, interests, or desires of the participant. The interpretations, emotions, memories, and desires elicited by watching a puppet show will be unique to each audience member.

Values and Interests:

Children may want to make a puppet for themselves or someone they know. The puppet can be made to represent someone in their life (mother, father, sibling, friend, etc.).

For each performance component, determine the level of challenge required to perform. (Mod = moderate, Max = maximum).	Level of Challenge		Comments (Indicate N/A if Not Applicable)
	Mod	Max	
A. Sensorimotor Component			
1. Sensory			
a. Awareness and Processing			
Visual		X	Awareness of color and placement of materials on sock. Cutting and gluing.
Tactile	X		Texture of materials.
Proprioception		X	Hand position and movement inside the sock to give the puppet "life."
b. Perceptual Skills			
Kinesthesia		X	Squeezing glue out of the bottle, and pressing materials on sock.
Form Constancy	X		Recognizing yarn in small pieces and puppet as representation of a life form.
Spatial Relations	X		Recognizing correct rotation of features.
2. Neuromuscular			
Strength	X		Putting sock on arm and holding arm up to draw on sock.
3. Motor			
Praxis		X	Constructional praxis to fabricate puppet. Postural praxis to move puppet in a particular predetermined way to give it movement and "life."
Laterality		X	Using dominant hand to draw, cut, and glue, and move puppet.
Bilateral Integration		X	One hand wears the sock, while the other is drawing. Holding the felt with one hand while cutting with the other.

For each performance component, determine the level of challenge required to perform. (Mod = moderate, Max = maximum).	Level of Challenge		Comments (Indicate N/A if Not Applicable)
	Mod	**Max**	
Fine Coordination/Dexterity		**X**	*Using pencil and grasping materials.*
Visual-Motor Integration		**X**	*Cutting, drawing, and gluing.*
B. Cognitive Integration and Cognitive Components			
Attention Span	**X**		*Completing task and waiting for the glue to dry.*
Sequencing	**X**		*Drawing before cutting before gluing. Acting out a story line.*
Concept Formation	**X**		*Creating image of puppet before beginning activity.*
Spatial Operations		**X**	*Putting sock on hand and facial features in proper place with correct rotation.*
C. Psychosocial Skills & Psychological Components			
1. Psychological	**X**		
Interests			*Client may enjoy activity.*
2. Social		**X**	
Self-Expression			*Own style and skills expressed.*
3. Self-management	**X**		
Coping Skills			*Cutting small shapes. Gluing materials on sock.*
Time Management	**X**		*Allowing time for glue to dry.*

Performance Context	
A. **Temporal Aspects**	Comments
Chronological Age	*Typically between the ages of 5 and 12, but can be enjoyed across the life span.*
Developmental	*Initiative thought phase to formal operational (Piaget).*
B. **Environmental**	
1. Physical	*Accessibility of materials.*
2. Social	*Numbers of students, friends, and siblings around and what they are doing.*
3. Cultural	*Popular activity in many cultures. Activity can be completed by both sexes.*

Adaptations, Grading, and Structuring:

Activity
1. *Paper, felt, or material puppet*
2. *Specified time constraints*
3. *Face drawn instead of cut out*
4. *Precut shapes used for facial features*
5. *Homemade puppet clothing to the puppet's actions*
6. *Writing of theater script*

Environment
1. *Number of peers present*
2. *Conducted in group*
3. *Theater stage production*

Personal Approach
1. *Vocals for puppet*
2. *Done as unilateral*
3. *Amount of "life" given to the puppet's actions*

Assistive and Adaptive Equipment:

1. *Adaptive scissors*
2. *Ruler with large print numbers*

Reference

Hettinger, J. (1996). Putting the person first. *OT Week, 10*(23), 10–11.

Occupational Performance Analysis Form–Short Form
Rachel Budney, Occupational Therapy Student, Class of 1998

Occupation
Role Performance: *Friend, Brother, Sister, Classmate(s), Parent, Grandparent*
Task: *Leisure and play activity, socialization, functional mobility, meal preparation and cleanup, and feeding and eating.*
Activity: *Tea party* Steps Required to Perform: 1. *Obtain teacup and saucer, small plate, napkin, spoon, and tea bag. Bring to table.* 2. *One person in the group should obtain prepared snacks from refrigerator.* 3. *Pour prewarmed water from teapot into teacup and pass teapot.* 4. *Tear open tea bag and place in teacup.* 5. *Pass snack tray around table.* 6. *Remove tea bag from teacup and wrap string around spoon to drain bag.* 7. *Use tongs to add sugar cubes and pitcher to pour cream (if desired).* 8. *Drink, eat, and socialize. (Topic is given.)* 9. *Clean up.* *The above steps describe the general American tea party. There are a variety of ways to adapt these steps to create a "tea" similar to the unique ceremonies or traditions of other nations.*
Materials, tools, and Equipment (availability, cost, source . . .): *Tea bags, snacks (prepared), sugar cubes, cream, napkins, table, chairs, stove or hot plate, teacups, saucers, teapot, small plates, spoons, tongs, cream pitcher, and tray.*
Safety Precautions and Contraindications: *Temperature of tea and/or food allergies.*
Time to Complete: *45 minutes*

The Person

Relevance and Meaningfulness: (historical or current personal and social relevance)

The origin of tea is credited to China, but historians find it impossible to agree on the validity of any early tea references. Tea legends, both written and oral, are inexhaustible and completely unreliable (Shalleck, 1971). Tea drinking spread to Japan with the creation of a tea ceremony that elevated tea drinking from a social pastime to an aesthetic cult. The Japanese Tea Ceremony, an outgrowth of an ancient Chinese rite, is a ritual of great exclusiveness; it sets standards of refinement for the arts, for literature, and for everyday life (Shalleck, 1971). The Japanese Tea Ceremony is still cultivated by Japanese Buddhist monks, the imperial family, and many middle-class housewives. After the year 1700, tea was introduced to the West (Schapira, 1975). London became the tea capital, initiating a custom of drinking five cups a day, along with English tea manners. Tea has also become an integral part of life for many Americans. Tea has made its unique mark in many cultures, each culture with its own history, custom, and ceremony.

Since America is becoming increasingly diverse, a "tea party" is an excellent therapeutic activity, lending itself to unique adaptations for various clients of different cultural backgrounds. Schapira (1975) describes the distinctive tea ceremonies and customs performed in countries such as Iran, Morocco, Tibet, Turkey, Great Britain, Australia, Canada, India, and Japan. A tea ceremony that is culturally parallel to a client's background would be an ideal therapeutic activity. Also, America is increasingly becoming a tea-drinking society, and tea is often associated with social gatherings or relaxation. Traditionally, tea drinking in America is accompanied by a light snack or sweet dessert and social interaction among friends. Herbal teas are popular as a result of the increasing awareness of health and natural products, and they are often served at the ever popular coffee bars. Today, not only are there restaurants performing the cultural tea ceremonies of other countries, but there are American restaurants and cafes serving a social tea to anxious customers needing a break.

In addition to their social and cultural variety, tea parties can be appropriate activities for people throughout the life span as a cooperative or individual activity. Tea parties differ in their significance to different people, and their meaningfulness may depend on personal heritage, family or peer group traditions, or past experiences. The tea brewing process, materials or equipment used, and people present during a party may also vary in their meaning and significance.

Values and Interests:

Children may value or be interested in having a tea party for social acceptance (cooperation and sharing stories); imaginative play (pretend guests or dolls); or functional purposes. Many individuals of all age groups enjoy this activity. Interest levels will vary, especially between the sexes.

For each performance component, determine the level of challenge required to perform. (Mod = moderate, Max = maximum).	Level of Challenge		Comments (Indicate N/A if Not Applicable)
	Mod	**Max**	
A. Sensorimotor Component			
1. Sensory			
a. Awareness and Processing Tactile		X	*Picking up utensils and snacks. Temperature: hot, cold.*
Proprioception		X	*Pouring tea and cream. Adding sugar cubes with tongs.*
Gustatory		X	*Drinking tea and eating snacks.*
b. Perceptual Skills Kinesthesia Kinesthesia		X	*Using appropriate force when pouring tea and cream. Drinking from a cup. Adding sugar cubes with tongs.*
Pain Response	X		*Hot tea (too hot!).*
Body Scheme	X		*Sitting, walking: awareness of position at all times.*
Depth Perception		X	*Pouring tea and cream. Reaching.*
2. Neuromuscular Range of Motion	X		*Walking. Reaching to cupboard and across table.*
Strength	X		*Lifting teapot.*
Postural Control	X		*Postural stability to maintain stability while sitting and walking.*
3. Motor Laterality		X	*Stirring, pouring cream, using tongs, and draining tea bag. Hand dominance required.*
Bilateral Integration		X	*Pouring tea (hold top on with one hand and pour with the other), draining tea bag, and passing things around table.*

For each performance component, determine the level of challenge required to perform. (Mod = moderate, Max = maximum).	Level of Challenge		Comments (Indicate N/A if Not Applicable)
	Mod	Max	
Praxis		X	*Opening tea bag. Draining tea bag, using tongs, and using two hands for pouring tea.*
Fine and Oral Motor Coordination		X	*Opening tea bag, stirring with small spoon, draining tea bag, and using tongs.*
B. Cognitive Integration and Cognitive Components *Attention Span*		X	*Sustain for entire quiet and table-top activity. Maintain awareness of the hot temperature of the tea.*
Concept Formation		X	*Telling personal stories and socializing.*
Spatial Operations	X		*Wrapping tea bag around spoon with string.*
C. Psychosocial Skills & Psychological Components 1. Psychological *Values*		X	*Important and meaningful holiday stories and traditions are shared.*
2. Social *Social Conduct*		X	*Interacting appropriately with others.*
Interpersonal Skills		X	*Appropriate verbal and nonverbal communication.*
3. Self-management *Coping Skills*	X		*Taking turns when talking.*
Self-Control	X		*Listening without interrupting.*

Performance Context

A. **Temporal Aspects**	Comments
Chronological Age	*Middle childhood: 5 to 8 years of age through older years.*
Life Cycle	*Play and socialization process.*
B. **Environmental**	
1. Physical	*Tea supplies. Room with relaxed environment.*
2. Social	*Small group of four to five girls. Parallel and/or cooperative play.*
3. Cultural	*Popular and significant activity for many cultures, with each having its specific style.*

Adaptations, Grading, and Structuring:

Activity
1. *Clients can prepare snacks.*
2. *Use a drink other than tea.*
3. *Vary the size of teacups, teapot, and utensils.*
4. *The nature of the tea set can vary from plastic to china.*
5. *Tea can be made from tea bags or loose tea.*

Environment
1. *Vary or limit diversity among clients.*
2. *Take clients to a restaurant for an ethnic or American tea.*

Personal Approach
1. *Assign discussion topic or promote casual conversation.*

Assistive and Adaptive Equipment:

1. *Provide built-up grips for utensils.*
2. *Provide reaching devices.*
3. *Provide straws.*

References

Schapira, J. (1975). *The book of coffee and tea.* New York: St. Martin's Press.

Shalleck, Jamie. (1971). *Tea.* New York: Viking Press.

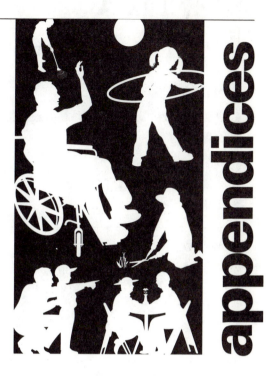

appendices

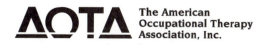

The American Occupational Therapy Association, Inc.

APPENDIX A

Occupational Performance Analysis Form[1]

Occupation
Role:
Task:

Activity:
 	
    Steps Required to Perform:
 	
    1.
 	
    2.
 	
    3.
 	
    4.
 	
    5.
 	
    6.
 	
    7.
 	
    8.
 	
    9.
 	
    10.

Materials, Tools, and Equipment (availability, cost, source . . .):
Safety Precautions and Contraindications:
Time to Complete:

[1]From "Uniform Terminology for Occupational Therapy," by the American Occupational Therapy Association, 1994, *American Journal of Occupational Therapy, 48,* pp. 1047–1054. Copyright 1994 by the American Occupational Therapy Association. Adapted with permission.

The Person

Relevance and Meaningfulness: (historical or current personal and social relevance)

Values and Interests:

For each performance component, determine the level of challenge required to perform. (Min = minimum, Mod = moderate, Max = maximum).	Level of Challenge			Comments (Indicate N/A if Not Applicable)
	Min	**Mod**	**Max**	
A. Sensorimotor Component				
1. Sensory				
a. Sensory Awareness				
b. Sensory Processing				
(1) Tactile				
(2) Proprioceptive				
(3) Vestibular				
(4) Visual				
(5) Auditory				
(6) Gustatory				
(7) Olfactory				

For each performance component, determine the level of challenge required to perform. (Min = minimum, Mod = moderate, Max = maximum).	Level of Challenge			Comments (Indicate N/A if Not Applicable)
	Min	**Mod**	**Max**	
c. Perceptual Skills				
(1) Stereognosis				
(2) Kinesthesia				
(3) Pain Response				
(4) Body Scheme				
(5) Right-Left Discrimination				
(6) Form Constancy				
(7) Position in Space				
(8) Visual-Closure				
(9) Figure Ground				
(10) Depth Perception				
(11) Spatial Relations				
(12) Topographical Orientation				
2. Neuromusculoskeletal				
a. Reflex				
b. Range of Motion				
c. Muscle Tone				
d. Strength				
e. Endurance				
f. Postural Control				
g. Postural Alignment				
h. Soft Tissue Integrity				

For each performance component, determine the level of challenge required to perform. (Min = minimum, Mod = moderate, Max = maximum).	Level of Challenge			Comments (Indicate N/A if Not Applicable)
	Min	**Mod**	**Max**	
3. Motor				
a. Gross Coordination				
b. Crossing the Midline				
c. Laterality				
d. Bilateral Integration				
e. Motor Control				
f. Praxis				
g. Fine Coordination/Dexterity				
h. Visual-Motor Integration				
i. Oral-Motor Control				
B. Cognitive Integration and Cognitive Components				
1. Level of Arousal				
2. Orientation				
3. Recognition				
4. Attention Span				
5. Initiation of Activity				
6. Termination of Activity				
7. Memory				
8. Sequencing				
9. Categorization				
10. Concept Formation				

For each performance component, determine the level of challenge required to perform. (Min = minimum, Mod = moderate, Max = maximum).	Level of Challenge			Comments (Indicate N/A if Not Applicable)
	Min	Mod	Max	
11. Spatial Operations				
12. Problem Solving				
13. Learning				
14. Generalization				
C. Psychosocial Skills and Psychological Components*				
1. Psychological				
a. Self-Concept				
2. Social				
a. Social Conduct				
b. Interpersonal Skills				
c. Self-Expression				
3. Self-Management				
a. Coping Skills				
b. Time Management				
c. Self-Control				

*Values, Interests, and Role Performance components are included at the beginning of the analysis form.

Performance Context

A. **Temporal Aspects**	Comments
1. Chronological	
2. Developmental	
3. Life cycle	
4. Disability Status	
B. **Environmental**	
1. Physical	
2. Social	
3. Cultural	

Adaptations, Grading, and Structuring:

Activity	Environment	Personal Approach
1.	1.	1.
2.	2.	2.
3.	3.	3.
4.	4.	4.
5.	5.	5.
6.	6.	6.

Assistive and Adaptive Equipment:

1.

2.

3.

4.

5.

APPENDIX B

Occupational Performance Analysis—Short Form[1]

Occupation
Role:
Task:
Activity: 　Steps Required to Perform: 　1. 　2. 　3. 　4. 　5.
Materials, Tools, and Equipment (availability, cost, source . . .):
Safety Precautions and Contraindications:
Time to Complete:

---

[1]From "Uniform Terminology for Occupational Therapy," by the American Occupational Therapy Association, 1994, *American Journal of Occupational Therapy, 48,* pp. 1047–1054. Copyright 1994 by the American Occupational Therapy Association. Adapted with permission.

The Person		

Relevance and Meaningfulness: (historical or current personal and social relevance)

Values and Interests:

For each performance component, determine the level of challenge required to perform. (Mod = moderate, Max = maximum).	Level of Challenge		Comments (Indicate N/A if Not Applicable)
	Mod	**Max**	
A. Sensorimotor Component 1. Sensory a. Awareness and Processing			
b. Perceptual Processing			
2. Neuromusculoskeletal			
3. Motor			
B. Cognitive Integration and Cognitive Components			

For each performance component, determine the level of challenge required to perform. (Mod = moderate, Max = maximum).	Level of Challenge		Comments (Indicate N/A if Not Applicable)
	Mod	**Max**	
C. Psychosocial Skills and Psychological Components 1. Psychological			
2. Social			
3. Self-Management			

Performance Context

	Comments
A. Temporal Aspects	
B. Environmental	
1. Physical	
2. Social	
3. Cultural	

Adaptations, Grading, and Structuring:

Activity	Environment	Personal Approach
1.	1.	1.
2.	2.	2.
3.	3.	3.

Assistive and Adaptive Equipment:

1.

2.

APPENDIX C

Occupational Performance Analysis Form
Canadian Student Version

Occupation
Role:
Task:
Activity: Steps Required to Perform: 1. 2. 3. 4. 5. 6. 7. 8. 9. 10.
Materials, Tools, and Equipment (availability, cost, source . . .):
Safety Precautions and Contraindications:
Time to Complete:

[1]Adapted from Appendix A, *Guidelines for the Client-Centred Practice of Occupational Therapy,* Health Canada, 1983, and Appendix A, Guidelines for Client-Centered Mental Health Practice, Health Canada, 1993. With permission of the Minister of Public Works and Government Services Canada, 1997.

The Person

Relevance and Meaningfulness: (historical or current personal and social relevance)

Values and Interests:

For each performance component, determine the level of challenge required to perform. (Min = minimum, Mod = moderate, Max = maximum).	Level of Challenge			Comments (Indicate N/A if Not Applicable)
	Min	Mod	Max	
Physical Components Sensation and Sensory Integration (touch, pain, pressure, vision, hearing, taste, vibration, proprioception, kinesthesis, and stereognosis)				
Visual Perception				
Range of Motion				
Strength and Muscle Tone (individual muscles or muscle groups)				
Coordination				
Balance and Posture				
Endurance				
Mental Cognition (memory, orientation, concentration, attention span, problem solving, decision making, intellect, insight, judgment, generalization)				

For each performance component, determine the level of challenge required to perform. (Min = minimum, Mod = moderate, Max = maximum).	Level of Challenge			Comments (Indicate N/A if Not Applicable)
	Min	**Mod**	**Max**	
Mood and Affect				
Behavior (appropriateness, self-control)				
Perception (awareness of reality)				
Thought Content (clarity, appropriateness, organization)				
Emotions (defenses)				
Body Image				
Volition (volition of thought and behavior)				
Sociocultural				
Cultural values, beliefs, language				
Involvement in community				
Interpersonal skills (dyadic and social skills)				
Management of social roles				
Family and friendship relationships				
Spiritual				
Sense of pleasure or purpose				
Inner motivation (sense of hopefulness or apathy)				
Feelings of power or helplessness				

389

The Environment	
	Comments
Physical Environment	
Social Environment	
Cultural Environment	
Political and Economic Environment	
Legal Environment	

Adaptations, Grading, and Structuring:

Activity	Environment	Personal Approach
1.	1.	1.
2.	2.	2.
3.	3.	3.
4.	4.	4.

Assistive and Adaptive Equipment:

1.	3.	5.
2.	4.	6.

APPENDIX D

Performance Component Analysis Tables

Canadian Student Version

Performance Component Analysis Tables–Canadian Students[1]

Physical Components	Infants			Children		Adults
			Riding a tricycle			
Sensation and Sensory Integration (touch, pain, pressure, vision, hearing, taste, vibration, proprioception, kinesthesis, and stereognosis)			*Mod* *Textured handles. Foot pedal pressure. Awareness of arm and leg position(s) and force without looking. Linear and angular vestibular. High visual demand.*			
Visual Perception			*Mod* *Requires depth perception, spatial relations, and position in space to negotiate the physical environment.*			
Range of Motion			*Mod-Max* *End range in hands. Midrange in shoulders, hips, and knees.*			
Strength and Muscle Tone (individual muscles or muscle groups)			*Mod* *Requires resistive strength (4/5 or greater in upper and 4/5 to 5/5 in lower extremities). Isometric contractions in fingers, isotonic in arms and legs.*			

[1]Adapted from Appendix A, *Guidelines for the Client-Centred Practice of Occupational Therapy*, Health Canada, 1983. With permission of the Minister of Public Works and Government Services Canada, 1997.

Performance Component Analysis Tables—Canadian Students, continued

	Infants	Children	Adults
		Riding a tricycle	
Coordination		*Min–Max* *Gross coordination of arms and legs to get on, off, and ride. Cylindrical grasp of handlebars.*	
Balance and Posture		*Mod* *Required to get on and off tricycle and sustain sitting.*	
Endurance		*Min* *Dependent on distance and surface quality.*	

Mental Component Analysis

Mental Components	Infants	Children		Adults	
		Riding a tricycle			
Cognition (memory, orientation, concentration, attention span, problem solving, decision making, intellect, insight, judgment, generalization)		*Mod* *Recall how to use and orient self to place. Sustain and divide attention.*			
Mood and Affect		*Min* *Not demanding of affect, but may positively influence.*			
Behavior (appropriateness, self-control)		*Min—Mod* *Relations with nonhuman environment. May require interpersonal skill and appropriate social conduct.*			
Perception (awareness of reality)		*Mod*			
Thought Content (clarity, appropriateness, organization)		*N/A*			

Mental Component Analysis, continued

	Infants	Children	Adults
		Riding a tricycle	
Emotions (defenses)		*Min* *Success may positively influence.*	
Body Image		*Min* *Engagement influences sensorimotor body image; success may influence self-image.*	
Volition (volition of thought and behavior)		*Min–Mod* *Engagement influences value and interest in activity and play.*	

Sociocultural and Spiritual Component Analysis

Sociocultural and Spiritual Components	Riding a tricycle	Infants	Children	Adults
Sociocultural Cultural Values, Beliefs, and Language			*Mod* *Relevance to cultural value of pediatric play.*	
Involvement in Community			*Min–Mod* *Engagement promotes access to and interaction with local community.*	
Interpersonal Skills (dyadic and social skills)			*Min* *Not required unless in group. Parallel activity.*	
Management of Social Roles			*Min*	
Family and Friendship Relationships			*Min–Mod* *May receive positive feed-back from family. New mobility may influence family dynamics (i.e., new safety considerations).*	

Sociocultural and Spiritual Component Analysis, continued

	Infants	Children		Adults
			Riding a tricycle	
Friendships			*Mod* Potentially provide sibling or peer play and bonding opportunity.	
Spiritual Component (sense of Pleasure or Purpose)			*Min–Max* Success may influence depending on volition and cultural significance of activity.	
Inner Motivation (sense of hopefulness or apathy)			*Min–Mod* Dependent on individual and his or her sociocultural traditions and environment.	
Feelings of Power and Helplessness			*Min–Mod* Dependent on individual and his or her history of personal play success and pressure from the sociocultural environment.	

APPENDIX E: UNIFORM TERMINOLOGY FOR OCCUPATIONAL THERAPY — THIRD EDITION

This is an official document of The American Occupational Therapy Association. This document is intended to provide a generic outline of the domain of concern of occupational therapy and is designed to create common terminology for the profession and to capture the essence of occupational therapy succinctly for others.

It is recognized that the phenomena that constitute the profession's domain of concern can be categorized, and labeled, in a number of different ways. This document is not meant to limit those in the field, formulating theories or frames of reference, who may wish to combine or refine particular constructs. It is also not meant to limit those who would like to conceptualize the profession's domain of concern in a different manner.

Introduction

The first edition of Uniform Terminology was approved and published in 1979 (AOTA, 1979). In 1989, *Uniform Terminology for Occupational Therapy—Second Edition* (AOTA, 1989) was approved and published. The second document presented an organized structure for understanding the areas of practice for the profession of occupational therapy. The document outlined two domains. **Performance areas** (activities of daily living [ADL], work and productive activities, and play or leisure) include activities that the occupational therapy practitioner emphasizes when determining functional abilities (**occupational therapy practitioner** refers to both registered occupational therapists and certified occupational therapy assistants). **Performance components** (sensorimotor, cognitive, psychosocial, and psychological aspects) are the elements of performance that occupational therapists assess and, when needed, in which they intervene for improved performance.

This third edition has been further expanded to reflect current practice and to incorporate contextual aspects of performance. **Performance areas, performance components,** and **performance contexts** are the parameters of occupational therapy's domain of concern. **Performance areas** are broad categories of human activity that are typically part of daily life. They are activities of daily living, work and productive activities, and play or leisure activities. **Performance components** are fundamental human abilities that—to varying degrees and in differing combinations—are required for suc- cessful engagement in performance areas. These components are sensorimotor, cognitive, psychosocial, and psychological. **Performance contexts** are situations or factors that influence an individual's engagement in desired and/or required performance areas.

Performance contexts consist of **temporal** aspects (chronological age, developmental age, place in the life cycle, and health status) and **environmental** aspects (physical, social, and cultural considerations). There is an interactive relationship among performance areas, performance components, and performance contexts. Function in performance areas is the ultimate concern of occupational therapy, with performance components considered as they relate to participation in performance areas. Performance areas and performance components are always viewed within performance contexts. Performance contexts are taken into consideration when determining function and dysfunction relative to performance areas and performance components, and in planning intervention. For example, the occupational therapist does not evaluate strength (a performance component) in isolation. Strength is considered as it affects necessary or desired tasks (performance areas). If the individual is interested in homemaking, the occupational therapy practitioner would consider the interaction of strength with homemaking tasks. Strengthening could be addressed through kitchen activities, such as cooking and putting groceries away. In some cases, the practitioner would employ an adaptive approach and recommend that the family switch from heavy stoneware to lighter-weight dishes, or use lighter-weight pots on the stove to enable the individual to make dinner safely without becoming fatigued or compromising safety.

Occupational therapy assessment involves examining performance areas, performance components, and performance contexts. Intervention may be directed toward elements of performance areas (e.g., dressing, vocational exploration), performance components (e.g., endurance, problem solving), or the environmental aspects of performance contexts. In the latter case, the physical and/or social environment may be altered or augmented to improve and/or maintain function. After identifying the performance areas the individual wishes or needs to address, the occupational therapist assesses the features of the environments in which the tasks will be performed. If an individual's job requires cooking in a restaurant as opposed to leisure cooking at home, the occupational therapy practitioner faces several challenges to enable the individual's success in different environments. Therefore, the third critical aspect of performance is the performance context, the features of the environment that affect the person's ability to engage in functional activities.

This document categorizes specific activities in each of the performance areas (ADL, work and productive activities, play or leisure). This categorization is based on what is considered "typical," and is not meant to imply that a particular individual characterizes personal activities in the same manner as someone else. Occupational therapy practitioners

embrace individual differences, and so would document the unique pattern of the individual being served, rather than forcing the "typical" pattern on him or her and family. For example, because of experience or culture, a particular individual might think of home management as an ADL task rather than "work and productive activities" (current listing). Socialization might be considered part of a play or leisure activity instead of its current listing as part of "activities of daily living," because of life experience or cultural heritage.

Examples of Use in Practice

Uniform Terminology—Third Edition defines occupational therapy's domain of concern, which includes performance areas, performance components, and performance contexts. While this document may be used by occupational therapy practitioners in a number of different areas (e.g., practice, documentation, charge systems, education, program development, marketing, research, disability classifications, and regulations), it focuses on the use of uniform terminology in practice. This document is not intended to define specific occupational therapy programs or specific occupational therapy interventions. Examples of how performance areas, performance components, and performance contexts translate into practice are provided below.

• An individual who is injured on the job may have the potential to return to work and productive activities, which is a performance area. In order to achieve the outcome of returning to work and productive activities, the individual may need to address specific performance components, such as strength, endurance, soft tissue integrity, time management, and the physical features of performance contexts, like structures and objects in his or her environment. The occupational therapy practitioner, in collaboration with the individual and other members of the vocational team, uses planned interventions to achieve the desired outcome. These interventions may include activities such as an exercise program, body mechanics instruction, and job site modifications, all of which may be provided in a work-hardening program.

- An elderly individual recovering from a cerebrovascular accident may wish to live in a community setting, which combines the performance areas of ADL with work and productive activities. In order to achieve the outcome of community living, the individual may need to address specific performance components, such as muscle tone, gross motor coordination, postural control, and self-management. It is also necessary to consider the sociocultural and physical features of performance contexts, such as support available from other persons, and adaptations of structures and objects within the environment. The occupational therapy practitioner, in cooperation with the team, utilizes planned interventions to achieve the desired outcome. Interventions may include neuromuscular facilitation, practice of object manipulation, and instruction in the use of adaptive equipment and home safety equipment. The practitioner and individual also pursue the selection and training of a personal assistant to ensure the completion of ADL tasks. These interventions may be provided in a comprehensive inpatient rehabilitation unit.

- A child with learning disabilities is required to perform educational activities within a public school setting. Engaging in educational activities is considered the performance area of work and productive activities for this child. To achieve the educational outcome of efficient and effective completion of written classroom work, the child may need to address specific performance components. These include sensory processing, perceptual skills, postural control, motor skills, and the physical features of performance contexts, such as objects (e.g., desk, chair) in the environment. In cooperation with the team, occupational therapy interventions may include activities like adapting the student's seating in the classroom to improve postural control and stability, and practicing motor control and coordination. This program could be developed by an occupational therapist and supported by school district personnel.

- The parents of an infant with cerebral palsy may ask to facilitate the child's involvement in the performance areas of activities of daily living and play. Subsequent to assessment, the therapist identifies specific performance components, such as sensory awareness and neuromuscular control. The practitioner also addresses the physical and cultural features of performance contexts. In collaboration with the parents, occupational therapy interventions may include activities such as seating and positioning for play, neuromuscular facilitation techniques to enable eating, facilitating parent skills in caring for and playing with their infant, and modifying the play space for accessibility. These interventions may be provided in a home-based occupational therapy program.

- An adult with schizophrenia may need and want to live independently in the community, which represents the performance areas of activities of daily living, work and productive activities, and leisure activities. The specific performance categories may be medication routine, functional mobility, home management, vocational exploration, play or leisure performance, and social interaction. In order to achieve the outcome of living independently, the individual may need to address specific performance components, such as topographical orientation; memory; categorization; problem solving; interests; social conduct; time management; and sociocultural features of performance contexts, such as social factors (e.g., influence of family and friends) and roles. The occupational therapy practitioner, in cooperation with the team, utilizes planned interventions to achieve the desired outcome. Interventions may include activities such as training in the use of public transportation, instruction in budgeting skills, selection and participation in social activities, instruction in social conduct, and participation in community reintegration activities. These interventions may be provided in a community-based mental health program.

• An individual with a history of substance abuse may need to reestablish family roles and responsibilities, which represent the performance areas of activities of daily living, work and productive activities, and leisure activities. In order to achieve the outcome of family participation, the individual may need to address the performance components of roles; values; social conduct; self-expression; coping skills; self-control; and the sociocultural features of performance contexts, such as custom, behavior, rules, and rituals. The occupational therapy practitioner, in cooperation with the team, utilizes planned interventions to achieve the desired outcomes. Interventions may include roles and values exercises, instruction in stress management techniques, identification of family roles and activities, and support to develop

family leisure routines. These interventions may be provided in an inpatient acute care unit.

Person–Activity–Environment Fit

Person–activity–environment fit refers to the match among the skills and abilities of the individual; the demands of the activity; and the characteristics of the physical, social, and cultural environments. It is the interaction among the performance areas, performance components, and performance contexts that is important and determines the success of the performance. When occupational therapy practitioners provide services, they attend to all of these aspects of performance and the interaction among them. They also attend to each individual's unique personal history. The personal history includes one's skills and abilities (performance components), the past performance of specific life tasks (performance areas), and experience within particular environments (performance contexts). In addition to personal history, anticipated life tasks and role demands influence performance.

When considering the person–activity–environment fit, variables such as novelty, importance, motivation, activity tolerance, and quality are salient. Situations range from those that are completely familiar to those that are novel and have never been experienced. Both the novelty and familiarity within a situation contribute to the overall task performance. In each situation, there is an optimal level of novelty that engages the individual sufficiently and provides enough information to perform the task. When too little novelty is present, the individual may miss cues and opportunities to perform. When too much novelty is present, the individual may become confused and distracted, inhibiting effective task performance.

Humans determine that some stimuli and situations are more meaningful than others. Individuals perform tasks they deem important. It is critical to identify what the individual wants or needs to do when planning interventions.

The level of motivation an individual demonstrates to perform a particular task is determined by both internal and external factors. An individual's biobehavioral state (e.g., amount of rest, arousal, tension) contributes to the potential to be responsive. The features of the social and physical environments (e.g., persons in the room, noise level) provide information that is either adequate or inadequate to produce a motivated state.

Activity tolerance is the individual's ability to sustain a purposeful activity over time. Individuals must not only select, initiate, and terminate activities, but they must also attend to a task for the needed length of time to complete the task and accomplish their goals.

The quality of performance is measured by standards generated by both the individual and others in the social and cultural environments in which the performance occurs. Quality is a continuum of expectations set within particular activities and contexts (see Figure 1).

Figure 1. Uniform Terminology for Occupational Therapy

UNIFORM TERMINOLOGY FOR OCCUPATIONAL THERAPY
THIRD EDITION OUTLINE

I. Performance Areas

A. Activities of Daily Living
  1. Grooming
  2. Oral Hygiene
  3. Bathing/Showering
  4. Toilet Hygiene
  5. Personal Device Care
  6. Dressing
  7. Feeding and Eating
  8. Medication Routine
  9. Health Maintenance
  10. Socialization
  11. Functional Communication
  12. Functional Mobility
  13. Community Mobility
  14. Emergency Response
  15. Sexual Expression
B. Work and Productive Activities
  1. Home Management
    a. Clothing Care
    b. Cleaning
    c. Meal Preparation/Cleanup
    d. Shopping
    e. Money Management
    f. Household Maintenance
    g. Safety Procedures
  2. Care of Others
  3. Educational Activities
  4. Vocational Activities
    a. Vocational Exploration
    b. Job Acquisition
    c. Work or Job Performance
    d. Retirement Planning
    e. Volunteer Participation
C. Play or Leisure Activities
  1. Play/Leisure Exploration
  2. Play/Leisure Performance

II. Performance Components

A. Sensorimotor Component
  1. Sensory
    a. Sensory Awareness
    b. Sensory Processing
      (1) Tactile
      (2) Proprioceptive
      (3) Vestibular
      (4) Visual
      (5) Auditory
      (6) Gustatory
      (7) Olfactory
    c. Perceptual Processing
      (1) Stereognosis
      (2) Kinesthesia
      (3) Pain Response
      (4) Body Scheme
      (5) Right-Left Discrimination
      (6) Form Constancy
      (7) Position in Space
      (8) Visual-Closure
      (9) Figure Ground
      (10) Depth Perception
      (11) Spatial Relations
      (12) Topographical Orientation
  2. Neuromusculoskeletal
    a. Reflex
    b. Range of Motion
    c. Muscle Tone
    d. Strength
    e. Endurance
    f. Postural Control
    g. Postural Alignment
    h. Soft Tissue Integrity
  3. Motor
    a. Gross Coordination
    b. Crossing the Midline
    c. Laterality
    d. Bilateral Integration
    e. Motor Control
    f. Praxis
    g. Fine Coordination/Dexterity
    h. Visual-Motor Integration
    i. Oral-Motor Control
B. Cognitive Integration and Cognitive Components
  1. Level of Arousal
  2. Orientation
  3. Recognition
  4. Attention Span
  5. Initiation of Activity
  6. Termination of Activity
  7. Memory
  8. Sequencing
  9. Categorization
  10. Concept Formation
  11. Spatial Operations
  12. Problem Solving
  13. Learning
  14. Generalization
C. Psychosocial Skills and Psychological Components
  1. Psychological
    a. Values
    b. Interests
    c. Self-Concept
  2. Social
    a. Role Performance
    b. Social Conduct
    c. Interpersonal Skills
    d. Self-Expression
  3. Self-Management
    a. Coping Skills
    b. Time Management
    c. Self-Control

III. Performance Contexts

A. Temporal Aspects
  1. Chronological
  2. Developmental
  3. Life Cycle
  4. Disability Status
B. Environmental Aspects
  1. Physical
  2. Social
  3. Cultural

Uniform Terminology for Occupational Therapy—Third Edition

Occupational therapy is the use of purposeful activity or interventions to promote health and achieve functional outcomes. **Achieving functional outcomes** means to develop, improve, or restore the highest possible level of independence of any individual who is limited by a physical injury or illness, a dysfunctional condition, a cognitive impairment, a psychosocial dysfunction, a mental illness, a developmental or learning disability, or an adverse environmental condition. **Assessment** means the use of skilled observation or evaluation by the administration and interpretation of standardized or nonstandardized tests and measurements to identify areas for occupational therapy services.

Occupational therapy services include, but are not limited to

1. the assessment, treatment, and education of or consultation with the individual, family, or other persons; or
2. interventions directed toward developing, improving, or restoring daily living skills, work readiness or work performance, play skills or leisure capacities, or enhancing educational performance skills;
3. providing for the development, improvement, or restoration of sensorimotor, oral-motor, perceptual or neuromuscular functioning; or emotional, motivational, cognitive, or psychosocial components of performance.

These services may require assessment of the need for and use of interventions such as the design, development, adaptation, application, or training in the use of assistive technology devices; the design, fabrication, or application of rehabilitative technology such as selected orthotic devices; training in the use of assistive technology, orthotic or prosthetic devices; the application of physical agent modalities as an adjunct to or in preparation for purposeful activity; the use of ergonomic principles; the adaptation of environments and processes to enhance functional performance; or the promotion of health and wellness (AOTA, 1993, p. 1117).

I. Performance Areas

Throughout this document, activities have been described as if individuals performed the tasks themselves. Occupational therapy also recognizes that individuals arrange for tasks to be done through others. The profession views independence as the ability to self-determine activity performance, regardless of who actually performs the activity.

A. Activities of Daily Living—
Self-maintenance tasks.

1. Grooming—Obtaining and using supplies; removing body hair (use of razors, tweezers, lotions, etc.); applying and removing cosmetics; washing, drying, combing, styling, and brushing hair; caring for nails (hands and feet), caring for skin, ears, and eyes; and applying deodorant.

2. Oral Hygiene—Obtaining and using supplies; cleaning mouth; brushing and flossing teeth; or removing, cleaning, and reinserting dental orthotics and prosthetics.

3. Bathing/Showering—Obtaining and using supplies; soaping, rinsing, and drying body parts; maintaining bathing position; and transferring to and from bathing positions.

4. Toilet Hygiene—Obtaining and using supplies; clothing management; maintaining toileting position; transferring to and from toileting position; cleaning body; and caring for menstrual and continence needs (including catheters, colostomies, and suppository management).

5. *Personal Device Care*—Cleaning and maintaining personal care items, such as hearing aids, contact lenses, glasses, orthotics, prosthetics, adaptive equipment, and contraceptive and sexual devices.

6. *Dressing*—Selecting clothing and accessories appropriate to time of day, weather, and occasion; obtaining clothing from storage area; dressing and undressing in a sequential fashion; fastening and adjusting clothing and shoes; and applying and removing personal devices, prostheses, or orthoses.

7. *Feeding and Eating*—Setting up food; selecting and using appropriate utensils and tableware; bringing food or drink to mouth; cleaning face, hands, and clothing; sucking, masticating, coughing, and swallowing; and management of alternative methods of nourishment.

8. *Medication Routine*—Obtaining medication, opening and closing containers, following prescribed schedules, taking correct quantities, reporting problems and adverse effects, and administering correct quantities by using prescribed methods.

9. *Health Maintenance*—Developing and maintaining routines for illness prevention and wellness promotion, such as physical fitness, nutrition, and decreasing health risk behaviors.

10. *Socialization*—Accessing opportunities and interacting with other people in appropriate contextual and cultural ways to meet emotional and physical needs.

11. *Functional Communication*—Using equipment or systems to send and receive information, such as writing equipment, telephones, typewriters, computers, communication boards, call lights, emergency systems, Braille writers, telecommunication devices for the deaf, and augmentative communication systems.

12. *Functional Mobility*—Moving from one position or place to another, such as in-bed mobility, wheelchair mobility, transfers (wheelchair, bed, car, tub, toilet, tub/shower, chair, floor). Performing functional ambulation and transporting objects.

13. *Community Mobility*—Moving self in the community and using public or private transportation, such as driving, or accessing buses, taxi cabs, or other public transportation systems.

14. *Emergency Response*—Recognizing sudden, unexpected hazardous situations, and initiating action to reduce the threat to health and safety.

15. *Sexual Expression*—Engaging in desired sexual and intimate activities.

B. Work and Productive Activities—*Purposeful activities for self-development, social contribution, and livelihood.*

1. *Home Management*—Obtaining and maintaining personal and household possessions and environment.

   a. *Clothing Care*—Obtaining and using supplies; sorting, laundering (hand, machine, and dry clean); folding; ironing; storing; and mending.

   b. *Cleaning*—Obtaining and using supplies; picking up; putting away; vacuuming; sweeping and mopping floors; dusting; polishing; scrubbing; washing windows; cleaning mirrors; making beds; and removing trash and recyclables.

   c. *Meal Preparation and Cleanup*—Planning nutritious meals; preparing and serving food;

opening and closing containers, cabinets and drawers; using kitchen utensils and appliances; cleaning up and storing food safely.

d. *Shopping*—Preparing shopping lists (grocery and other); selecting and purchasing items; selecting method of payment; and completing money transactions.

e. *Money Management*—Budgeting, paying bills, and using bank systems.

f. *Household Maintenance*—Maintaining home, yard, garden, appliances, vehicles, and household items.

g. *Safety Procedures*—Knowing and performing preventive and emergency procedures to maintain a safe environment and to prevent injuries.

2. Care of Others—Providing for children, spouse, parents, pets, or others, such as giving physical care, nurturing, communicating, and using age-appropriate activities.

3. Educational Activities—Participating in a learning environment through school, community, or work-sponsored activities, such as exploring educational interests, attending to instruction, managing assignments, and contributing to group experiences.

4. Vocational Activities—Participating in work-related activities.

a. *Vocational Exploration*—Determining aptitudes; developing interests and skills, and selecting appropriate vocational pursuits.

b. *Job Acquisition*—Identifying and selecting work opportunities, and completing application and interview processes.

c. *Work or Job Performance*—Performing job tasks in a timely and effective manner; incorporating necessary work behaviors.

d. *Retirement Planning*—Determining aptitudes; developing interests and skills; and selecting

appropriate avocational pursuits.

e. *Volunteer Participation*—Performing unpaid activities for the benefit of selected individuals, groups, or causes.

C. Play or Leisure Activities—*Intrinsically motivating activities for amusement, relaxation, spontaneous enjoyment, or self-expression.*

1. Play or Leisure Exploration—Identifying interests, skills, opportunities, and appropriate play or leisure activities.

2. Play or Leisure Performance—Planning and participating in play or leisure activities. Maintaining a balance of play or leisure activities with work and productive activities, and activities of daily living. Obtaining, utilizing, and maintaining equipment and supplies.

II. Performance Components

A. Sensorimotor Component—
The ability to receive input, process information, and produce output.

1. Sensory

a. *Sensory Awareness*—Receiving and differentiating sensory stimuli.

b. *Sensory Processing*—Interpreting sensory stimuli:

(1) *Tactile*—Interpreting light touch, pressure, temperature, pain, and vibration through skin contact/receptors.

(2) *Proprioceptive*—Interpreting stimuli originating in muscles, joints, and other internal tissues that give information about the position of one body part in relation to another.

(3) *Vestibular*—Interpreting stimuli from the inner ear receptors regarding head position and movement.

(4) *Visual*—Interpreting stimuli through the eyes, including peripheral vision and acuity,

and awareness of color and pattern.

(5) *Auditory*—Interpreting and localizing sounds, and discriminating background sounds.

(6) *Gustatory*—Interpreting tastes.

(7) *Olfactory*—Interpreting odors.

c. *Perceptual Processing*—Organizing sensory input into meaningful patterns.

(1) *Stereognosis*—Identifying objects through proprioception, cognition, and the sense of touch.

(2) *Kinesthesia*—Identifying the excursion and direction of joint movement.

(3) *Pain Response*—Interpreting noxious stimuli.

(4) *Body Scheme*—Acquiring an internal awareness of the body and the relationship of body parts to each other.

(5) *Right–Left Discrimination*—Differentiating one side from the other.

(6) *Form Constancy*—Recognizing forms and objects as the same in various environments, positions, and sizes.

(7) *Position in Space*—Determining the spatial relationship of figures and objects to self or other forms and objects.

(8) *Visual-Closure*—Identifying forms or objects from incomplete presentations.

(9) *Figure Ground*—Differentiating between foreground and background forms and objects.

(10) *Depth Perception*—Determining the relative distance between objects, figures, or landmarks and the observer, and changes in planes of surfaces.

(11) *Spatial Relations*—Determining the position of objects relative to each other.

(12) *Topographical Orientation*—Determining the location of objects and settings and the route to the location.

2. Neuromusculoskeletal

a. *Reflex*—Eliciting an involuntary muscle response by sensory input.

b. *Range of Motion*—Moving body parts through an arc.

c. *Muscle Tone*—Demonstrating a degree of tension or resistance in a muscle at rest and in response to stretch.

d. *Strength*—Demonstrating a degree of muscle power when movement is resisted, as with objects or gravity.

e. *Endurance*—Sustaining cardiac, pulmonary, and musculoskeletal exertion over time.

f. *Postural Control*—Using righting and equilibrium adjustments to maintain balance during functional movements.

g. *Postural Alignment*—Maintaining biomechanical integrity among body parts.

h. *Soft Tissue Integrity*—Maintaining anatomical and physiological condition of interstitial tissue and skin.

3. Motor

a. *Gross Coordination*—Using large muscle groups for controlled, goal-directed movements.

b. *Crossing the Midline*—Moving limbs and eyes across the midsagittal plane of the body.

c. *Laterality*—Using a preferred unilateral body part for activities requiring a high level of skill.

d. *Bilateral Integration*—Coordinating both body sides during activity.

e. *Motor Control*—Using the body in functional and versatile movement patterns.

f. *Praxis*—Conceiving and planning a new motor act in response to an environmental demand.

g. *Fine Coordination/Dexterity*—Using small muscle groups for controlled movements, particularly in object manipulation.

h. *Visual-Motor Integration*—Coordinating the interaction of information from the eyes with body movement during activity.

i. Oral-Motor Control—Coordinating oropharyngeal musculature for controlled movements.

B. Cognitive Integration and Cognitive Components—*The ability to use higher brain functions.*

1. **Level of Arousal**—Demonstrating alertness and responsiveness to environmental stimuli.

2. **Orientation**—Identifying person, place, time, and situation.

3. **Recognition**—Identifying familiar faces, objects, and other previously presented materials.

4. **Attention Span**—Focusing on a task over time.

5. **Initiation of Activity**—Starting a physical or mental activity.

6. **Termination of Activity**—Stopping an activity at an appropriate time.

7. **Memory**—Recalling information after brief or long periods of time.

8. **Sequencing**—Placing information, concepts, and actions in order.

9. **Categorization**—Identifying similarities of and differences among pieces of environmental information.

10. **Concept Formation**—Organizing a variety of information to form thoughts and ideas.

11. **Spatial Operations**—Mentally manipulating the position of objects in various relationships.

12. **Problem Solving**—Recognizing a problem, defining a problem, identifying alternative plans, selecting a plan, organizing steps in a plan, implementing a plan, and evaluating the outcome.

13. **Learning**—Acquiring new concepts and

14. **Generalization**—Applying previously learned concepts and behaviors to a variety of new situations.

C. Psychosocial Skills and Psychological Components—*The ability to interact in society and to process emotions.*

1. **Psychological**
   a. *Values*—Identifying ideas or beliefs that are important to self and others.
   b. *Interests*—Identifying mental or physical activities that create pleasure and maintain attention.
   c. *Self-Concept*—Developing the value of the physical, emotional, and sexual self.

2. **Social**
   a. *Role Performance*—Identifying, maintaining, and balancing functions one assumes or acquires in society (e.g., worker, student, parent, friend, religious participant).
   b. *Social Conduct*—Interacting by using manners, personal space, eye contact, gestures, active listening, and self-expression appropriate to one's environment.
   c. *Interpersonal Skills*—Using verbal and nonverbal communication to interact in a variety of settings.
   d. *Self-Expression*—Using a variety of styles and skills to express thoughts, feelings, and needs.

3. **Self-Management**
   a. *Coping Skills*—Identifying and managing stress and related factors.
   b. *Time Management*—Planning and participating in a balance of self-care, work, leisure, and rest activities to promote satisfaction and health.
   c. *Self-Control*—Modifying one's own behavior in response to environmental needs, demands, constraints, personal aspirations, and feedback from others.

III. Performance Contexts

Assessment of function in performance areas is greatly influenced by the contexts in which the individual must perform. Occupational therapy practitioners consider performance contexts when determining feasibility and appropriateness of interventions. Occupational therapy practitioners may choose interventions based on an understanding of contexts, or may choose interventions directly aimed at altering the contexts to improve performance.

A. Temporal Aspects

1. **Chronological**—Individual's age.

2. **Developmental**—Stage or phase of maturation.

3. **Lifecycle**—Place in important life phases, such as career cycle, parenting cycle, or educational process.

4. **Disability status**—Place in continuum of disability, such as acuteness of injury, chronicity of disability, or terminal nature of illness.

B. Environment

1. **Physical**—Nonhuman aspects of contexts. Includes the accessibility to and performance within environments having natural terrain, plants, animals, buildings, furniture, objects, tools, or devices.

2. **Social**—Availability and expectations of significant individuals, such as spouse, friends, and caregivers. Also includes larger social groups which are influential in establishing norms, role expectations, and social routines.

3. **Cultural**—Customs, beliefs, activity patterns, behavior standards, and expectations accepted by the society of which the individual is a member. Includes political aspects, such as laws that affect access to resources and affirm personal rights. Also includes opportunities for education, employment, and economic support.

References

American Occupational Therapy Association. (1979). *Occupational therapy product output reporting system and uniform terminology for reporting occupational therapy services.* Bethesda, MD: Author.

American Occupational Therapy Association. (1989). Uniform terminology for occupational therapy—Second edition. *American Journal of Occupational Therapy, 43,* 808–815.

American Occupational Therapy Association. (1993). Association policies—Definition of occupational therapy practice for state regulation (Policy 5.3.1). *American Journal of Occupational Therapy, 47,* 1117–1121.

Prepared by

The Terminology Task Force
Winifred Dunn, PhD, OTR, FAOTA
Chairperson; Mary Foto, OTR, FAOTA
Jim Hinojosa, PhD, OTR, FAOTA
Barbara Schell, PhD, OTR/L, FAOTA
Linda Kohlman Thomson, MOT, OTR, FAOTA
Sarah D. Hertfelder, MEd, MOT, OTR/L, Staff
Liaison for Commission on Practice
Jim Hinojosa, PhD, OTR, FAOTA, Chairperson

Adopted by the Representative Assembly July 1994

This document replaces the following documents, all of which were rescinded by the 1994 Representative Assembly: *Occupational Therapy Product Output Reporting System* (1979), *Uniform Terminology for Reporting Occupational Therapy Services—First Edition* (1979), "Uniform Occupational Therapy Evaluation Checklist" (1981, *American Journal of Occupational Therapy, 35,* 817–818), and "Uniform Terminology for Occupational Therapy—Second Edition" (1989, *American Journal of Occupational Therapy, 43,* 808–815).

Appendix F: Uniform Terminology— Third Edition: Application to Practice

Introduction

This document was developed to help occupational therapists apply *Uniform Terminology—Third Edition* to practice. The original grid format (Dunn, 1988) enabled occupational therapy practitioners to systematically identify deficit and strength areas of an individual and to select appropriate activities to address these areas in occupational therapy intervention (Dunn & McGourty, 1990). For the third edition, the profession is highlighting **contexts** as another critical aspect of performance. A second grid provides therapy practitioners with a mechanism to consider the contextual features of performance in activities of daily living (ADL), work and productive activity, and play or leisure. **Performance Areas** and **Performance Components** (see Figure A) focus on the individual. These features are imbedded in the **Performance Contexts** (see Figure B).

On the original grid (Dunn, 1988), the horizontal axis contains the Performance Areas of Activities of Daily Living, Work and Productive Activities, and Play or Leisure Activities (see Figure A). These Performance Areas are the functional outcomes that occupational therapy addresses. The vertical axis contains the Performance Components, including Sensorimotor Components, Cognitive Components, and Psychosocial Components. The Performance Components are the skills and abilities that an individual uses to engage in the Performance Areas. During an occupational therapy assessment, the occupational therapy practitioner determines an individual's abilities and limitations in the Performance Components and how they affect the individual's functional outcomes in the Performance Areas.

The first application document (Dunn & McGourty, 1989) described how to use the original Uniform Terminology grid with a variety of individuals. It is quite useful to introduce these concepts. However, the third edition of *Uniform Terminology* contains some changes in the Performance Areas and Performance Components lists. Be sure to check for the terminology currently approved in the third edition before applying this information in current practice environments.

With the addition of Performance Contexts into *Uniform Terminology*, occupational therapy practitioners must consider how to interface what the individual wants to do (i.e., performance area) with the contextual features that may support or block performance. Figure B illustrates the interaction of Performance Areas and Performance Contexts as a model for therapists' planning.

The grid in Figure B can be used to analyze the contexts of performance for a particular individual. For example, when working with a toddler with a developmental disability who needs to learn to eat, the occupational therapy practitioner would consider all the Performance Contexts features as they might affect this toddler's ability to master eating. Unlike the grid in Figure A, in which the occupational therapy practitioner selects both Performance Areas (i.e., what the individual wants or needs to do) and the Performance Component (i.e., a person's strengths and needs), in this grid (Figure B) the occupational therapy practitioner only selects the Performance Area. After the Performance Area is identified through collaboration with the individual and significant others, the occupational therapy practitioner considers *all* Performance Contexts features as they might affect performance of the selected task.

Figure A. Uniform Terminology Grid (Performance Areas and Performance Components)

PERFORMANCE COMPONENTS	PERFORMANCE AREAS																						
	Activities of Daily Living	Grooming	Oral Hygiene	Bathing/Showering	Toilet Hygiene	Personal Device Care	Dressing	Feeding and Eating	Medication Routine	Health Maintenance	Socialization	Functional Communication	Functional Mobility	Community Mobility	Emergency Response	Sexual Expression	Work and Productive Activities	Home Management	Care of Others	Educational Activities	Vocational Activities	Play or Leisure Activities	Play/Leisure Exploration	Play/Leisure Performance

A. Sensorimotor Component

Sensory
  Sensory Awareness
  Sensory Processing
    (1) Tactile
    (2) Proprioceptive
    (3) Vestibular
    (4) Visual
    (5) Auditory
    (6) Gustatory
    (7) Olfactory
  Perceptual Processing
    (1) Stereognosis
    (2) Kinesthesia
    (3) Pain Response
    (4) Body Scheme
    (5) Right-Left Discrimination
    (6) Form Constancy
    (7) Position in Space
    (8) Visual-Closure
    (9) Figure Ground
    (10) Depth Perception
    (11) Spatial Relations
    (12) Topographical Orientation
Neuromusculoskeletal
  Reflex
  Range of Motion
  Muscle Tone
  Strength
  Endurance
  Postural Control
  Postural Alignment
  Soft Tissue Integrity
Motor
  Gross Coordination
  Crossing the Midline
  Laterality
  Bilateral Integration
  Motor Control
  Praxis
  Fine Coordination/Dexterity
  Visual-Motor Integration
  Oral-Motor Control

Figure A. Uniform Terminology Grid (Performance Areas and Performance Components) (continued)

PERFORMANCE AREAS

Performance Areas (columns): Activities of Daily Living, Grooming, Oral Hygiene, Bathing/Showering, Toilet Hygiene, Personal Device Care, Dressing, Feeding and Eating, Medication Routine, Health Maintenance, Socialization, Functional Communication, Functional Mobility, Community Mobility, Emergency Response, Sexual Expression, Work and Productive Activities, Home Management, Care of Others, Educational Activities, Vocational Activities, Play or Leisure Activities, Play/Leisure Exploration, Play/Leisure Performance

PERFORMANCE COMPONENTS

B. Cognitive Integration and Cognitive Components

1. Level of Arousal
2. Orientation
3. Recognition
4. Attention Span
5. Initiation of Activity
6. Termination of Activity
7. Memory
8. Sequencing
9. Categorization
10. Concept Formation
11. Spatial Operations
12. Problem Solving
13. Learning
14. Generalization

C. Psychosocial Skills and Psychological Components

1. Psychological
   a. Values
   b. Interests
   c. Self-Concept
2. Social
   a. Role Performance
   b. Social Conduct
   c. Interpersonal Skills
   d. Self-Expression
3. Self-Management
   a. Coping Skills
   b. Time Management
   c. Self-Control

Figure B. Uniform Terminology Grid (Performance Areas and Performance Contexts)

PERFORMANCE AREAS

Performance Areas (columns):
- Activities of Daily Living
- Grooming
- Oral Hygiene
- Bathing/Showering
- Toilet Hygiene
- Personal Device Care
- Dressing
- Feeding and Eating
- Medication Routine
- Health Maintenance
- Socialization
- Functional Communication
- Functional Mobility
- Community Mobility
- Emergency Response
- Sexual Expression
- Work and Productive Activities
- Home Management
- Care of Others
- Educational Activities
- Vocational Activities
- Play or Leisure Activities
- Play/Leisure Exploration
- Play/Leisure Performance

PERFORMANCE CONTEXTS

A. Temporal Aspects
- Chronological
- Developmental
- Life Cycle
- Disability Status

B. Environment
- Physical
- Social
- Cultural

Intervention Planning

Intervention planning occurs both within the general domain of concern of occupational therapy (i.e., uniform terminology) and by considering the profession's theoretical frames of reference that offer insights about how to approach the problem. In Figure A, the occupational therapy practitioner considers the Performance Areas that are of interest to the individual and the individual's strengths and concerns within the Performance Components. The intervention strategies would emerge from the cells on the grid that are placed at the intersection of the Performance Areas and the targeted Performance Components (strength and/or concern). For example, if a child needed to improve sensory processing and fine coordination for oral hygiene and grooming, an occupational therapy practitioner might select a sensory integrative frame of reference to create intervention strategies, such as adding textures to handles and teaching the child sand and bean digging games. Dunn and McGourty (1989) discuss this in more detail.

When using Figure B, the occupational therapy practitioner considers the Performance Contexts features in relation to the desired Performance Area. The occupational therapy practitioner would analyze the individual's temporal, physical, social, and cultural contexts to determine the relevance of particular interventions. For example, if the child mentioned above was a member of a family in which having messy hands from sand play was unacceptable, the occupational therapy practitioner would consider alternate strategies that are more compatible with their life-style. For example, perhaps the family would be more interested in developing puppet play. This would still provide the child with opportunities to experience the textures of various puppets and the hand movements required to manipulate the puppets in play context, without adding the messiness of sand. When occupational therapy practitioners consider contexts, interventions become more relevant and applicable to individual's lives.

Case Example 1

Sophie is a 75-year-old woman who was widowed 3 years ago, is recovering from a cerebrovascular accident (CVA), and has been transferred from an acute care unit to an inpatient medical rehabilitation unit. Prior to her admission, she was living in a small house in an isolated location and has no family living nearby. She was driving independently and frequently ran errands for her friends. She is adamant in her goal to return to her home after discharge. All of her friends are quite elderly and are not able to provide many resources for support.

Sophie and the team collaborated to identify her goals. Sophie decided that she wanted to be able to meet her daily needs with little or no assistance. Almost all of the Performance Areas are critical in order to achieve the outcome of community living in her own home. Being able to cook all of her meals, bathe independently, and have alternative transportation available is necessary. Because of their significant impact on the patient's function in the Performance Areas, some of the Performance Components that may need to be addressed are figure ground, muscle tone, postural control, fine coordination, memory, and self management.

In the selection of occupational therapy interventions, it is critical to analyze the elements of Performance Contexts for the individual. The physical and social elements of her home environment do not support returning home without modifications to her home and additional social supports being established. Railings must be added to the front steps, and provision of and instruction

in the use of a tub seat and instruction in the use of specialized transportation may need to occur. If this same individual had been living in an apartment in a retirement community prior to her CVA, the contexts of performance would support a return home with fewer environmental modifications being needed. Being independent in cooking might not be necessary due to meals being provided, and the bathroom might already be accessible and safe. If the individual had friends and family available, the social support network might already be established to assist with shopping and transportation needs. The occupational therapy interventions would be different due to the contexts in which the individual will be performing. Interventions must be selected with the impact of the Performance Contexts as an essential element.

Case Example 2

Malcolm is a 9-year-old boy who has a learning disability that causes him to have a variety of problems in the school. His teachers complain that he is difficult to manage in the classroom. Some of the Performance Components that may need to be addressed are his self-control, such as interrupting, difficulty sitting during instruction, and difficulty with peer relations. Other children avoid him on the playground, because he does not follow rules, does not play fair, and tends to anger quickly when confronted. The Performance Component impairment with concept formation is reflected in his sloppy and disorganized classroom assignments.

The critical elements of the Performance Contexts are the temporal aspect of age appropriateness of his behavior and the social environmental aspect of his immature socialization. The significant cultural and temporal aspects of his family are that they place a high premium on athletic prowess.

The occupational therapy practitioner intervenes in several ways to address his behavior in the school environment. The occupational therapy practitioner focuses on structuring the classroom environment and facilitating consistent behavioral expectations for Malcolm by educational personnel. She also consults with the teachers to develop ways to structure activities that will support his ability to relate to other children in a positive way.

In contrast, another child with similar learning disabilities, but who is 12 years old and in the 7th grade might have different concerns. Elements of the Performance Contexts are the temporal aspect of the age appropriateness of his behavior and the social environmental context of school where bullying behavior is unacceptable and in which completing assignments is expected. In addressing the cultural Performance Contexts, the occupational therapy practitioner recognizes from meeting with parents that they have only average expectations for academic performance but value athletic accomplishments.

Since teachers at his school consider completion of home assignments to be part of average performance, the occupational therapy practitioner works with the child and parents on time management and reinforcement strategies to meet this expectation. After consultation with the coach, she works with the father to create activities to improve his athletic abilities. When occupational therapy practitioners consider family values as part of the contexts of performance, different intervention priorities may emerge.

Prepared by

The Terminology Task Force
Winifred Dunn, PhD, OTR, FAOTA, Chairperson
Mary Foto, OTR, FAOTA
Jim Hinojosa, PhD, OTR, FAOTA
Barbara A. Boyt Schell, PhD, OTR/L, FAOTA
Linda Kohlman Thomson, MOT, OTR, OT (C), FAOTA
Sarah D. Hertfelder, MEd, MOT, OTR/L, Staff Liaison for The Commission on Practice
Jim Hinojosa, PhD, OTR, FAOTA, Chairperson

This document replaces the 1989 document *Application of Uniform Terminology to Practice* that accompanied the "Uniform Terminology for Occupational Therapy—Second Edition" (*American Journal of Occupational Therapy, 43,* 808–815).

APPENDIX G

Occupational Performance Profile		
Occupations	**Person**	**Contexts**
Roles	Values, Interests, and Goals	Temporal
Tasks and Activities	Performance Components	Social
Activities of Daily Living	Sensorimotor Components	
Work and Productive Activities	Cognitive Integration and Cognitive Components	Cultural
Play or Leisure Activiites	Psychological and Psychosocial Components	Physical

Occupational Performance Profile–Canadian Version		
Occupations	**The Individual**	**Environment**
Roles	Goals and Priorities	Social
Tasks and Activities	Performance Components	
Self Care	Spiritual Component	
		Physical
	Physical Components	
Productive Activities		
		Cultural
	Mental Component	
Leisure		
	Sociocultural Components	Political/Economic

APPENDIX H: CLIENT GOALS FORM

Long-term goals specify the purpose or aim of intervention or a program and identify the limitations in occupational performance areas that will be addressed. These goals are developed in collaboration with the occupational therapy service consumer or others who act on their behalf. Goals define the domain (e.g., socialization) and direction (e.g., increase or decrease) of change that is expected to occur by the end of intervention.

Short-term objectives relate directly to goals and specify the impairment task or context, that must change in order to achieve the expected functional outcome. Objectives specify the direction and degree of change in measurable terms and delineate expected time frames (American Occupational Therapy Association, 1995). Objectives generally do not specify the methods that will be employed.

Client Goals
Long-Term Goal #1
Short-Term Objective #1A
Short-Term Objective #1B
Long-Term Goal #2
Short-Term Objective #2A
Short-Term Objective #2B
Long-Term Goal #3
Short-Term Objective #3A
Short-Term Objective #3B

Reference

American Occupational Therapy Association. (1995). Elements of clinical documentation (Revision). *American Journal of Occupational Therapy, 49,* 1032–1035.

APPENDIX I: POSITION PAPER: OCCUPATION

Concern with the occupational nature of human beings was fundamental to the establishment of occupational therapy. Since the time of occupational therapy's founding, the term occupation has been used to refer to an individual's active participation in self-maintenance, work, leisure, and play (AOTA, 1993; Bing, 1981; Levine, 1991; Meyer, 1922). Within the literature of the field, however, the meaning of occupation has been ambiguous because the term has been used interchangeably with other concepts. This paper's intent is to distinguish the term occupation from other terms, to summarize traditional beliefs about its nature and its therapeutic value, and to identify factors that have impeded the study and discussion of occupation.

The Dynamic, Multidimensional Nature of Occupations

Occupations are the ordinary and familiar things that people do every day. This simple description reflects, but understates, the multidimensional and complex nature of daily occupation.

Occupations can be broadly explained as having both performance and contextual dimensions because they involve acts within defined settings (Christiansen, 1991; Nelson, 1988; Rogers, 1982). In that they frequently extend over time, occupations have a temporal dimension (Kielhofner, 1977; Meyer, 1922). Further, in that engagement in occupation is seen to be driven by an intrinsic need for mastery, competence, self-identity, and group acceptance, occupations have a psychological dimension (Brown, 1986; Burke, 1977; Christiansen, 1994; DiMatteo, 1991; Fidler & Fidler, 1979, 1981; White, 1971). Since occupations are often associated with a social or occupational role and are therefore identifiable in the culture, they have social and symbolic dimensions (Mosey, 1986; Fidler & Fidler, 1983;

Frank, 1994). Finally, because they are infused with meaning within the lives of individuals, occupations have spiritual dimensions (Clark, 1993; Mattingly & Fleming, 1993). The term spiritual is used here to refer to the nonphysical and nonmaterial aspects of existence. In this sense, it is postulated that daily pursuits contribute insight into the nature and meaning of a person's life.

This multidimensional view of occupations and their central place in the experience of living was recognized early in the profession's history. Influenced by the pragmatic philosophies of John Dewey and William James (Breines, 1987) which related well-being to an individual's participation in the world around him or her, early theorists such as Tracy (1910), Dunton (1918), and Slagle (1922) contended that doing things favorably influenced interest and attention, provided relaxation, promoted moral development, reenergized the individual, normalized habits, and conferred a physical benefit (Upham, 1918). Adolph Meyer (1922) asserted that, for healthy people, daily living unfolds in a natural and balanced pattern of occupational pursuits that bring both satisfaction and fulfillment. He noted that occupations have a performance or doing component, as well as a spiritual or personal meaning component. Meyer recognized that through daily occupations, people organized their lives in terms of time and made meaning of their existence as human beings. Meyer believed that the organizing, self-fulfilling characteristics of occupations could make them an important mechanism of adaptation. He postulated that the individual could affect his or her state of health through occupations selected and performed each day. This view has been a principle of many conceptual frames of reference developed by occupational therapy scholars since that time (Christiansen, 1991; Kielhofner, 1993; Reilly, 1962).

In summary, occupational therapy scholars agree that human occupations have emotional, cognitive, physical, spiritual, and contextual dimensions, all of which are related to general well-being. However, occupational therapy scholars have not been able to agree on the specific concepts regarding these dimensions, or on specific terms to name them.

Distinguishing Between Occupation and Related Terms

The physical and mental abilities and skills required for satisfactory engagement in a given occupational pursuit constitute the performance dimension of human occupation, often referred to in the occupational therapy literature as occupational performance. The performance dimension of occupations is that aspect which has received the most study and attention in the history of the field. This may explain why the terms function and purposeful activity have been used as synonyms for engagement in occupation (Henderson, et. al., 1991).

Occupations, because of their intentional nature, always involve mental abilities and skills, and typically, but not always, have an observable physical or active dimension. Whether one is laying bricks or practicing meditation exercises, one can be said to be "doing" something. Only one of these occupations, however, requires observable physical action. Whether physical or mental in nature, the behaviors necessary for completion of tasks in daily occupations can be analyzed according to specific components related to moving, perceiving, thinking, and feeling. Various occupational performance components have been described and defined within the *Uniform Terminology for Occupational Therapy—Third Edition* (AOTA, 1994).

Position papers on function and purposeful activity have been developed by the American Occupational

Therapy Association (AOTA), and it is important to clarify the differences in meaning between these terms and the term occupation. The AOTA has proposed that when occupational therapists use the term function, they refer to an individual's performance of activities, tasks, and roles during daily occupations (occupational performance) (AOTA, in press). Purposeful activity has also been recognized as a term to describe engagement in the tasks of daily living, with the use of this term emphasizing the intentional, goal-directed nature of such engagement (AOTA, 1993). In this paper, it is proposed that reference to human occupation necessarily encompasses the required human capacities to act on the environment with intentionality in a given pursuit, as well as the unique organization of these pursuits over time and the meanings attributed to them by doers as well as those observing them.

In summary, occupations have performance, contextual, temporal, psychological, social, symbolic, and spiritual dimensions; whereas, function in its specific use denotes primarily the performance dimension. While the term purposeful activity recognizes multiple dimensions and emphasizes intentionality, it is viewed as a term that does not capture the richness of human enterprise embodied in the word occupation. It is asserted that while all occupations constitute purposeful activity, not all purposeful activities can be described as occupations.

Therapeutic Benefits of Occupations

Since Adolph Meyer's (1922) philosophical essay, many scholarly papers have been written about the therapeutic value of occupations (Clark, 1993; Cynkin & Robinson, 1990; Englehardt, 1977; Reilly, 1962; Yerxa, 1967). These have identified a broad scope of benefits, ranging from the facilitation of habilitation, adaptation, and self-actualization to improvements in motor control and sensory processing. While there is growing evidence to support some of these claims, additional research is needed before it can be demonstrated that other benefits are likely valid.

Because occupation is an extremely complex phenomenon and has not been subjected to rigorous research until recently, many questions about its nature and its relationship to health and well-being remain unanswered. This emphasizes the need for further study. Current beliefs and theories about occupation should be regarded as incomplete and evolving.

Forces Advancing and Impeding the Study and Discussion of Occupation

One of the problems inhibiting the study of occupations is how to clearly, logically, and consistently describe different levels and types of occupations. Used here, the term levels refers to the complexity of a given occupation. For example, while getting dressed and driving to work are readily interpretable as organized sets of actions that may partially comprise a typical day, each of these involves a variety of specific and definable behaviors, such as buttoning a shirt or turning an ignition key, which are less complex. Even occupational behaviors of greater complexity, such as dressing or driving, are nested within clusters of activity that comprise and are recognized as part of larger sets of organized behavior within cultures, such as pursuing a career. This phenomenon of nesting, where simple acts can be identified as parts of more complex sets of acts, is a dimension of occupations that relates to their organization over time and can be viewed as reflecting varying levels of complexity.

The English language has words associated with occupations, such as actions, tasks, and projects, which imply differences in complexity. Evans (1987) and Kielhofner (1993) have been among those who have described the hierarchical nature of occupations, and others (Christiansen, 1991; Nelson, 1988) have suggested that it would be useful if specific terms for human enterprise denoted different levels of this hierarchy. However, there is little agreement among scholars in occupational therapy or in the social sciences for how these terms ought to be used to describe varying levels of complexity in occupational behavior.

Similar difficulties exist in describing types or categories of occupations. Certain categories of occupations have gained conventional usage by occupational therapists and are recognized in contemporary culture. These include work, self-care (or self-maintenance), play, and leisure.

Studies of human beings in different cultures have shown similarities in time use according to these general categories (Christiansen, in press). However, while general categories of occupations are recognized across cultures, the specific tasks that constitute each category and the delineation of categories vary across individuals. The classification of a given task within a larger category seems to be dependent upon the context in which it is performed. For example, sewing may be viewed as work by some and classified as leisure by others. Similarly, most occupational pursuits seem to have both a general or cultural meaning attributed by participants and observers as well as a specific and personal meaning known only to the performer (Nelson, 1988; Rommetveit, 1980). Consider, for example, that getting dressed is viewed as a necessary and practical aspect of daily life in most cultures, but assumes symbolic importance when it is performed without assistance for the first time by the 3-year-old child, or by an adult mastering use of a new prosthetic arm. Dressing in anticipation of a ceremony or developmental milestone, such as high school graduation or a wedding, imbues the act with special significance. Over time, the experiences embedded in daily occupations assume collective meaning and are interpreted as essential parts of a person's self-narrative or life story (Bruner, 1990; Clark, 1993; Mattingly & Fleming, 1993).

Research on Occupations and Research in Occupational Therapy

It is useful to recognize that research on occupations should be distinguished from research in occupational therapy (Mosey, 1992). In the first instance, inquiry is directed toward understanding the nature of the typical daily occupations in which people engage; that is, what people do, how they do it, and why they do it. The study of occupational therapy, conversely, concerns itself with the effect of occupation on health, development of frames of reference that facilitate the identification and remediation of occupational dysfunction, and other topical issues of significance to this science-based profession.

Research for both areas has been impeded by the lack of conventional definitions for terms related to occupation. This, in turn, has contributed to disagreements about the proper concern of practice and the appropriate focus of research (Christiansen, 1981, 1991; Kielhofner & Burke, 1977; Mosey, 1985, 1989; Rogers, 1982; and Shannon 1977). Recently, occupational science has emerged as an area of study concerned with understanding humans as occupational beings (Clark, et. al., 1991; Yerxa, et. al., 1989). As additional research enables us to learn more about the nature of occupations and their

potential as a means for promoting and restoring health and well-being, it is likely that there will be continued discussion on the use of terminology to describe specific concepts.

This paper has attempted to identify distinctions among current terms relating to human occupation. As our understanding of occupations advances, more concepts and terms will evolve. It is important to continue to develop knowledge about occupations to facilitate our further understanding of an important, complex, and rich aspect of human life. In this way, the profession of occupational therapy will better appreciate the vision of its founders, more clearly understand its current state, and more likely realize the potential embodied in occupations as touchstones of human existence.

References

American Occupational Therapy Association. (1993). Position paper: Purposeful activity. *American Journal of Occupational Therapy, 47,* 1081–1082.

American Occupational Therapy Association. (1994). Uniform terminology for occupational therapy—third edition. *American Journal of Occupational Therapy, 48,* 1047–1059.

American Occupational Therapy Association. Occupational performance: Occupational therapy's definition of function. *American Journal of Occupational Therapy, 49,* 1019–1020.

Bing, R. (1981). Occupational therapy revisited: A paraphrastic journey. *American Journal of Occupational Therapy, 35,* 499–518.

Breines, E. (1987). Pragmatism as a foundation for occupational therapy. *American Journal of Occupational Therapy, 41,* 522–525.

Brown, R. (1986). *Social psychology* (2nd ed.). New York: Free Press.

Bruner, J. (1990). *Acts of meaning.* Cambridge, MA: Harvard University Press.

Burke, J.P. (1977). A clinical perspective on motivation: Pawn versus origin. *American Journal of Occupational Therapy, 31,* 254–258.

Christiansen, C. (1981). Toward resolution of crisis: Research requisites in occupational therapy. *Occupational Therapy Journal of Research, 1,* 115–124.

Christiansen, C. (1991). Occupational therapy: Intervention for life performance. In C. Christiansen & C. Baum (Eds.), *Occupational therapy: Overcoming human performance deficits* (p. 143). Thorofare, NJ: Slack.

Christiansen, C. (1994). A social framework for understanding self–care intervention. In C. Christiansen (Ed.), *Ways of living: Self-care strategies for special needs* (pp. 1–26). Bethesda, MD: American Occupational Therapy Association.

Christiansen, C. (In press). Three perspectives on balance in occupation. In F. Clark & R. Zemke (Eds.), *Occupational science: The first five years.* Philadelphia: F. A. Davis.

Clark, F. A. (1993). Occupation embedded in a real life: Interweaving occupational science and occupational therapy. *American Journal of Occupational Therapy, 47,* 1067–1078.

Clark, F. A., Parham, D., Carlson, M. E., Frank, G., Jackson, J., Pierce, D., Wolfe, R. J., & Zemke, R. (1991). Occupational science: Academic innovation in the service of occupational therapy's future. *American Journal of Occupational Therapy, 45,* 300–310.

Cynkin S., & Robinson, A. M. (1990). *Occupational therapy and activities health: Toward health through activities.* Boston: Little, Brown.

DiMatteo, M. R. (1991). *The psychology of health, illness, and medical care: An individual perspective.* Pacific Grove, CA: Brooks-Cole.

Dunton, W. R. (1918). The principles of occupational therapy. *Public Health Nurse, 10,* 316–321.

Englehardt, H. T. (1977). Defining occupational therapy: The meaning of therapy and the virtues of occupation. *American Journal of Occupational Therapy, 31,* 666–672.

Evans, A. K. (1987). National speaking: Definition of occupation as the core concept of occupational therapy. *American Journal of Occupational Therapy, 41,* 627–628.

Fidler, G. S. (1981). From crafts to competence. *American Journal of Occupational Therapy, 35,* 567–573.

Fidler, G. S., & Fidler, J. W. (1979). Doing and becoming: Purposeful action and self actualization. *American Journal of Occupational Therapy, 32,* 305–310.

Fidler, G. S., & Fidler, J. W. (1983). Doing and becoming: The occupational therapy experience. In G. Kielhofner (Ed.), *Health through occupation* (pp. 267–280). Philadelphia: F.A. Davis.

Frank, G. (1994). The personal meaning of self–care. In C. Christiansen (Ed.), *Ways of living: Self-care strategies for special needs* (pp. 27–49). Bethesda, MD: American Occupational Therapy Association.

Henderson, A., Cermak, S., Coster, W., Murray, E., Trombly, C., & Tickle-Degnen, L. (1991). The issue is: Occupational science is multidimensional. *American Journal of Occupational Therapy, 45*, 370372.

Kielhofner, G. (1977). Temporal adaptation: A conceptual framework for occupational therapy. *American Journal of Occupational Therapy, 31*, 235–242.

Kielhofner, G. (1993). *Conceptual foundations of occupational therapy.* Philadelphia: F.A. Davis.

Kielhofner, G., & Burke, J.P. (1977). Occupational therapy after sixty years: An account of changing identify and knowledge. *American Journal of Occupational Therapy, 31*, 675–689.

Levine, R. (1991). Occupation as a therapeutic medium. In C. Christiansen & C. Baum (Eds.), *Occupational therapy: Overcoming human performance deficits* (pp. 592–631). Thorofare, NJ: Slack.

Mattingly, C., & Fleming, M. (1993). *Clinical reasoning.* Philadelphia: F. A. Davis.

Meyer, A. (1922). The philosophy of occupational therapy. *Archives of Occupational Therapy, 1*, 1–10.

Mosey, A. C. (1985). A monistic or pluralistic approach to professional identity. *American Journal of Occupational Therapy, 39*, 504–509.

Mosey, A. C. (1986). *Psychosocial components of occupational therapy.* New York: Raven.

Mosey, A. C. (1989). The proper focus of scientific inquiry in occupational therapy: Frames of reference. *Occupational Therapy Journal of Research, 9*, 195–201.

Mosey, A. C. (1992). Partition of occupational science and occupational therapy. *American Journal of Occupational Therapy, 46*, 851–855.

Nelson, D. L. (1988). Occupation: Form and performance. *American Journal of Occupational Therapy, 42*, 633–641.

Reilly, M. (1962). Occupation can be one of the great ideas of 20th century medicine. *American Journal of Occupational Therapy, 16*, 1–9.

Rogers, J. (1982). The spirit of independence: The evolution of a philosophy. *American Journal of Occupational Therapy, 36*, 709–715.

Rommetveit, R. (1980). On meanings of acts and what is meant and made known by what is said in a pluralistic social world. In M. Brenner (Ed.), *The structure of action* (pp. 108–149). Oxford: Basil Blackwell.

Shannon, P. D. (1977). The derailment of occupational therapy. *American Journal of Occupational Therapy, 31*, 229–234.

Slagle, E. C. (1922). Training aids for mental patients. *Archives of Occupational Therapy, 1*, 11–17.

Tracy, S. (1910). *Studies in invalid occupations: A manual for nurses and attendants.* Boston: Whitcomb & Barrows.

Upham, E. G. (1918). *Ward occupations in hospitals. Federal Board for Vocational Education Bulletin 25.* Washington, DC: Government Printing Office.

White, R. W. (1971). The urge towards competence. *American Journal of Occupational Therapy, 25*, 271–274.

Yerxa, E. (1967). Authentic occupational therapy. *American Journal of Occupational Therapy, 21*, 1–9.

Yerxa, E., Clark, F., Frank, G., Jackson, J., Parham, D., Pierce, D., Stein, C., & Zemke, R. (1989). An introduction to occupational science: A foundation for occupational therapy in the 21st century. In J. Johnson & E. Yerxa (Eds.), *Occupational science: The foundation for new models of practice* (pp. 1–18). New York: Haworth.

Authors

Charles Christiansen, EdD, OTR, OT(C), FAOTA
Florence Clark, PhD, OTR, FAOTA
Gary Kielhofner, DrPH, OTR, FAOTA
Joan Rogers, PhD, OTR, FAOTA
with contributions from
David Nelson, PhD, OTR, FAOTA
for Commission on Practice
Jim Hinojosa, PhD, OTR, FAOTA, Chairperson

Adopted by the Representative Assembly April 1995

Previously published and copyrighted by the American Occupational Therapy Association in 1995 in the *American Journal of Occupational Therapy, 49*, 1015–1018.

APPENDIX J: OCCUPATIONAL PERFORMANCE: OCCUPATIONAL THERAPY'S DEFINITION OF FUNCTION

Fidler and Fidler (1963) define function as *doing;* Trombly (1993) promotes the use of *occupational function;* and function can describe a performance (i.e., functional strength, functional range of motion, and functional skills). The word *function* can mean role, use, activity, capacity, job, position, pursuit, or place (Landau & Bogus, 1977). The many ways in which the word *function* is used, or implied, may contribute to confusion regarding occupational therapy's unique role in addressing function. Although there may be some confusion about the use of terms, there is no confusion about the sense of purpose held by occupational therapy practitioners as they address the functional needs of the clients they serve.

Occupational therapy uses the word *function* interchangeably with performance and occupational performance because occupational therapy's domain is the function of the person in his or her occupational roles. The concept of function is implicit, rather than explicit, in many of the frames of reference used by occupational therapy practitioners as they focus on strategies to overcome deficits that impair the function of the individual. Occupational therapy practitioners help people address challenges or difficulties that threaten or impair their ability to perform activities and tasks that are basic to the fulfillment of their roles as worker, parent, spouse or partner, sibling, and friend to self or others.

In order to understand how occupational therapy uses *function,* it is necessary to review the historical roots of occupational therapy. Occupational therapy emerged as a developing profession in the years during and following World War I. The theoretical writings of Adolph Meyer (1922) and others were

Figure 1. Planning for children with physical disabilities: Identifying and changing disabling environments through participatory research.

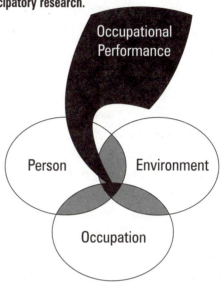

Doctoral dissertation, University of Waterloo, Waterloo, Canada. Reproduced with permission of Law, M. (1993).

initially influenced by the then emerging school of American psychology whose "functional approach" focused on the process of adaptation to the environment rather than to the structure of the organism (Boring, 1950). The founders of occupational therapy were committed to the importance of occupation and the preservation of function (Peloquin, 1991), and early clinical efforts focused on the role of work and productivity to maintain or improve function (Hopkins, 1988). The concept of function and occupation remains at the core of occupational therapy today. However, more recently, the interaction of the functional and structural approaches has emerged, and function is viewed as the interaction of neural and physiological mechanisms, behavior, and environment. This interaction is critical to understanding the effect of occupation on health (Almli, 1993), as the function of the individual is supported in a dynamic relationship between the person, his or her occupation, and the environment (see Figure 1). The unique term used by occupational therapists to express function is *occupational performance.* "Occupational performance reflects the individual's dynamic experience of engaging in daily occupations within the environment" (Law & Baum, 1994, p.12).

The concept of function has always been a central focus of occupational therapy and remains so. Other professions are beginning to recognize its importance and are placing increased value on function. Fisher (1992) acknowledged that the common goal of promoting functional independence is shared by occupational therapy, physical therapy, nursing, social work, psychology, and medicine, among others. A shift is occurring from a focus on pathology to a focus on function as one of the primary indicators of treatment effectiveness (Ware, 1993). This shift also brings to the forefront the issues that occupational therapy has always valued—the person's capacity to function in a community context.

Occupational therapy's emphasis on function is broader than the function of a human organ [or body part] (Christiansen, 1991). It goes far beyond the loss or abnormality of the anatomical structure or function as defined by *impairment* (NCMRR, 1993); or the lack of ability to perform an action or activity in the manner considered normal as defined by *functional limitation* (NCMRR). Occupational therapy views the individual as performing activities and roles within a social, cultural, and physical environment as defined by ability, or with a limitation—*disability* (NCMRR). The occupational therapy practitioner addresses the function of the individual at the occupational performance level where the environmental supports and barriers, the individual's skills, and the individual's occupational demands interact (see Figure 2).

Figure 2. A Person-Environment-Occupation Model of Occupational Performance.

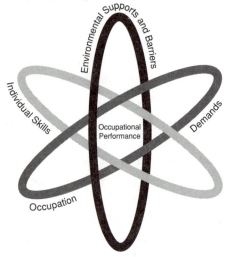

From "The Person-Environment-Occupation Model: A Transactive Approach to Occupational Performance," by M. Law, B. Cooper, S. Strong, D. Stewart, P. Rigby, & L. Letts, 1996. *Canadian Journal of Occupational Therapy, 63,* pp. 9–23. Copyright 1996 by the Canadian Association of Occupational Therapists (CAOT). Reproduced with permission of CAOT Publications.

Since 1917, occupational therapy has focused its services to enhance the function of individuals with, or threatened with, disability. Its practitioners have focused their efforts on function by using interventions to improve the occupational performance of persons who lack the ability to perform an action or activity considered necessary for their everyday lives. This is accomplished through a joint effort of the person and the clinician, where the person's problems, strengths, and assets are identified; followed by therapeutic interventions, educational strategies, access to resources, and environmental adaptations, so the person can accomplish his or her goals (Law & Baum, 1994). The unique contribution of occupational therapy is that the practitioner creates the opportunity for individuals to gain the skill and confidence to accomplish activities and tasks that are meaningful and productive, and in doing so, increases their occupational performance, thus their function.

References

Almli, C. R. (1993, June). *Motor system, development, and neuroplasticity: Implications of theory and practice in occupational therapy.* AOTF Research Colloquium, Seattle, WA.

Boring, E. G. (1950). *A history of experimental psychology* (2nd ed.). Englewood Cliffs, NJ: Prentice Hall.

Christiansen, C. (1991). Occupational therapy intervention for life performance. In C. Christiansen & C. M. Baum (Eds.), *Occupational therapy: Overcoming human performance deficits* (pp. 3–43). Thorofare, NJ: Slack.

Fidler, G. & Fidler, J. (1963). *Occupational therapy: A communication process in psychiatry.* New York: Macmillan.

Fisher, A. G. (1992). The foundation-functional measures, part 1: What is function, what should we measure, and how should we measure it? *American Journal of Occupational Therapy, 46,* 183–185.

Hopkins, H. L. (1988). An historical perspective on occupational therapy. In H. L. Hopkins & H. D. Smith (Eds.), *Willard and Spackman's occupational therapy* (pp. 16–37) (7th ed.). Philadelphia: Lippincott.

Landau, S. I., & Bogus, R. J. (1977). *The Doubleday Roget's thesaurus in dictionary form* (p. 278). Garden City, NY: Doubleday.

Law, M. (1993). *Planning for children with physical disabilities: Identifying and changing disabling environments through participatory research.* Doctoral dissertation, University of Waterloo, Waterloo, Canada.

Law, M., & Baum, C. M. (1994). *Creating the future: A joint effort.* St. Louis: Authors (Program in Occupational Therapy, Washington University School of Medicine, 4567 Scott Avenue, St. Louis, MO 63110).

Law, M., Cooper, B., Letts, L., Rigby, P., Stewart, S., & Strong, S. (1994). *A model of person-environment interactions: Application to occupational therapy.* Unpublished manuscript, McMaster University, Hamilton, Canada.

Meyer, A. (1922). The philosophy of occupational therapy. *Archives of Occupational Therapy, 1*(1), 1–10.

NCMRR. (1993). *Research plan for the National Center for Medical Rehabilitation Research,* (National Institutes of Health Publication No. 93-3509). Washington, DC: U.S. Government Printing Office.

Peloquin, S. M. (1991). Occupational therapy service: Individual and collective understanding of the founders, part 1. *American Journal of Occupational Therapy, 45,* 352–360.

Trombly, C. (1993). The issue is—Anticipating the future: Assessment of occupational function. *American Journal of Occupational Therapy, 47,* 253–257.

Ware, J. E. (1993). Measures for a new era of health assessment. In A. L. Stewart & J. E. Ware (Eds.), *Measuring functioning and well-being* (pp. 3–12). Durham, NC: Duke University Press.

Authors

Carolyn Baum, PhD, OTR, FAOTA
Dorothy Edwards, PhD
and the faculty of the Program in Occupational Therapy, Washington University School of Medicine, St. Louis, Missouri for Commission on Practice
Jim Hinojosa, PhD, OTR, FAOTA, Chairperson

Adopted by the Representative Assembly April 1995
Previously published and copyrighted by the American Occupational Therapy Association in 1995 in the *American Journal of Occupational Therapy, 49,* 1019–1020.

APPENDIX K: POSITION PAPER: PURPOSEFUL ACTIVITY

The American Occupational Therapy Association, Inc., submits this paper to clarify the use of the term purposeful activity, a central focus of occupational therapy throughout its history. People engage in purposeful activity as part of their daily life routines, in the context of occupational performance (Resolution C, 1979). Occupation refers to active participation in self-maintenance, work, leisure, and play. Purposeful activity refers to goal-directed behaviors or tasks that comprise occupations. An activity is purposeful if the individual is an active, voluntary participant and if the activity is directed toward a goal that the individual considers meaningful (Evans, 1987; Gilfoyle, 1984; Mosey, 1986; Nelson, 1988). The purposefulness of an activity lies with the individual performing the activity and with the context in which it is done (Henderson et al., 1991). The meaning of an activity is unique to each person, influenced by his or her life experiences (Mosey, 1986; Pedretti, 1982), life roles, interests, age, and cultural background, as well as the situational context in which the activity occurs. Occupational therapy practitioners are committed to the use of purposeful activity to evaluate, facilitate, restore, or maintain individuals' abilities to function in their daily occupations.

Occupational therapists use activities to evaluate an individual's capacities to meet the functional demands of his or her environment and daily life. Based on an evaluation, the occupational therapy practitioner, in collaboration with the individual, designs activity experiences that offer the individual opportunities for effective action. Purposeful activities assist and build upon the individual's abilities and lead to achievement of personal functional goals. Purposeful activity provides opportunities for persons to achieve mastery of their environment, and successful performance promotes feelings of personal competence (Fidler & Fidler, 1978). A person who is involved in purposeful activity directs attention to the goal rather than to the processes required for achievement of the goal. Engagement in purposeful activity within the context of interpersonal, cultural, physical, and other environmental conditions requires and elicits coordination among the individual's sensory motor, cognitive, and psychosocial systems. Purposeful activity may involve the independent use of complex cognitive processes, such as premeditation, reflection, planning, and use of symbolic cues. Conversely, it may involve less complex processes and take place in an environment of external structure, support, and supervision (Allen, 1987; Henderson et al., 1991). Engagement in purposeful activity provides direct and objective feedback of performance both to the occupational therapy practitioner and the individual.

The therapeutic purposes for which purposeful activity is used include mastery of a new skill, restoration of a deficient ability, compensation for functional disability, health maintenance, or prevention of dysfunction. To use purposeful activity therapeutically, an occupational therapy practitioner analyzes the activity from several perspectives. First, the activity is examined to identify its component parts to determine which skills and abilities are necessary to complete the task. Second, it is examined in terms of the context in which it will be performed. Third, the practitioner considers the person's age, occupational roles, cultural background, gender, interests, and preferences that may influence the meaningfulness of the activity for the individual. All this information is considered together to assist the occupational therapy practitioner in synthesizing (i.e., adapting, grading, and combining) activities for therapeutic purposes for a particular individual.

Purposeful activities cannot be prescribed based on analysis of their inherent characteristics alone; rather, by definition, prescription of purposeful activity is individual-specific. An occupational therapy practitioner grades or adapts a chosen activity for an individual to promote successful performance or elicit a particular response. Grading activities challenges the patient's abilities by progressively changing the process, tools, materials, or environment of a given activity to gradually increase or decrease performance demands. These incremental modifications are made in response to the individual's dynamic changes and provide opportunities for gradual development of skill and related therapeutic benefits. The grading of activities is accomplished by modifying the sequence, duration, or procedures of the task; the individual's position; the position of the tools and materials; the size, shape, weight, or texture of the materials; the nature and degree of interpersonal contact; the extent of physical handling by the occupational therapy practitioner during performance; or the environment in which the activity is attempted. Supportive or assistive devices or techniques may be used to enhance the effectiveness of an activity or to facilitate performance (Henderson et al., 1991; Pedretti & Pasquinelli, 1990). Such techniques or devices are considered facilitative or preparatory to performance of purposeful activity and engagement in occupations.

If the therapy goal is to enhance a performance component so that an individual can engage in an occupational performance area, the selected activity and environmental conditions are manipulated to present graded challenges to the specific skills required. When an individual's successful completion of a task is a priority, occupational therapy practitioners adapt the task and the environment to facilitate performance. Adaptation is a process that

changes an aspect of the activity or the environment to enable successful performance and accomplish a particular therapeutic goal. Adaptation of a task may require the use of assistive devices and techniques or grading strategies.

Occupational therapy education provides the necessary background for using activities as therapeutic modalities by instructing the student about behavioral and biological sciences related to the use and meaning of activity, about the nature of purposeful activity, about the process of activity analysis and synthesis, and about the application of activity to therapeutic problems within occupational therapy frames of reference.

In summary, purposeful activity occurs within the context of work, self-care, play, and leisure activities and is used therapeutically to evaluate, facilitate, restore, or maintain individuals' abilities to function competently within their daily occupations. The occupational therapy practitioner's commitment to those he or she serves is to guide them in the use of purposeful activities so as to empower them to enhance the quality of their being in the daily reality where they live as parents, children, students, homemakers, workers, or retirees (Reilly, 1966).

References

Allen, C. K. (1987). Activity: Occupational therapy's treatment method. *American Journal of Occupational Therapy, 41,* 563–575.

Evans, A. K. (1987). Nationally speaking: Definition of occupation as the core concept of occupational therapy. *American Journal of Occupational Therapy, 41,* 627–628.

Fidler, G. S. & Fidler, J. W. (1978). Doing and becoming: Purposeful action and self actualization. *American Journal of Occupational Therapy, 32,* 305–310.

Gilfoyle, E. (1984). Eleanor Clark Slagle Lectureship, 1984: Transformation of a profession. *American Journal of Occupational Therapy, 38,* 575–584.

Henderson, A., Cermak, S., Coster, W., Murray, E., Trombly, C., & Tickle-Degnen, L. (1991). The issue is—Occupational science is multidimensional. *American Journal of Occupational Therapy, 45,* 370–372.

Mosey, A. C. (1986). *Psychosocial components of occupational therapy.* New York: Raven Press.

Nelson, D. L. (1988). Occupation: Form and performance. *American Journal of Occupational Therapy, 42,* 633–641.

Pedretti, L. W. (1982). *The compatibility of current treatment methods in physical disabilities with the philosophical base of occupational therapy.* Presentation at the American Occupational Therapy Association Annual Conference, Philadelphia, May 1982.

Pedretti, L. W., & Pasquinelli, S. (1990). A frame of reference for occupational therapy in physical dysfunction. In L.W. Pedretti & B. Zoltan (Eds.), *Occupational therapy practice skills for physical dysfunction* (pp. 1–17). St. Louis, MO: Mosby.

Reilly, M. (1966). The challenge of the future to an occupational therapist. *American Journal of Occupational Therapy, 20,* 221–225.

Resolution C, 531-79. The philosophical base of occupational therapy. *American Journal of Occupational Therapy, 33,* 785.

Authors

Jim Hinojosa, PhD, OTR, FAOTA
Joyce Sabari, PhD, OTR
Lorraine Pedretti, MS, OTR
with contributions from
Mark S. Rosenfeld, PhD, OTR
Catherine Trombly, ScD, OTR/L, FAOTA
for Commission on Practice
Jim Hinojosa, PhD, OTR, FAOTA, Chairperson

Approved by the Representative Assembly April 1983

Revised and approved by the Representative Assembly June 1993

Previously published and copyrighted by the American Occupational Therapy Association in the *American Journal of Occupational Therapy, 47,* 1081–1082.

APPENDIX L: BROADENING THE CONSTRUCT OF INDEPENDENCE

Occupational therapy practice supports a broad view of independence and defines independence as the ability to take responsibility for one's own role performance needs and desires. In order to acknowledge the variety of ways individuals accomplish the necessary and desirable tasks in their lives, it is essential to embrace a broad view.

Occupational therapy practitioners understand and value not only the independent performance of tasks, but also the use of adaptations or alternative methods to support independent task performance. The value of independence to individuals varies, depending on their social and cultural contexts. The profession recognizes independence as a state of self-determination. Occupational therapy practitioners value the right of individuals to choose their preferred level of independence relative to their life role activities and the context in which they are performed. Individuals are independent when they perform tasks themselves, when they perform tasks in an adapted environment, and when they appropriately oversee task completion by others on their own behalf. Individuals in each of these situations are considered equally independent because they are responsible for identifying what they want and need to do, and are capable of getting the tasks completed. In accordance with this view of independence, the profession supports the following:

• Individuals select a variety of strategies to manage their responsibilities so that they can continue to perform necessary and desired tasks.

• There are a variety of ways for individuals to be independent. Many people hire and supervise others to perform necessary household tasks. Some people do this because of time constraints.

Other people do this due to physical limitations. Each of these individuals is considered equally independent in managing household demands. For example, individuals are not considered less independent in meal preparation if they use a step stool or a reaching device in the process of preparing meals.

• Adaptations should be viewed as resourceful and convenient for all individuals, regardless of their current disability status.

• Individuals are considered resourceful when they have the needed devices or strategies available to them in their environments to support independent functioning.

• Individuals should not be stigmatized by the use of devices or strategies to support their unique approaches to independence. For example, individuals are not considered less independent if they use a datebook or other memory devices to keep an appointment.

• In rating performance, some systems differentiate independent performance from less independent performance based solely on the use of adaptive devices and amount of human assistance required. Although such systems may provide useful information, they do not document the ingenuity or motivation of individuals to use supportive resources.

This document reaffirms occupational therapy practitioners' commitment to support a broad definition of independence for all members of society. This inclusive view recognizes that all of society is strengthened when individuals are viewed as functional members of that society, regardless of how they perform their chosen endeavors.

Bibliography

World Health Organization (WHO). (1980).
International classification of impairments, disabilities, and handicaps: A manual of classification relating to the consequences of disease. Albany, NY: WHO Publications.

Prepared by

Winifred Dunn, PhD, OTR, FAOTA
Mary Foto, OTR, FAOTA
Jim Hinojosa, PhD, OTR, FAOTA
Barbara A. Boyt Schell, PhD, OTR, FAOTA
Linda Kohlman Thomson, MOT, OTR, OT(C), FAOTA
Sarah D. Hertfelder, MEd, MOT, OTR, FAOTA, Staff Liaison for Commission on Practice
Jim Hinojosa, PhD, OTR, FAOTA, Chairperson

Adopted by the Representative Assembly April 1995

Previously published and copyrighted by the American Occupational Therapy Association in 1995 in the *American Journal of Occupational Therapy, 49*, 1014.

APPENDIX M: MATERIAL SUPPLIERS

Material Suppliers

This list of suppliers is not intended to be exhaustive, nor does it represent endorsements by the author or the American Occupational Therapy Association.

Activity or Special Product Suppliers

Earthquake Survival, Lost at Sea, and Wilderness Survival are available from:

Pfeiffer & Company

An imprint of Jossey-Bass, Inc., Publishers
350 Sansome Street, 5th Floor
San Francisco, CA
800-274-4434
FAX: 800-605-2665

Art and Craft Suppliers

Craft Time, Inc.

PO Box 93706
Atlanta, GA 30377
404-873-2028
FAX: 404-874-5148

Dick Blick Art Materials & Craft Supplies

PO Box 1267
Galesburg, IL 61402-1267
800-447-8192

Fire Mountain Gems

28195 Redwood Highway
Cave Junction, OR 97523-9304
888-347-3436
FAX: 888-347-3329

Nasco Arts & Crafts

901 Janesville Avenue
PO Box 901
Fort Atkinson, WI 53538-0901
800-558-9595

S & S

PO Box 513
Colchester, CT 06415-0513
800-243-9232
FAX: 800-566-6678

Vanguard Crafts, Inc.

PO Box 340170
Brooklyn, NY 11234-0003
718-377-5188
FAX: 718-692-0056

Woodworker's Supply, Inc.

1108 North Glenn Road
Casper, WY 82601
800-645-9292

APPENDIX N: TASK ANALYSIS COURSE MODULE

Appendix N includes course objectives, accreditation references, a class schedule, case summary, and resource material to assist occupational therapy educators who plan to use *Task Analysis: An Occupational Performance Approach* within a course.

Course Objectives

Upon completion of the readings and learning exercises in this text, the occupational therapy student will:

1. Describe the historical relevance of occupation to the occupational therapy profession.
2. Illustrate and explain an occupational performance theoretical model.
3. Identify, describe, and apply some of the theories underlying the use of purposeful activity.
4. Define and compare the constructs of (a) impairments, disabilities, and handicaps; (b) roles, tasks, and activities; (c) occupation, occupational performance, and function; (d) meaningful and purposeful activity; and (e) independence.
5. Identify and define the domains of concern to the occupational therapy practitioner as defined in *Uniform Terminology for Occupational Therapy,* (1994).
6. Explain the concept person-activity-environment (PAE) fit; identify the variables that affect PAE fit; and describe the relevance of PAE fit to the process of occupational therapy evaluation and intervention.
7. Explain the term **task analysis** and describe its use during client screening, evaluation, program planning, intervention, and reevaluation.
8. Explain and give examples of how task analysis is used to contribute to the health and wellness of individuals and communities.
9. Analyze the activities of daily living, productive work, play, and leisure pursuits of pediatric, adolescent, and adult client cases to understand their previous or current occupational performance profiles and begin to predict potential future profiles.
10. Develop and apply logical thinking, critical analysis, creativity, problem solving, clinical observations, and task analysis skills to evaluate client cases. Select and design purposeful, therapeutic activities to address intervention goals and priorities.
11. Describe the relevance of habituation, lifestyle, and a balance of occupations to health and wellness.
12. Develop and apply skills in teaching and working with others through small group tasks, collaborative team projects, group discussions, and oral presentations.
13. Conclude that an individual's roles, tasks, and developmental issues change across the life span, and that participation in selected tasks and meaningful activities can restore, reinforce, and enhance role functioning, adaptation, health, and wellness.

Accreditation Criteria

Completion of the readings, assignments, and learning exercises in this text will assist educational programs in providing the following curriculum content areas as recommended by the accreditation essentials of the American Occupational Therapy Association (1991a; 1991b):

Registered Occupational Therapist
(Section II B): 1.b., 2.b., 3.b.(1), 3.b.(3), 3.b.(4), 3.b.(5), 3.c.(1), 3.c.(2), 3.c.(3), 3.d.(1)(a), 3.d.(2)(b), 3.d.(3)(a), 3.d.(3)(f).

Occupational Therapy Assistant (Section II B): 1.b., 2.b., 2.c., 2.d., 2.e., 3.a., 3.b., 3.c.(1), 3.c.(2), 3.c.(3), 3.d.(1)(a), 3.d.(1)(c), 3.d.(2)(a), 3.d.(2)(b), 3.d.(3)(a), 3.d.(3)(f), 3.g.(1), 3.g.(2).

Course Schedule

The following schedule provides a suggested outline for completion of the chapters and learning assignments in this text. The schedule assumes that students attend a task analysis course for $1^1/_2$ to 2 hours twice per week. This text was developed for use over two courses that span 1 academic year. Adaptations to the schedule will be required for those programs that offer shorter courses.

The cases within this text have been sequenced to increase in complexity. The cases within the pediatric section require use of the Occupational Performance Analysis Form (OPAF), while the adolescent, adult, and seniors section use the Occupational Performance Analysis—Short Form (OPA-SF). Although the cases or age clusters can be used out of sequence, students must practice using the OPAF before the OPA-SF.

Many of the cases require students to identify and define therapy goals and objectives. While some guidance is provided on the Client Goals Form, instructors of students in registered occupational therapy and certified occupational therapy assistant programs will have different expectations of their students and provide assistance as required.

Traditional activity analysis courses provide the opportunities for students to learn different media, crafts, and so forth. Expectations are that the cases within this text will provide a realistic context for the incorporation of these activities. The range of media offered to students for a particular case will depend on the educational objectives of the instructor.

Specific cases found within *Task Analysis: An Occupational Performance Approach* can also be incorporated into other courses such as pediatrics, geriatrics, physical medicine practice, mental health practice, therapeutic techniques, and so on. The chapter titled "Worker Rehabilitation and the Biomechanical Approach: The Case of Rick" is also appropriate for use in an industrial medicine or kinesiology course. The chapter titled "Accessible Senior Centers: The Volunteer Agency" is appropriate for use in a course in which students are required to assume a consultant role to maintain or improve the health of a community.

Topic	Class 1	Class 2
Task Analysis: An Occupational Performance Approach		
Introduction to Task Analysis	Task Analysis: Historical and Contemporary Perspectives	Task Analysis: The Contribution of Occupational Therapy to Health
Analysis of People, Occupations, and Lifestyles	Occupational Performance Profiles	Occupational Performance Areas
Performance Component Analysis	Sensorimotor Performance Components	Neuromuscular and Motor Performance Components
	Cognitive Performance Components	Psychosocial and Psychological Performance Components
Performance Context Analysis	Physical Environment	Temporal Aspects and Social and Cultural Environments
Purposeful Activities	Purposeful Modifications and Adaptations	Occupational Performance Analysis Form
Children		
Occupational Performance Analysis Form	Purposeful Play	Children's Cultural Crafts and Games
Pediatric Client Cases	Leisure Activities: Bob	Educational Activities: Tina
	Switch Access to Learning: Sidney	Childhood Occupations: Miguel

Topic	Class 1	Class 2
Adolescents		
Occupational Performance Analysis— Short Form	Adolescent Activities, Crafts, and Games	
Adolescent Client Cases	In Search of Self and others: Ali, Barb, Carl, and Dana	Activities of Daily Living: Sylvie and Laureal
	Computer Access to Education: Greg	Adolescent Occupations: Daniel
Adults		
Occupational Performance Analysis	Adult Activities, Crafts, and Games	
Adult Client Cases	Arts and Literature: Laurie	Activities of Daily Living: Dawn
	Worker Rehabilitation and the Biomechanical Approach: Rick	
	Driving, Sports, and Recreation: Jeff	
	Adult Occupations: Rena	
Seniors		
Older Adult Client Cases	Home Improvement: Nelson	Dining Out: Wayne and Minnie
	Dining In: Rhonda	Crafts for Assessment and Intervention
	The Case of Maureen	The Case of Bert
	Senior Occupations: Gladys	
Accessible Seniors Center Project		

Case Summary

Case	Age	Diagnoses	Issues
Bob	4	Developmental delay	Clumsiness in play and delayed acquisition of certain preacademic concepts.
Tina	6	Developmental delay	Difficulty performing certain educational activities and learning certain preacademic concepts.
Sidney	7	Spastic cerebral palsy and mental retardation	Use of switches and assistive technology devices to learn and participate in student role.
Miguel	5	Down's syndrome	Independently complete case analysis and design intervention. Children's activities of daily living.
Ali, Barb, Carl, and Dana	13 to 17	Adjustment disorder, bulimia, depression, and attempted suicide in adolescents	Design of individual and group therapy sessions to address psychosocial and psychological needs.
Sylvie and Laureal	17 and 19	Depression; traumatic brain injury	Meal preparation and social group cooking project.
Greg	15	Muscular dystrophy	Use of assistive technology devices to ensure computer access.
Daniel	14	Spastic cerebral palsy and mental retardation	Transitioning from student to worker role. Job analysis.
Laurie	40	Depression	Adjustment to traumatic injury and the effects of personal causation, self-efficacy, and self-concept on adaptation.
Dawn	52	Hip replacement	Requires training and adaptive equipment to promote independence in self-care.
Rick	28	Back injury and fractured wrist	Work site evaluation and job analysis of a rehabilitation engineer who makes adapted equipment.

Case Summary, continued

Case	Age	Diagnoses	Issues
Jeff	32	Traumatic brain injury and high thoracic spinal cord injury	Task analysis of driving or a selected sport and adaptations to ensure participation.
Rena	40	Cerebral vascular accident	Single parent of two boys. Independently complete case analysis and design intervention.
Nelson	65	Diabetic and amputee	Return to productive roles, home management tasks, and leisure interests. Detection and prevention of depression.
Wayne and Minnie	70s	Parkinson's disease and fracture	Maintain functional and community mobility. Prevent falls and maintain health of caregiver.
Rhonda	89	Cerebral vascular accident	Task analysis of feeding and eating.
Maureen	77	Alzheimer's disease	Select activities, crafts, or game to contribute to cognitive evaluation and consult to recreational activities staff.
Bert	75	Multiple cerebral infarcts with hemiplegia, aphasia, and cognitive impairment	Select activities, crafts, or game to contribute to cognitive evaluation and consult to recreational activities staff.
Gladys	78	Rheumatoid arthritis	Facilitate independence, maintain caregiver health, and introduce the contribution of activity analysis to sexuality.
Accessible Seniors Center: The Volunteer Agency			Develop a proposal for a seniors day program to promote the health of the elder community.

Resources

Students will be required to consult many of the resource materials used by occupational therapy clinical practitioners. Each student should be provided with supplier catalogues from major suppliers of activities of daily living and assistive technology devices. The books and periodicals listed in the Learning Resources should be made available to students.

References

American Occupational Therapy Association (AOTA). (1991a). *Essentials and guidelines for an accredited educational program for the occupational therapist.* Bethesda, MD: Author.

AOTA. (1991b). *Essentials and guidelines for an accredited educational program for the occupational therapy assistant.* Bethesda, MD: Author.

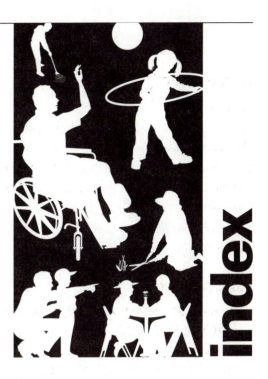

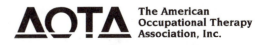
The American
Occupational Therapy
Association, Inc.

A